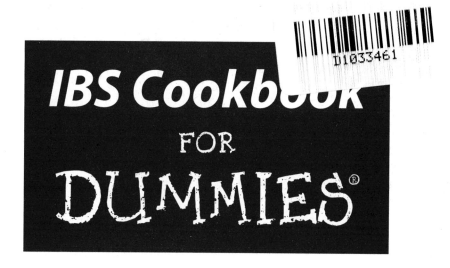

IBS Cookbook
FOR
DUMMIES®

**by Carolyn Dean, MD, ND,
and L. Christine Wheeler, MA**

WILEY

Wiley Publishing, Inc.

IBS Cookbook For Dummies®

Published by
Wiley Publishing, Inc.
111 River St.
Hoboken, NJ 07030-5774
www.wiley.com

WILEY

About the Authors

Carolyn Dean, MD, ND, is known as "The Doctor of the Future," but it began in her teens when she read all the health literature she could get her hands on. When no one wanted to take her advice about nutrition and exercise, she decided to become a doctor — then they'd have to listen! She graduated with her MD in 1978 from Dalhousie University in Halifax, Nova Scotia, did her internship at Mount Sinai in Toronto, and graduated from the Ontario College of Naturopathic Medicine (now the Canadian College of Naturopathic Medicine). She has been dedicated to the practice of natural medicine and helping patients and clients take charge of their health ever since.

Carolyn is the author and coauthor of 18 books, including *IBS For Dummies* (Wiley), *The Magnesium Miracle* (Ballantine Books), and *The Yeast Connection and Women's Health* (Square One Publishers). Carolyn offers an online newsletter and a 48-week Internet health program called *Future Health Now!* Her goal isn't about telling people to take handfuls of supplements; it's about diet, lifestyle, and cultivating a great attitude!

As the Medical Director of the Nutritional Magnesium Association (www.nutritionalmagnesium.org), Carolyn helps educate the public about the benefits of magnesium. She also offers a wellness telephone consultation service. With her dual degrees in medicine and naturopathic medicine, she's able to choose the best from both worlds for clients from around the world. You can join Carolyn's newsletter and health program and find out more about her myriad projects at www.drcarolyndean.com.

Christine Wheeler, MA, divides her professional life between writing and editing books on health and natural wellness and being a Certified Emotional Freedom Techniques (EFT) Practitioner. She's ghostwritten four titles she can't tell you about, but her work with her sister Carolyn is out in the open. They coauthored *IBS For Dummies* (Wiley) and the book you are holding in your hands.

Christine is also an expert in helping people who fear public speaking and experience performance anxiety and has cocreated the successful audio program *Eliminating Your Fear of Public Speaking: Finding Your Voice with EFT,* which you can find at www.tappingvancouver.com.

As an EFT Practitioner, Christine has helped countless people resolve the emotional and physical pain and symptoms associated with having IBS and other illnesses and conditions. She works with clients in person in her private practice in Vancouver, Canada, and in phone consultations with people from all over the world. You can find her at www.christinewheeler.com.

Dedication

Carolyn places dedications on the heads of Bob and all her new friends on Maui who have made writing a book in paradise quite blissful.

Christine dedicates this book, and any words she writes, to Ken.

Authors' Acknowledgments

Huge thanks go to the team of experts at Wiley starting with Stacy Kennedy, our Acquisitions Editor, who knew it was time for our first book to have an offspring. To Alissa Schwipps, Senior Project Editor, thank you for your patience, guidance, and great ideas as we navigated through writing our first cookbook. Thanks also to Copy Editor Megan Knoll who made great suggestions, and our recipe editors Emily Nolan and Connie Sarros who provided very colorful feedback.

Thank you to our agent, Jack Sach of BookEnds, who knew we had a cookbook in us and encouraged us to let it out.

We have such appreciation for our chefs who have contributed their beautiful recipes in the hopes of helping people who are dealing with intestinal disorders. Their passion for their work fueled our passion for this book. An extra special thanks goes to our healing chef, Colleen Robinson, who tirelessly helped us to adapt recipes to make them friendlier and friendlier for people with IBS. Chefs Shannon Leone and Angela Elliott get a standing ovation for turning over their kitchens and cookbooks to us; your contributions are invaluable.

Thank you to our past readers, clients, and patients who have shared with us how reading and using *IBS For Dummies* helped them with their condition. We were happy to have the opportunity to write another book for all of you.

Carolyn: A special thanks to Wiley for the six months of nonstop fun with my sister Chris. And to my dear friends Barbara Ann and J.W. who showered me with perspective. My husband of 40 years still asks me "Carolyn, do we eat asparagus?", so we just fasted our way through this cookbook!

Christine: I'd like to thank my sister Carolyn for making me love books as a kid and for making me love *writing* books now. To my great friend Rob Egger, thanks for knowing exactly when to phone, text, email, or make me go to a movie. In so many ways, I'm grateful for my partner Ken for the love, encouragement, and laughter and for cooking meals while I was writing a cookbook.

Publisher's Acknowledgments

We're proud of this book; please send us your comments at http://dummies.custhelp.com. For other comments, please contact our Customer Care Department within the U.S. at 877-762-2974, outside the U.S. at 317-572-3993, or fax 317-572-4002.

Some of the people who helped bring this book to market include the following:

Acquisitions, Editorial, and Media Development

Senior Project Editor: Alissa Schwipps

Acquisitions Editor: Stacy Kennedy

Copy Editor: Megan Knoll

Assistant Editor: Erin Calligan Mooney

Editorial Program Coordinator: Joe Niesen

Technical Editor: Barbara B. Bolen, PhD

Senior Editorial Manager: Jennifer Ehrlich

Editorial Assistants: Jennette ElNaggar, David Lutton

Art Coordinator: Alicia B. South

Photographer: T. J. Hine Photography, Inc.

Food Stylist: Lisa Bishop

Cover Photos: © T. J. Hine Photography, Inc.

Cartoons: Rich Tennant (www.the5thwave.com)

Composition Services

Project Coordinator: Katherine Crocker

Layout and Graphics: Carl Byers, Christine Williams

Proofreaders: Cindy Ballew, Melissa Cossell

Indexer: Rebecca R. Plunkett

Publishing and Editorial for Consumer Dummies

    Diane Graves Steele, Vice President and Publisher, Consumer Dummies

    Kristin Ferguson-Wagstaffe, Product Development Director, Consumer Dummies

    Ensley Eikenburg, Associate Publisher, Travel

    Kelly Regan, Editorial Director, Travel

Publishing for Technology Dummies

    Andy Cummings, Vice President and Publisher, Dummies Technology/General User

Composition Services

    Debbie Stailey, Director of Composition Services

Contents at a Glance

Recipes at a Glance

Soups

Salads

Table of Contents

Introduction

*I*f you picked up this book, that means you are ready for a change. How many times have you said to yourself, I really want to find out what foods my body loves; I really need to clean up my diet; I really don't need to eat all this junk food; I know what makes me feel worse and I keep on doing it? We feel your pain; you are not alone. But you'll find this book to be an easy and even fun way to explore a new way of eating for your IBS.

A lot of people struggle with IBS at some point or the other in their lifetimes, so you're not alone in your quest for IBS solutions. Both of us have had many bouts of IBS over the last 20 years, but we're both able to control our symptoms by avoiding wheat, limiting dairy and sugar, and doing Emotional Freedom Techniques (EFT) for the stress and emotional factors that can contribute to IBS. With our training (Christine's in EFT and Carolyn's in medicine and nutrition), and the fact that we both fancy ourselves as comedians, we hope to give you a memorable resource with creative ideas for what to eat and how to cook it in order to keep IBS at bay. For example, we advise eating organic foods if at all possible. Genetically modified grains, corn, and soy seem to be the wave of the future, but these genetic experiments are associated with gut disturbance in animals. The only way to avoid them is to buy organic. As you find out about IBS-friendly food, we assure you that you'll be able to befriend food again.

About This Book

We've written *IBS Cookbook For Dummies* as a companion to *IBS For Dummies* (Wiley). But here we take a closer look at the role food and food preparation can play in both triggering and managing your IBS. Our goal is to show you that not all foods, or even all foods you may expect, are off limits — you just have to know your individual body to recognize what it can and can't handle.

You don't have to read this book from start to finish — unless you want to, of course. (When we read a *For Dummies* book, we go straight to the cartoons at the beginning of each part. Then when we're laughing we know we're in the best frame of mind for learning!) Jumping around in a *For Dummies* book is great exercise, so we've set it up so that you can start reading this book anywhere you want. Simply look over the index or table of contents and then proceed to the chapter that tells you exactly what you need to know.

By the way, we take full responsibility for all jokes, puns, silly alliteration, and bathroom humor. It's the part of the job we love most.

Conventions Used in This Book

The following conventions are used throughout the text to make things consistent and easy to understand:

- ✔ All Web addresses appear in `monofont`.

- ✔ New terms appear in *italics* and are closely followed by an easy-to-understand definition.

- ✔ **Bold** highlights the action parts of numbered steps as well as keywords in some bulleted lists.

- ✔ IBS-D stands for IBS-diarrhea, and IBS-C stands for IBS-constipation.

- ✔ When you see the acronym *SCD,* it stands for the Specific Carbohydrate Diet™, which is specifically formulated for intestinal conditions. You can read more about it in Chapter 3.

Here are a few more conventions that apply to the recipes:

- ✔ Eggs are large.

- ✔ Pepper is freshly ground black pepper unless otherwise specified.

- ✔ Butter is unsalted.

- ✔ Sugar is granulated unless otherwise noted.

- ✔ Stevia is a natural noncaloric sweetener.

- ✔ All herbs are fresh unless dried herbs are specified.

- ✔ All temperatures are Fahrenheit. (Check out Appendix A for information about converting temperatures to Celsius.)

- ◔ If vegetarian recipes are your thing, look for recipes preceded by this tomato icon, which signals that a dish contains no meat.

Many cookbooks pride themselves on including esoteric ingredients they gather from all parts of the globe. Not us; you can find all our ingredients in your local grocery store, health food store, or online. We pride ourselves on having contributing chefs, cooks and food lovers who have provided us with IBS-friendly recipes that will appeal to your taste buds no matter what your stage and degree of IBS. Some recipes will provide more guidance than others but we think each one will be easy to follow whether you are a cooking maven or newbie.

We've tried our best to make these recipes as consistent with each other as possible, but they do come from several different sources, so they may not all have the same level of detail or guidance.

What You're Not to Read

We'd love you to read every word of our book, but if you just want to get in and out with the info you need, we flag some interesting but nonessential information that you can skip if you're in a hurry. You can come back to it later on as you become addicted to our lovely book.

- ✔ **Text in sidebars:** *Sidebars* are shaded boxes that usually give detailed examples or stories about our IBS clients with all the personal data removed so they won't be embarrassed and we won't be sued.

- ✔ **Anything with a Technical Stuff icon:** This icon indicates information that the scientist in you would love but that isn't necessary on the first reading.

- ✔ **The stuff on the copyright page:** No kidding. You'll find nothing of interest here unless you're inexplicably enamored by legal language and Library of Congress numbers.

Foolish Assumptions

We can actually be quite accurate with our assumptions about who is reading this book because we've both suffered the symptoms of IBS. You may not identify with every one of the following descriptions, but if even one of them makes sense to you, this book is for you:

- ✔ You've seen umpteen doctors and given them your money, time, and parts of your dignity, but none of them have given you relief.

- ✔ You're looking for support and reinforcement because those around you think your problem is in your head, not your bowels.

- ✔ You have to wake up at least one hour earlier than you want to in the morning to make sure your gut isn't going to play any tricks on you on your drive to work.

- ✔ You're tired of missing every important family gathering, or spending them in the bathroom.

- ✔ You've become a genius at covering up abdominal pain that would take down a Marine.

- ✔ You find yourself gazing longingly at the incontinence products in the drugstore.

- ✔ You know someone with IBS and want to be able to provide support (and possibly snacks).

How This Book Is Organized

Earlier in this introduction, we mention our love for the cartoons that begin each part in a *For Dummies* book. Of course, the cartoons are just the tip of the iceberg. Each part is chock full of valuable information, so here we give you an overview of what information you can find in this book and where.

Part I: You Are What You Eat: Food and IBS

What goes in must come out, but when you have IBS you can't help but wonder what the foods you eat are doing along the way. This part helps you identify your symptoms and some simple ways you can treat them with natural medicines and foods.

You find out about foods that are thought to trigger IBS and how to determine what foods trigger you.

Finally, we show you how to transition to an IBS-friendly diet, clear your kitchen of unfriendly foods, and stock up on better options.

Part II: Eating For Your Intestinal Health

We're excited to share more than 100 recipes for every meal of the day as well as snacks, soups, salads, drinks, and desserts, including options that mimic some old comfort-food favorites so you can enjoy them again safely. We provide these recipes with IBS-friendliness in mind, but you can expect many of them to become favorites of the whole family.

Part III: Simple Solutions for Specific Situations

Some IBS circumstances require special considerations. For example, even just leaving the house can be a challenge if you have IBS, so here you get some great tips for eating safely when you can't be in your own kitchen, whether you're out with friends or headed to an event. Parents of IBS kids can find a whole chapter of recipes and tips to help them help children make the transition to a more IBS-friendly diet.

Part IV: The Part of Tens

Some of the most important points in the book are condensed into these four chapters. They remind you to avoid certain foods and common eating traps, show you how to make the foods you do eat a little more digestible, and tip you off to the underdiscussed (at least in our opinion) problem of yeast overgrowth.

Part V: Appendixes

These four appendixes give conversion info for those of the metric persuasion, show you how to substitute more friendly alternatives to certain triggers, identify the fiber contents of many common foods, and help you find triggers where they may be hiding in foods and ingredient lists.

Icons Used in This Book

To make this book easier to read and simpler to use, we include some icons that can help you find and fathom key ideas and information.

This icon appears whenever an idea or item can save you time, money, or stress when taking care of your IBS.

Any time you see this icon, you know the information that follows is so important it's worth reading more than once.

This icon flags information that highlights dangers to your health or well-being.

This icon appears next to information that's interesting but not essential. Don't be afraid to skip these paragraphs.

Where to Go from Here

This book is organized so that you can start wherever you want and find cross references to other chapters for the complete story. If you're still feeling lost, we have a few suggestions about where to begin. If you want a primer on food and IBS or want to let your spouse or partner in on what's brewing in your gut, read Chapter 1. If you're ready for the recipes, dive into Part II to find out what's cooking. If you have a child with IBS, Chapter 15 is a good starting point.

Of course, you can always go straight through from start to finish. But be forewarned: When you see how much fun we had, you may find yourself reading the book from cover to cover, laughing uproariously at all our jokes.

Part I
You Are What You Eat: Food and IBS

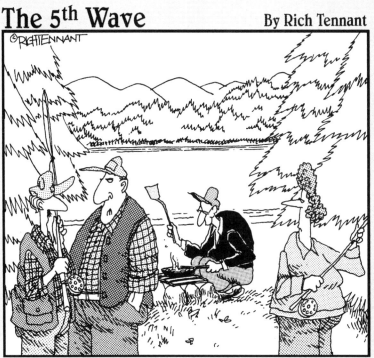

"Don't use that excuse on me, Wayne. Ain't no good reason why a man with IBS can't help himself to some of Earl's fried mealworms."

In this part . . .

Reconciling your body's need for food and your IBS's intolerance of many foods can be difficult, so in this part we help you break down your new eating plan. Chapter 1 gives you an overview of food's relationship with IBS. All IBS sufferers are different, so Chapter 2 helps you determine your own personal triggers, which can be the opposite of your best friend's. In Chapter 3, we help you transition toward an IBS-friendlier diet that's based on your needs; Chapter 4 shows you how to support that diet with a properly stocked kitchen. Finally, Chapter 5 gives you tips on calming your stomach when you have a flare-up despite your best attempts.

Chapter 1

IBS, Food, and You

In This Chapter
▶ Understanding the cause, effects, and triggers of IBS
▶ Watching out for similar conditions
▶ Exploring nutritional and medical treatments for IBS

*R*emember the day you found out that you may have IBS? Maybe your doctor offered you the diagnosis along with a prescription for the appropriate intestinal accelerant or depressant. Or maybe you surfed the Internet from your perch on the toilet, entered your list of symptoms into the search engine, and came up with IBS. Either way, finding that diagnosis likely brought some relief because you finally knew that you weren't alone (or crazy) — IBS is real!

Lots of people with IBS try to tough it out on their own without seeking medical treatment (according to some, about 70 percent). We've seen the lists of books our clients have read, the Web sites they've surfed, and the support groups they've attended. We hear your cries of frustration as you sit in front of 17 Web pages that all offer conflicting information about what to do, feel, eat, wear, think, take, and expect for IBS.

Feeling powerless? Well, one major way to take control of your IBS symptoms and your general health is to pay attention to the food you eat, and this chapter shows you just how to do that by providing you with an overview of IBS and how what you eat can affect it.

Following the Food Trail: How Food Is Supposed to Travel through Your System

Irritable bowel syndrome isn't all in your head, but it can make you feel crazy and out of control when it strikes. Most medical professionals agree that IBS doesn't cause any structural changes in the gut, which is why it's still called a syndrome and not a disease. What IBS does specifically (besides making your life miserable) is change the form and frequency of your bowel movements. No matter the name, know that you can regain control of your body and soothe your IBS symptoms simply by changing what and how you eat. But to do that, you first need to understand how the human body breaks down food so that you can recognize what your body *isn't* doing that's causing you so much discomfort. For even more details on the biology of IBS, check out our *IBS For Dummies* (Wiley).

When you chew food, saliva coats the particles with enzymes that begin the digestive process. Sounds disgusting, but it's very effective because carbs do start breaking down in your mouth. Chewing activates the stomach acid that gets to work on each bite you swallow, focusing on the protein. When your stomach acid sufficiently breaks down a meal, your body sends the mass of pulp out the other end of the stomach into the small intestine. Lipase fat enzymes from the pancreas and bile from the liver attack fats while amylase (an enzyme from the pancreas) continues the digestion of carbs.

The proper muscular movement of gastrointestinal tract (GIT) muscles propels everything through the various stages of digestion and absorption in the small intestine. By the time food reaches the large intestine, it should no longer be food but rather fibers and debris from microorganisms that now have to be excreted. The trip through the large intestine is designed to absorb any extra fluids, but if food particles remain because your small intestine hasn't properly digested them, microorganisms have a feast and can cause the symptoms of gas, bloating, and constipation or diarrhea associated with IBS.

Recognizing IBS' Common Cause and Triggers

The main issues with the GIT aren't unique to IBS. Anyone can suffer gut symptoms but in IBS, the symptoms never seem to stop. The following sections give you clues about what likely causes IBS and the triggers you can avoid to lessen the likelihood of an IBS attack.

Causing IBS

The only medically accepted cause of IBS is a history of having a previous gut infection. In surveys of people with IBS, the only common association that stands out is an intestinal infection, whether that's stomach flu, food poisoning, traveler's diarrhea, or something else. Whether the infectious organisms or the antibiotics used to treat the infection are the underlying cause is still unclear. The solution, which we talk about in Chapter 5, is to be sure and take probiotics whenever you have a gut infection or take an antibiotic.

Certain people may just be susceptible to IBS, so they may go on to develop chronic symptoms after an acute infection. But medical research isn't complete enough to confirm that theory because we don't know the criteria for being susceptible to IBS.

Triggering an attack

By definition, a *trigger* is something that initiates a process or a reaction. Certain factors may trigger symptoms of IBS in some people. If that sounds vague, that's because it is — each person is unique, and though you and your neighbor may have similar IBS symptoms, your triggers probably aren't the same.

- ✔ **The food you eat:** Yes, sad to say, food is a trigger for IBS. But what type of food triggers you and what type of reaction it triggers is very individual, so Chapter 2 helps you sort out your own personal triggers so that you can use Chapter 3 to put together a friendlier diet.

- ✔ **How you eat:** If you don't chew your food properly, or if you drink too much liquid with your meals, your food remains partially undigested and is fodder for intestinal microorganisms. Not enough hydrochloric acid in your stomach and/or not enough pancreatic enzymes can create similar circumstances. Also, eating large meals might cause the intestinal sphincters between your small and large intestine to open too soon and rush your undigested food through and cause diarrhea.

- ✔ **Previous negative reactions to foods:** If you've had a negative reaction to a food in the past, your brain may decide that that particular food is never going to be good for you and set off alarm bells the next time you're even in its presence. The food doesn't even have to pass your lips before your stomach starts to tighten up as if it's going to war. And the really nasty part of this whole story is that the food in question may not have even caused your symptoms in the first place.

- ✔ **Emotions:** Foods and emotions, especially stress, can trigger the release of serotonin in the gut, leading to some of your symptoms. This connection occurs because an amazingly high 90 percent of the serotonin feel-good hormone in the body arises from the gut.

Stress comes in many forms. In fact, one aspect of IBS can be an uncontrollable urge to control. That may sound like an oxymoron, but it may explain why a loss of control in the intestines is often paralleled by a loss of control in life. Diarrhea is a complete loss of intestinal control, and constipation is a clamping down to try to maintain control, resulting in cramps, pain, and distention. Chapter 5 outlines more details about stress's effects on the gut.

✔ **Yeast:** Alone or in combination, the overuse of antibiotics, a high-sugar diet, stress, cortisone, hormones, and other factors can all lead to an overgrowth of yeast in your gut, which can cause some nasty effects. For more info on yeast overgrowth, flip to Chapter 18.

✔ **Antibiotics:** Although sometimes they're necessary to kill dangerous bad bacteria and can be life saving, they can also take out the good bacteria in your system. Actually, these drugs aren't too smart; they are supposed to kill off bad bacteria that are causing your symptoms, but instead they mow down every bacteria in their path, throwing the healthy gut flora completely out of balance and opening the door for yeast to migrate from the large intestine to the small intestine, causing symptoms of gas, bloating, and stool changes. Chapter 18 gives you the skinny on the potential problems with antibiotics and yeast.

Take antibiotics when you need them and you can replace the good bacteria with probiotics as we discussed in Chapter 5.

How What You Eat Affects Your IBS

The GIT is always at work moving food through your body while distinguishing between safe and unsafe foods. If you've ever had food poisoning or too much to drink, you know what happens when your GIT rejects the toxic food or drink from your body — usually either vomiting or diarrhea.

Most sources agree that certain foods and even the mere act of eating can trigger symptoms of IBS, but nobody really says why or how that happens. Here's Carolyn's theory after spending 30 years working with patients who have IBS:

Your hard working GIT has evolved through the ages and seen many, many foods, both natural and artificial. If you think back just two or three generations in your own family, you likely have a very different diet than your great-grandparents did. In fact, grandma's comfort food probably had very simple ingredients, and what she mixed together in her homemade chocolate cake recipe is very different than the ingredients on the box of chocolate cake mix sitting in your cupboard.

Food has evolved from these simpler times into tastier, sweeter, richer, easier to prepare, more convenient versions with longer shelf lives. As a result, more foods are prepackaged with lots of added sugar, food additives, fats, and preservatives. Cooks and entrepreneurs have created restaurants that get inexpensive, filling, and tasty food into your system within moments of ordering it, even if that food's nutritional value may be questionable. Your GIT can become so overwhelmed by the variety of sugars, fats, grains, dairy, and food additives you're pumping into it that your system may either latch on to a food as toxic and use diarrhea to dump it or get confused and startled into constipation.

Differentiating from Inflammatory Bowel Disease (IBD)

IBD stands for Inflammatory Bowel Disease, which encompasses Crohn's disease and ulcerative colitis. IBD is a defined disease with definite signs and symptoms. To diagnose IBD, scopes look for signs of tissue inflammation and ulceration. X-rays taken after you take barium can help define areas of narrowing and ulceration. Bleeding and excessive mucus in the stools are the defining symptoms that differentiate IBD from IBS.

Some suggest that IBS may continue worsening and turn into IBD if you don't treat it properly with diet and probiotics. We don't say this to scare you but rather to encourage you to take charge of your condition now instead of putting it off or ignoring it altogether.

Considering Other Ailments Masquerading as IBS

The main four conditions that mimic IBS and can also be triggers for IBS if not treated are celiac disease, yeast overgrowth, lactose intolerance, and food sensitivities and allergies. They all have so many symptoms in common with IBS that you have to understand their subtleties and do some food avoidance and challenging testing (described in Chapter 2) to determine whether your IBS is really one of these ailments. This process of food elimination lets you find out whether your IBS symptoms are really from gluten, yeast overgrowth, lactose intolerance, and food sensitivities or allergies.

Celiac disease

Celiac disease is a genetic condition caused by an immune response to *gluten,* a protein found mainly in three grains (wheat, rye, and barley) and contaminating another grain (oats).

Oats don't actually contain gluten, but they're invariably farmed, stored, and/ or milled in facilities that also handle wheat, rye, and barley, so they can be contaminated with tiny trace amounts of gluten — still enough to trigger some people with celiac disease. Some oats are grown, stored, and milled in isolation and bear the gluten-free symbol.

The immune system attacks the gluten, damaging the intestines and impairing their absorption of food. The main symptoms of celiac disease include (but aren't limited to) the following:

- ✔ GI symptoms
- ✔ Headaches
- ✔ Poor concentration
- ✔ Infertility
- ✔ Weight loss or gain
- ✔ Depression
- ✔ Muscle, joint, or bone pain
- ✔ Anemia
- ✔ Fatigue

The treatment for celiac disease is simple: Avoid gluten grains and products that use these grains.

Yeast overgrowth

Yeast is a type of fungus, a cousin to mold and mildew in the form of tiny round buds that grow naturally on your skin and in your intestines. Yeast buds don't have mouths or stomachs — they grow into their food, absorbing sugars in the form of table sugar, milk sugar, fruit sugar, and glucose molecules from simple carbohydrates like bread. When a round yeast bud grows to a critical size, it can no longer absorb enough food through its surface to reach the center, so it breaks off into smaller buds that form their own colonies.

Antibiotics can contribute to yeast overgrowth because they kill all gut bacteria, including the good stuff, leaving room for yeast to take over.

Symptoms of yeast overgrowth include

- ✔ Chronic fatigue
- ✔ Allergies, sinusitis, and asthma
- ✔ Vaginitis or prostatitis

You can starve out yeast by avoiding sugar, wheat, and dairy; see Chapter 18 for more on controlling yeast overgrowth.

Lactose intolerance

Lactose (milk sugar) is what makes milk taste a bit sweet. Up to 75 percent of adults worldwide have diminished capacity to digest dairy products, so lactose intolerance isn't a rare condition. Experts estimate that about 50 million Americans feel the effects of lactose intolerance, and that figure doesn't count the millions who suffer occasionally when they load up on lactose. The reactions occur because undigested dairy becomes fodder for intestinal organisms that feed and breed off your waste. It can also attract water, which makes your stools very runny. The symptoms of lactose intolerance are very much like the symptoms for IBS:

- ✔ Abdominal pain and bloating
- ✔ Constipation
- ✔ Diarrhea (usually very runny)
- ✔ Alternating constipation and diarrhea
- ✔ Cramps
- ✔ Gas
- ✔ Nausea and vomiting

To determine whether your condition is lactose intolerance or dairy-triggered IBS, you can take a lactose tolerance blood test or a hydrogen breath test (lactose intolerance creates an excess of hydrogen in the breath). Your doctor first takes a preliminary reading of either your blood glucose or the amount of hydrogen in your breath, depending on which test you're taking. After you drink a liquid containing lactose, you repeat the test and compare the results. If your blood glucose has suddenly become elevated or your hydrogen breath reading has spiked, you are diagnosed with lactose intolerance, not IBS.

The best way to treat lactose intolerance? Avoiding lactose. In Appendix D, we list many foods that may contain lactose so you can make more informed food choices.

Food allergies and food sensitivities

Food allergies and sensitivities are two separate animals that can both cause IBS-like symptoms. The medical definition of a *food allergy* is a reaction to food causing an immediate reaction with swelling of mucus membranes and a positive IgE blood test showing elevated antibody levels. Strawberries, shellfish, and nuts are some of the big food allergy culprits; if you have an allergy and eat an offending food, your body releases histamines and other chemicals, causing hives, itching, and swelling that can occasionally be life-threatening. Only 1 percent of adults and 3 percent of children suffer IgE food allergies; naturally, if you have a food allergy, you want to identify and avoid that food.

Chronic food allergies can take up to 48 hours to appear, so associating them with food intake can be difficult unless you do the avoidance and challenge testing we talk about in Chapter 2. Dairy, wheat, soy, and corn are common IgG food allergies, and a positive test shows a higher level of IgG antibodies. Unfortunately, most doctors only recognize IgE food allergies and not the IgG kind, so you often have to do the dietary testing yourself to make your own diagnosis. Many nutritionally oriented doctors perform the IgG allergy tests to determine food allergies, but Carolyn finds that the food avoidance and challenge testing works just as well or even better.

You can take IgG food allergy blood tests, but if you have a leaky gut (which we discuss in Chapter 18), molecules of undigested food can be absorbed from the gut into the bloodstream. Your immune system attacks those molecules with IgG antibodies and can give you a false positive IgG test result for just about every food you're eating.

Food sensitivities are foods that you may have identified as unique triggers for your symptoms without any clear medical reason. The designation *food sensitivity* is more in the realm of inability to digest a particular food, with symptoms of mucus, nausea, or upset stomach after eating. You may burp after a pizza due to inability to digest green peppers, or dairy products may give you mucus and you find yourself clearing your throat after drinking a milkshake. Many foods that cause symptoms in people with IBS are labeled food sensitivities. That's where a food diary and avoiding and challenging foods become very important tools. (Head to Chapter 2 for guidance on creating a food diary.)

Treating Your Symptoms With Nutrition: What an IBS-Friendly Diet Looks Like

The definition of *medicine* as Carolyn learned it in medical school is the diagnosis of disease and the treatment of disease symptoms with drugs. We'd rather show you ways of treating IBS to relieve the condition, but there may be times when you need symptomatic treatment. The following sections give you tips on controlling your symptoms with diet, natural remedies, and medicine.

To get a good visual of an IBS-friendly diet, take a look at the color section near the middle of this book. A diet that provides you and your sensitive stomach with delicious, safe foods doesn't have a lot of garbage associated with it. We're talking about the ingredients and the packaging here — if you're eating fat-laden cuisine out of a bag, wrapper, or cardboard container that's going to end up in your trash can, it's very likely not IBS-friendly. If you've prepared the meal yourself from fresh ingredients, your gut is far more likely to thank you later. After you identify your personal triggers (see Chapter 2), Chapter 3 shows you how to transition away from triggers and trash and into a healthy-yet-tasty alternative.

To get you started on this friendly path, check out the recipes in Part II — 120 delightful dishes for your mouth and your stomach.

Supplementing a Healthy Diet

Whether or not you have IBS, supplements are important to create and maintain a healthy body. Many doctors argue that you can get all your vitamins and minerals from a healthy, balanced diet, but that's becoming harder and harder as heavy industrialized farming strips minerals from the soil without properly replacing them.

Don't assume that enriched foods — bread products with B vitamins, sugared yogurt with probiotics, milk with extra calcium — are totally healthy. The synthetic supplements manufacturers add don't completely make up for the actual nutrition that's been refined, processed, and bleached away.

If you have IBS-C, your colon is holding a lot of waste hostage in your body. You need a good antioxidant supplement to counteract the toxicity and a probiotic to fight off the fiendish bacteria roaming your body. IBS-D sufferers may often have the sense that they're losing their lunches before they've had time to absorb it. As a result, their bodies may be depleted of necessary nutrients, and a good-quality multivitamin is essential.

Studies that say vitamins are dangerous or ineffective are usually testing synthetic supplements and not the food-based nutrients that come from nature. And no supplement is an acceptable replacement for improving your diet and lifestyle.

Making magnesium your new best friend

Magnesium tops our list as the number one supplement for anyone because it's crucial for your health, it's simple to take, it's inexpensive, and it's effective in the proper forms whether you have IBS-C or IBS-D. Magnesium is necessary for the proper function of more than 325 different enzymes in the body, and maintaining adequate magnesium levels can ease the pain and spasms of IBS symptoms and make having such an illness a little less uncomfortable. The symptoms of magnesium deficiency include muscle spasms, palpitations, hypertension, insomnia, migraines, PMS, depression, and anxiety and panic attacks. Another major symptom is moderate fatigue — not just general tiredness but rather a distinct lack of energy that, when coupled with IBS, compromises your body's healing resources.

Most people don't think of having a magnesium deficiency because the symptoms are associated with so many other conditions. But being deficient in magnesium can affect your overall health because you're operating your body without all its vital components. And most doctors don't recognize a magnesium deficiency because no test in standard lab work accurately identifies it.

Magnesium is a great natural laxative, so it's very helpful if you have IBS-C to take a magnesium citrate powder in water or a magnesium dimalate tablet if you would rather swallow a pill. Recent research has also turned up two forms of magnesium that work for IBS-D: magnesium oil and angstrom-sized magnesium. The following list covers these and other helpful forms of magnesium.

> ✔ **Magnesium oil:** Although it's not technically an oil, magnesium chloride highly concentrated in distilled water has a slightly oily consistency. You spray or rub the oil on your skin, so it doesn't reach your intestines and cause a laxative effect (unless you bathe in a few gallons of it). Research shows that applying a solution of magnesium oil to your skin restores levels within your tissues in four to six weeks. The minimum daily dose is 400 milligrams or about 20 sprays if you're using a spray

bottle. You can dilute the oil with distilled water if it burns or tingles slightly; leave the oil on all day, or wash it off after at least 30 minutes if you prefer.

✔ **Angstrom minerals:** Good things come in small packages, and the smaller the magnesium particle, the more likely it's able to pass through the miniscule openings in the cell walls. Fortunately, magnesium and other minerals come in atom-sized packages called *angstrom*. The dosage for angstrom minerals is between five and ten times less than the common brands on the shelf. It comes in liquid form, and a dose is about 40 milligrams (2 tablespoons) twice a day taken with or without food in a small glass of water.

On her blog, Carolyn has gotten numerous testimonials from people who have switched to angstrom minerals (especially magnesium) and found enormous benefits. One woman wrote, "The (angstrom) magnesium works much faster that the taurate capsules. Sleeping even better, relaxed muscles, just calmer. I will continue taking this form of magnesium from now on." If you're looking for angstrom, the source we trust is www.completeh2ominerals.com.

✔ **Magnesium from food:** Seaweed and chocolate both have very high amounts of magnesium. We know how exciting the chocolate part sounds, but remember that we're talking about the 100-percent raw, bitter chocolate called *cacao*. Even so, Carolyn's Chocolate Banana Cream Pudding (see the recipe in Chapter 13) is a delicious magnesium supplement containing banana (33 milligrams for 4 ounces), coconut milk (100 milligrams per cup) and raw chocolate (100 milligrams for 2 tablespoons).

Other foods rich in magnesium are nuts, seeds, deep green leafy vegetables, and whole grains. You may think that these foods are off limits, but that's not the case. Our Basic Seed or Nut Pâté (see the recipe in Chapter 7) is a blend of nuts or seeds, lemon juice, sea salt, and garlic and is extremely high in magnesium. Deep green leafy vegetables may be a stretch for you but consider juicing greens or even blending your salad to a consistency that your tummy can tolerate.

Making room for other important vitamins and minerals

We don't deal too deeply with supplements in this book because our focus is on treating your IBS with food, but we want to make you aware of the most beneficial nutrients for your gut. The most important nutrients after magnesium are vitamin D, zinc, calcium, and vitamin A. Of course, you could make a case for any of the other 44 vitamins and minerals, but the following list just aims to get you started on the basics.

- ✔ **Vitamin D:** Vitamin D research is in its infancy, but so far it has shown that vitamin D affects most of the body's tissues. Current research links vitamin D deficiency with 17 different types of cancer (including breast cancer) and many other illnesses like osteoporosis, heart disease and juvenile diabetes. According to Dr. Soram Khalsa, author of *The Vitamin D Revolution* (HayHouse) having adequate vitamin D intake (2,000 IU a day year round) provides you with overall health benefits that may translate into the lessening of your IBS symptoms. Vitamin D is very difficult to get in your diet; in order to get 2,000 IU a day, you would have to drink 20 glasses of milk or eat 10 cans of tuna, but as vitamin D3, it's an easy-to-take supplement that may speed up the healing of damaged tissues and cells. Sun exposure does give you lots of vitamin D, but only at certain times of the day and certain times of the year.

- ✔ **Zinc:** Researchers say that fast-healing humans have high levels of zinc in their tissues. Almost 100 body enzymes depend on zinc to make them work properly; that's less than the 325 powered by magnesium (see the preceding section), but it's still pretty impressive. Many of these enzymes deal with tissue growth and repair and may just help those with leaky gut (which we discuss in Chapter 18). Sunflower seeds, pumpkin seeds, and oysters are good sources of zinc; our Basic Seed or Nut Pâté in Chapter 7 helps you easily obtain your daily dose of zinc (which in tablet form is 10 to 15 milligrams and in liquid angstrom form is 20 milligrams per day).

- ✔ **Calcium:** Calcium is the most abundant mineral in the body, helping to create your bones and teeth. It's also the most commonly used mineral supplement. Calcium is crucial for heart health because it makes muscles, including the heart muscle, contract. It neutralizes acidity in the body, activates enzymes, promotes cell division, and allows the transport of nutrients through cell membranes.

Although it's famously associated with dairy products, better sources for those with dairy triggers are whole grains, nuts, and seeds. Despite dairy concerns, yogurt is a good source of calcium and its beneficial probiotics may also slow down diarrhea. You can find dairy and non-dairy yogurt recipes in Chapter 6.

You may see calcium recommended as a treatment for IBS because of its tendency to cause constipation, but we must warn you of the dangers of taking too much calcium. Carolyn receives reports from doctors and clients who tell her they are developing complications (including gall stones, kidney stones, and magnesium deficiency) possibly caused by overuse and overprescription of over-the-counter calcium tablets.

Excess calcium sticks around in the body, building up in tissues and throwing your magnesium levels out of balance. Carolyn now only recommends 20 milligrams of calcium liquid angstrom supplement twice a day.

✔ **Vitamin A:** Vitamin A is important for healthy skin — both your outside skin and the inside skin of your lungs and gut. If you have vitamin A deficiency, symptoms of IBS-D can worsen because the mucus membranes of the gut are not as strong and healthy. At the same time, diarrhea can cause loss of vitamin A. Supplemental vitamin A usually comes from cod liver oil, but some food sources include colorful (dark green, yellow, orange, and red) vegetables and fruits, including spinach, pumpkins, peppers, squash, carrots, yellow peaches, apricots, papayas, and mangoes. It's also found in high amounts in egg yolks, although some folks with IBS may be avoiding those (see Chapter 6). The recommended daily intake for vitamin A is 3,000 IU, but we suggest at least 5,000 IU per day, which you can usually get in 1 teaspoon of cod liver oil.

Using digestive supplements to help digest your food

When we give people the choice to chew each bite of food 40 times or take a digestive supplement, they usually go for the supplement, but we wish people would choose chewing (or at least chewing *and* a supplement). Chewing well lets you do one-third of your digesting in your mouth with salivary enzymes. Plus, it also alerts the rest of the GIT to get ready for dinner. If your food isn't well-chewed and fully digested as it makes its way through the digestive tract, some of it reaches the intestines in particle sizes that are difficult to absorb, leaving fodder for microorganisms to power up on so they can set off your symptoms later.

✔ **Digestive enzymes:** Most digestive enzymes contain amylase, betaine hydrochloride, lipase, and peptidase, and the vegetarian formulas contain bromelain and papain from pineapple and papaya. Take one or two in the middle or at the end of your meal to help relieve symptoms of gas, bloating, and belching. Another remedy that is effective and less expensive is to take 1 to 3 teaspoons of organic apple cider vinegar in 4 ounces of water before and/or during a meal.

✔ **Probiotics:** Countless recent studies have shown the importance of *probiotics* (good bacteria) for the GIT in promoting fermentation to assist digestion and maintaining an appropriate pH in the large intestine to deter invading bacteria. Probiotics are the answer to the good bacteria vacuum created by antibiotics; bifidus and lactobacillus acidophilus are examples of helpful probiotics you can take. The optimum dosage range for probiotics is from 2 to 10 billion active cells daily. Make sure the label on your product guarantees this number through the expiration date.

✔ **Herbs:** Many herbs have been used for centuries to treat gut symptoms and assist digestion. The best herbs for the gut are *demulcents,* or substances that have the ability to form a soothing film over a mucus membrane to protect enzyme function and areas that absorb nutrients. You get the very gooey picture of that process when you think of slippery elm bark, aloe vera, Irish moss, and the newest protein powder on the block, chia seeds. Jelly-like and cooling, they're anti-inflammatory and soothing.

Be sure to use aloe vera and not the laxative aloe latex products. The safest aloe vera we know is George's Aloe.

Here are some suitable herbs that can help take the spasm and bloating out of the gut, making digesting food and absorbing nutrients much easier. Check out *IBS For Dummies* (Wiley) for more information:

- **Peppermint oil:** Relaxes the intestines and relieves bloating

- **Fennel:** Antispasmodic that eliminates gas and bloating

- **Ginger:** Antispasmodic that relieves nausea and indigestion

- **Chamomile:** Antispasmodic and anti-inflammatory that relieves anxiety

- **Caraway:** Antispasmodic that relieves gas and aids digestion

- **Anise:** Relieves gas and bloating, settles the bowel, and has antifungal properties

- **Oregano:** Relieves nausea, vomiting, diarrhea, and muscle spasms and has antifungal and antibacterial properties

- **Angelica root *(dong quai)*:** Relieves intestinal cramps, gas, and bloating

- **Bitter herbs such as bitter orange peel, gentian root, artichoke leaf, areca seed, and dandelion root:** Stimulate gastric juices and increase bile production

- **Areca seed:** Relieves abdominal distention and constipation and has antiparasitic properties

Beginning the Healing Process

Adopting an IBS friendly diet begins at home — right in your own kitchen. Although thinking about everything you have to do may feel overwhelming right now, remember to be patient with yourself and know that you're at the beginning of your healing process and in charge of how fast or slow you move through this transition.

Everything seems a bit easier when you break it down into steps, so one of the first things to do is get the offending foods out of your kitchen (or at least your line of vision). Chapter 4 shows you how to chuck the junk and stock up on IBS-friendly foods, whether you live alone or with others who don't have IBS.

The shopping tips in Chapter 4 are especially helpful as you load up on the ingredients for the recipes in Part II. Whether you are new to the kitchen or a seasoned cook, the recipes are easy to follow and feature easy-to-find, IBS-friendly ingredients. The recipes may even show you some new ways to cook and prepare food.

But there's also life outside your kitchen, and we've got lots of tips for eating away from home in Chapter 14. Whether it's lunch at the office, dinner at a restaurant, or a family gathering, our tips help you prepare for safe and fun meals. You are on the path to a healthier way to eat.

Chapter 2

Finding Your Intestinal Triggers

*T*here's no template for the care and feeding of IBS, which is why it's important for you to find out what's eating you as you embark on this IBS adventure. In this chapter, we explain the sensitivities that people can have to dairy, gluten, sugar, fructose, and insoluble fiber; we then show you how to safely experiment with your diet so you can determine whether these IBS triggers are aiming for your intestines.

In this chapter, we provide very specific guidelines on challenging three of the traditional four food groups in order to help you identify your triggers. In case you've forgotten, the four are meat, dairy, grains, and fruits and veggies; meat is off the hook in this chapter. Armed with this knowledge, you can start exploring the many food substitutions and recipes that we outline for you. (Check out Appendix B for a quick reference list of trigger food substitutions.) If you've been living with IBS for many years, we assure you that there are many more options and substitutions than existed even ten years ago.

We want to be clear right from the beginning that we know we're jumping into very dangerous territory by telling you to avoid certain foods. These may be the foods you crave, eat every day, and can't wait to enjoy after a long day at work. It's hard to believe that your favorite comfort food may be causing you such intestinal discomfort, but the relief you'll feel by cutting it out of your diet and exploring new recipes that don't trigger IBS will be well worth the effort.

Identifying Trigger Foods

No doubt you know of some foods that clearly aren't your friends and are fairly easy to avoid, but there are likely to be some IBS culprits lurking in your current diet. You know the ones we're talking about — remember that painful reminder when you ate the spicy sausage and drank beer at your weekend picnic?

An IBS trigger may also be described as food sensitivity. (Some people talk about food intolerance, but since lactose intolerance and fructose intolerance (malabsorption) are genuine diseases, we use the word *sensitivity* instead for clarity.) There are many different symptoms of food sensitivity, including headaches and achy joints that don't even seem to affect the gastrointestinal (GI) tract. You may be treating such symptoms with prescription medications when simple food avoidance can bring you permanent relief. We provide a list of symptoms of food sensitivity in the section "Listening to your body" later in this chapter.

An *intolerance* is an inability of the natural digestive processes to break down a food substance, leading to symptoms. Lactose intolerance and fructose intolerance are two examples. An *allergy,* on the other hand, is a condition wherein an immune system response causes antibodies to be released in response to a particular food. A *food sensitivity* is another designation of your body rejecting a food. It doesn't necessarily show up on allergy tests, and the most common way to diagnose it is to do food avoidance and challenging, which we cover in the individual trigger foods sections later in this chapter. Celiac disease, on the other hand, is an auto-immune reaction to gluten and not an intolerance, allergy, or sensitivity, although you can have gluten intolerance, gluten allergy, or gluten sensitivity.

Knowing the top five trigger foods

Knowledge is power. We've spoken to many IBS sufferers who would prefer to remain in denial than admit that their favorite treat was causing some of their IBS symptoms. But knowing the top trigger foods gives you power over your diet and food intake, and some simple substitutions can be a treat for your taste buds while calming your colon. We hope the recipes in this book will help alleviate the anxiety that may be churning as you consider eliminating anything from your diet.

The top five foods that trigger IBS are

- ✔ Dairy
- ✔ Wheat
- ✔ Sugar
- ✔ Fructose
- ✔ Insoluble fiber

The most common reaction that IBS sufferers have when we tell them to avoid dairy or wheat or fruit (a source of fructose) is disbelief. How can the staff of life (wheat) or the milk you were raised on be bad for you? And apart from the forbidden apple, fruit is usually considered a healthy snack. However, in the context of IBS you may not be able to digest these foods to a degree where your body is comfortable with them, meaning they gang up on your intestines and cause problems that you may not even recognize.

We feel your pain. At one time or another, we've sadly turned our backs on all these foods and food groups and lived to write about it. And you will, too. Well, maybe not write about it, but you can tell your grandchildren that you survived.

Listening to your body

Remember that weekend treat mentioned earlier, when the spicy sausage and beer intermingled to become a fermenting cauldron in your gut? That was your body saying no!

People become so accustomed to having burpy, gassy, churning reactions to everyday foods that they don't even consider that these foods may be contributing to IBS. So you don't listen to the sounds your gut is making because you really don't want to admit that you're having a reaction. We want you to become accustomed to hearing and feeling the signs and signals that your body is giving you and to become more aware of the impact of food on your system.

Here's a comprehensive list of food sensitivity symptoms, courtesy of www.foodintol.com.

- ✔ **Respiratory symptoms:** Coughing, sneezing, wheezing, asthma, ear infections, snoring, sleep apnea, pneumonia, bronchitis

- ✔ **Immune system symptoms:** Catching colds and infections easily, mouth ulcers, yeast fungal infections

- ✔ **Neural (nervous system) symptoms:** Poor coordination, clumsiness, headaches, migraines, depression, memory problems, intellectual difficulties, dementia

- ✔ **Skin, hair and nails:** Eczema, psoriasis, dermatitis, hives, rosacea, rashes, hair loss, split and cracked nails, poor complexion, dandruff

- ✔ **Metabolism problems:** Moodiness, weight gain, weight loss, chills, thyroid disease, cravings, addictions

- ✔ **Musculoskeletal symptoms:** Stiff muscles or joints, tendonitis, arthritis, bone thinning, bone fractures, osteoporosis

> ✔ **Malabsorption:** Extreme tiredness and lack of energy, difficulty concentrating, vitamin deficiencies, iron deficiency, anemia, calcium deficiency
>
> ✔ **Gastro symptoms:** Irritable bowel syndrome (IBS), diarrhea, constipation, indigestion, esophageal reflux, stomach ulcers, bowel cancer
>
> ✔ **Genital and reproductive symptoms:** Vaginitis, urinary tract infections, infertility, difficulty conceiving, miscarriage

You're looking for signs like these not because you're a glutton for punishment but so you can avoid the particular food combinations that resulted in such symptoms the next time.

Making a food diary

If your memory seems to get conveniently wiped out after every IBS food attack, we suggest you record the events surrounding your meal in a food diary. Write down your observations as close to the event as possible so that they're fresh in your mind. Describe the symptoms and discomfort in detail so that you're also aware of other triggers like stress, exhaustion, and tension. Otherwise, you may just blame the food and end up limiting your diet unnecessarily.

If you eat out a lot, use a small notebook that you can carry around in your pocket or purse. If it's not handy, you won't use it. If people ask you what you're doing you can tell them you're writing the Great American Novel, channeling a winning lottery number, or calculating the square root of pi. They'll never bother you again.

On one side of the page, list everything you eat and the time you eat it. On the other side, record whatever symptoms arise during the day along with the time.

When reviewing your food diary, you're looking for patterns; you may be surprised to find a correlation between what you eat and how you feel. Your spicy sausage and beer is only one of many revealing moments. Another may be that bagel with lox and cream cheese that you have once a week when you have a meeting in a particular neighborhood; luckily there's a restroom handy to deal with the cramping and diarrhea that seems to hit you out of the blue. Another connection may be the fried chicken that your mother makes for Sunday dinners; no cramping, just many trips to the restroom. Or you may find that your aunt's lasagna with three layers of three different cheeses stoppers you up for a week. In the case of lactose intolerance, your symptoms may come after two hours or even as soon as 30 minutes after eating. If constipation is your symptom for lactose intolerance, you may not notice it until you get up in the morning and your usual arising BM never arrives.

Suddenly you're amazed that your intolerance for certain foods has gone unnoticed for decades. While you're working on your food diary, you may hear an item on TV, read an article in a magazine, go online, or read this book, and it's like a giant light bulb goes off. You know beyond a shadow of a doubt that wheat and dairy are no longer your friends. You finally come to grips with the realization that eating bread and bagels and pizza and toasted cheese sandwiches are what's doing you in.

Identifying a food allergy, sensitivity, or food intolerance can be exciting, because there's an implied promise that if you stop eating certain foods that could be bothering you, you have a good chance of dumping your IBS symptoms.

Asking your ancestors

You don't just inherit genes from your ancestors; you inherit their food choices, eating habits, and recipes as well. In addition to inheriting your mother's eyes, you may also have inherited her intolerance for certain kinds of foods. Take a few moments to think about what food-related issues have been handed down through the generations in your family.

Interviewing your folks about food may be an interesting topic for your next family gathering. For example, you may have grown up with limited access to milk, cheese, and ice cream if dairy wasn't a favored food group in your house. But when you get out on your own and decide that you love drinking milkshakes and eating cheese pizza regularly, you may discover that you can't digest dairy products properly. Gas, bloating, diarrhea and/or constipation can be your reward for not following family tradition. On the other hand, if you grew up eating toast and cereal for breakfast, sandwiches for lunch, and rolls at dinner, you never got away from bread. The abdominal cramps that were only soothed by your mother's hand on your tummy could have been from all that wheat bread. And it wasn't until you decided to go on a diet in your 20s and take bread out of your menu that your stomach didn't rumble anymore.

The most common inherited reaction to food is *celiac disease,* which is an immune system response triggered by the consumption of gluten protein found in wheat, rye, barley, and often contaminating oats. Even though many members of one family suffer gastrointestinal symptoms, they may not even know they have celiac disease. Sometimes it takes a very inquisitive person determined to get to the bottom of his symptoms to solve the puzzle for the whole family.

Dairy as a Trigger Food

Humans are the only mammals to continue drinking milk after weaning, but as they wean off milk, most people experience a decrease in the amount of lactase enzyme necessary to digest dairy. Lactose, the sugar in milk, requires enzymes to break it down during digestion. Small amounts may cause no problems, but it's the larger load that the body can't handle.

Whether they do it consciously or unconsciously, many people recognize that dairy doesn't agree with them early on in life, so they avoid dairy products. Perhaps the avoidance is instinctive given that ancestry seems to influence a person's ability to digest dairy. But for those who crave creamy treats like ice cream and cheesecake, dairy-related IBS symptoms are one inheritance they'd rather give back.

Dairy and IBS

The connection between dairy and IBS can take the form of lactose intolerance and the insufficiency of lactase enzymes leading to the incomplete digestion of dairy leading to GI symptoms. Another connection and cause of symptoms may be an allergy or intolerance to the casein protein in dairy. This section delves into these possible sources of symptoms.

Lactose intolerance

Lactose intolerance symptoms primarily impact the GI tract. Lactase enzyme is designed to decode the lactose molecule into its two designer molecules: glucose and galactose. If that magic interaction doesn't occur — that is, if you're one of millions of people who don't produce lactase enzymes — lactose continues merrily along the superhighway of your gut wreaking havoc in its path. The chaos is due to bacteria and yeast in your large intestine feasting on undigested milk sugar, resulting in many IBS-like symptoms.

Symptoms of lactose intolerance include abdominal bloating, distention, pain and cramping, audible bowel noises, diarrhea, flatulence (passing gas), and sometimes nausea. As we outline in Chapter 1, these symptoms can be confused with an intestinal infection or celiac disease or be labeled IBS or IBD (inflammatory bowel disease).

Symptoms differ at different ages. Children with lactose intolerance may also have failure to thrive because one of their main sources of nutrients isn't being absorbed and they're losing nutrients due to diarrhea. Remember the childhood birthday parties where cake and ice cream (or ice cream cake) were the main attraction? Imagine how scary and embarrassing those are for a child who's blindsided by a need to rush to the bathroom while the other kids are pinning the tail on the donkey.

Adults may have the symptoms we list along with an urgency to evacuate the bowels. As we note earlier in the chapter, the timing can be from 30 minutes to two hours after a meal containing lactose.

According to the National Digestive Diseases Information Clearinghouse (NDDIC), 30 to 50 million Americans are lactose intolerant. But different cultures experience different levels of intolerance. 90 to 100 percent of Asian Americans, 80 percent of African Americans, and 15 percent of Caucasians suffer from the condition. Folks of northern European descent have even lower rates of lactose intolerance.

The symptoms associated with lactose intolerance are often related to the amount of dairy consumed and vary from one individual to another. If you eat dairy as the bulk of your meal or snack instead of it being a small portion of your meal, you may have a more difficult time digesting it. However, having milk or cheese as part of a full meal, which allows for a longer digestion time, give your limited lactase enzymes more time to do their work. Some dairy products also contain less lactose and are often easier to tolerate. Chapter 17 shows you more ways to make dairy easier to digest.

Casein allergy or intolerance

Casein is a milk protein, whereas lactose is a milk sugar. The symptoms of a casein allergy or intolerance are more difficult to identify as coming from dairy. Symptoms can include GI symptoms (vomiting, heartburn, abdominal pain, diarrhea, gas, and bloating) and also eczema, hives, asthma, and shortness of breath.

If you've taken the dairy challenge (see "Taking the dairy challenge" later in this chapter) and have finally narrowed down your IBS symptoms to dairy after avoiding it for two weeks, you may think that drinking and eating lactose-free products or taking lactase enzyme pills will solve your IBS problems. However, if your symptoms return in spite of lactose-eliminating precautions, casein may be the culprit.

Many foods that are advertised as "nondairy" or "dairy-free" still contain casein, and it may be found in high-protein or protein-enriched products. But casein can be hard to recognize on an ingredient list because it goes by several different names. Look for casein (obviously) but also sodium caseinate, galactose, sodium lactylate, lactose, lactalbumin, and other names that begin with or feature *lact–*.

Eating dairy-free

Dairy products are used in many processed and packaged foods, such as cereals, muffin and pancake mixes, stuffing, and meat extenders. Make reading labels your new hobby, and pay extra attention to understanding and spotting the many hidden names of dairy. The dairy vocabulary includes *whey, whey powder, clarified butter, ghee, artificial butter flavor, curds, lactose, hydrolysates, lactalbumin, lactoglobulin,* and *lactulose.*

We understand that you may shy away from the idea of giving up dairy products. Not only is dairy a staple in many households, with milk topping most grocery shopping lists, but dairy is also a comfort food and a treat. Many people grew up enjoying milk and cookies after school and a glass of milk before bedtime. But we assure you that this book provides alternatives to dairy that will become even better comfort foods because they won't disrupt your digestion.

For example, our favorite dairy substitute is nut pâté. Different nuts and seeds offer different flavors, and using more salt mimics the sharpness of aged cheese. Incorporating lemon, lime, pineapple, or coconut in the pâté recipe provides tartness or a sweet taste. Turn to Chapter 7 for our pâté recipes.

Nut milks are also high on the list of substitutions, and they come in so many different flavors: almond, cashew, macadamia, hazelnut, pecan, Brazil nut, and walnut. Almond milk can be low in calories and provide a subtle, creamy flavor in cereals, smoothies, and even your coffee.

Soy products are another viable alternative to dairy. Soy is processed and packaged into an unimaginable assortment of products, including cheese, yogurt, and milk. We strongly recommend that you use organic soy products because they haven't been genetically modified.

Rice products such as rice milk and processed rice cheese can fill your dairy gap. Rice cheese comes in many varieties complete with the ability to melt just the way cheese should.

Variety is the spice of life, so rotating several dairy substitutes may be just what you need. Try nut products one day, soy the second, and rice the third for a three-day rotation; most nutritionists recommend this strategy because most foods are out of your digestive tract after three days and won't build up a sensitivity.

Concern about calcium

A common question that people have when they imagine a life without dairy is, "How will I get enough calcium?" No doubt you grew up hearing that dairy is high in calcium, and it is. However, the high temperature of dairy pasteurization binds calcium to milk protein, making the calcium difficult to absorb. Several servings of dairy a day are necessary to obtain enough calcium, but people with lactose or casein intolerance just aren't able to get their calcium in this way. What's left out of the calcium story is magnesium. Dairy is low in magnesium, so if dairy is your main source of calcium, you're creating a relative deficiency in magnesium.

Calcium and magnesium levels are both high in green leafy vegetables, nuts and seeds, seaweed, beans, and fish with edible bones (salmon and sardines), so you can turn to these foods instead of dairy for your daily dose of calcium as well as magnesium.

Taking the dairy challenge

If you haven't already done so, get yourself a nice notebook to use as a food diary. We recommend that you keep track of your typical food and beverage intake (and your physical and emotional symptoms) diligently for at least a week before taking the dairy challenge. This preparation gives you a great benchmark because you track the effect your current, typical diet has on your IBS symptoms.

If you find yourself resisting the dairy challenge, or if you think that dairy couldn't possibly be the culprit in your IBS, please reconsider and make the commitment to yourself to do this challenge. Given the statistics, there's a possibility that dairy is involved in your IBS symptoms.

The dairy challenge involves avoiding dairy — and only dairy — for two weeks in order to determine whether these foods are causing your IBS symptoms. If you avoid all possible trigger foods at once, not only are you severely limiting your food choices, but you may become hungry and discouraged and drop the whole experiment.

Why two weeks, you ask? You typically need three to four days to clear a substance from your system and then another few days for your body to start repairing any damage the offending food may have caused.

Start by stocking your kitchen with dairy substitutes and giving your dairy products and foods containing dairy (read those labels and refer to the earlier section "Eating dairy-free") to your best friend (who hopefully doesn't have IBS). We suggest that you start on a weekend, and for two weeks, use your food diary to track your diet details and the physical and emotional symptoms that you notice after eating. After about a week, you may already notice the relief of a dairy-free diet. If not, don't worry; avoiding dairy is only part of the exercise.

The challenge part of the experiment comes at the end of two weeks. Make it a Saturday so you have Sunday to recover, if necessary, and stay close to home, especially if diarrhea is your body's chosen reaction to trigger foods. Then simply indulge in all the dairy foods we made you stop eating for two weeks, and record the results. Have a large glass of milk for breakfast. After a few hours, eat several pieces of cheese. Have some ice cream after dinner. During the two-week challenge, your body got used to being without dairy. Now that there's the equivalent of a three-car pileup of milk, cheese, and ice cream careening down the superhighway of your intestines, you'll be the first to know if dairy is doing you in.

If you discover that your symptoms never really left and are exactly the same as they were before you eliminated dairy from your diet, dairy probably isn't contributing to your IBS symptoms, and the search continues.

However, you may discover that eating dairy again after two weeks off makes you feel worse, so you can decide to moderate your dairy intake. Rotate dairy choices, and use the substitutes that you're now familiar with, having enjoyed them during the challenge.

The next food you should avoid and challenge is gluten (see the following section). Depending on your reaction to the dairy challenge, you can continue eating dairy or rotate it while eliminating gluten.

Gluten in Grains as a Trigger Food

Gluten is a combination of two proteins, gliadin and glutenin, that occur in grains such as wheat, rye, barley, and, to a lesser extent, oats. Its elastic and stretchy nature helps make bread dough rise, but gluten also gives rise to many IBS symptoms in people who have an autoimmune reaction to this protein, which turns to poison in their systems.

Linking autism and food intolerance

In a vulnerable segment of the population (perhaps as much as 10 percent), a particular gene sequence can be damaged by heavy metals, antibiotics, alcohol, and acetaminophen. This vulnerable gene sequence is found in people with autism and Alzheimer's, and it's the template for creating the kinase enzyme PI3, which the body requires to help digest and absorb gluten and casein. When not completely digested, casein and gluten produce brain-disrupting hallucinogens or brain depressants.

Not surprisingly, there's a high incidence of IBS and bowel disorders in the autistic population. A therapeutic diet for autism eliminates foods that are poisoning sufferers. Until researchers can figure out how to effectively splice genes, diet is the most effective treatment. Medical experience with gluten and casein intolerance in autism has lead to more research and has helped doctors understand the ramifications of genetic conditions like celiac disease.

In Carolyn's medical practice, she's seen a spectrum of gluten intolerance from mild and moderate symptoms to fully developed celiac disease. (*Celiac disease,* also called *gluten enteropathy,* is an inherited condition that occurs in about 1 percent of the population.) Some people don't even know they have celiac disease and put up with mild to moderate symptoms, going from doctor to doctor trying to find the cause.

Gluten and IBS

Celiac disease is a genetic condition that causes the immune system to attack gluten in the diet. However, you can have gluten intolerance or a gluten allergy and not suffer from celiac disease. Unfortunately, celiac disease is often called gluten intolerance, which leads to some confusion; having the abnormal genetic component is the key to celiac disease. Fortunately, the symptoms of gluten intolerance and allergy usually aren't as severe as those of celiac disease and are usually confined to the gastrointestinal tract. In Chapter 1, we outline how to sort out the symptoms of IBS, celiac disease, gluten intolerance, and gluten allergy.

According to the NDDIC, celiac disease affects people in all parts of the world. It was originally thought to be a rare childhood condition but is now identified as a genetic disorder. More than 2 million people (1 in 133 people) in the United States have the disease. The incidence increases to 1 in 22 people for those who have a first-degree relative — a parent, sibling, or child — diagnosed with celiac disease.

As we point out in Chapter 1, gluten triggers an immune response that flattens out the absorptive fingers, called *villi,* in the small intestine in people who suffer from celiac disease. Flattened villi can't reach out and grab nutrients from your food. With hampered absorption, you can develop malnutrition and vitamin deficiencies. Following is a list of some other serious implications of celiac disease:

- ✔ Weight loss and muscle wasting, which can occur from poor absorption of protein, fats, and even carbohydrates
- ✔ Anemia and fatigue resulting from improper absorption of iron and vitamin B12
- ✔ Edema (fluid retention) of the lower legs caused by protein deficiency
- ✔ Nerve symptoms of tingling and numbness resulting from B1 and B12 deficiencies
- ✔ Muscle cramping due to magnesium deficiency
- ✔ An itchy rash due to B vitamin deficiency
- ✔ Arthritis and osteoporosis resulting from magnesium and calcium deficiencies

Symptoms of celiac disease, gluten intolerance, and gluten allergy are very close to those of IBS. Abdominal pain and bloating, diarrhea, and constipation are mutually shared symptoms, but gas and stool that clears the house with its odor and oily, mucus-filled, floating stools (with high fat content) are unique to celiac disease. Some people can develop even more widespread symptoms, such as tooth discoloration, joint pain, mouth ulceration, hypoglycemia, nosebleed, short stature, amenorrhea (skipped menstrual period), infertility, miscarriage, and seizures.

In celiac disease, the most difficult symptoms to reconcile are the behavioral changes. In children the range of emotions can be from complete withdrawal to violent outbursts. Adults can experience depression. In Carolyn's medical practice, she's witnessed the transformation of many people whose depression, melancholy, and exhaustion lifted after avoiding wheat for just one week.

Even a decade ago, the incidence of celiac disease was thought to be 1 in 5,000 people; now it's increased to 1 in 100. How can this happen if celiac disease is a genetic condition? The celiac gene comes from one or both parents. If you have two defective genes, one from each of your parents, you're sure to develop celiac disease. Some researchers speculate that the increased consumption of wheat gluten products may be causing celiac disease to express itself in people who have only one defective gene, thus explaining the increased incidence of this condition.

Eating gluten-free

In addition to wheat bran and germ, semolina flour, and couscous, among others, you may be surprised to find out that food products such as binders and fillers commonly found in processed meat; soy sauce; malt found in beer, coffee, and cocoa mix; soft cheese; licorice; and cough drops contain gluten. It may not be too hard to cut out some or all of the items, but what grains can you eat on a gluten-free diet? The many tasty alternatives include quinoa, corn, millet, rice, buckwheat, sorghum, amaranth, teff, wild rice, and Indian rice grass. We include lots of recipes using some of these substitutes in Chapter 12.

If you've done some research and suspect that you have celiac disease, you should *not* begin a gluten-free diet before you're diagnosed by a doctor. As soon as you avoid gluten, your intestines begin to heal, and the gliadin and glutenin antibodies disappear. When you go for diagnosis testing, the results won't be accurate. Instead, avoid the biggest gluten offender, wheat, for one week, keep up your food diary, and check to see if your symptoms are altered. If they are, you can keep eating gluten grains until you have your blood test or small intestine biopsy.

If you're diagnosed with celiac disease, the prescribed treatment is avoidance of wheat, rye, barley, and oats for the rest of your life. Removing the damaging gluten from scraping and irritating your intestines allows the intestinal villi to heal and stay vital and healthy for the proper absorption of nutrients.

Taking the gluten challenge

If you think you may still have difficulty with gluten but don't suspect that you have celiac disease and aren't diagnosed with that condition, you may have a gluten allergy and can undertake a gluten challenge much like the dairy challenge explained in the earlier section "Taking the dairy challenge" to determine whether gluten triggers your IBS symptoms.

Spend at least one week documenting your normal diet in your food diary, and then eliminate wheat from your diet completely for two weeks. (We start with wheat because it's the most common of the gluten foods and the one that we've found people to be most intolerant of.) Continue to chronicle your food intake and your physical and emotional symptoms to reflect the change in your diet.

After two weeks, you may introduce wheat back into your diet, ideally in a simple form — perhaps biscuits or pasta rather than yeast bread. Again, we suggest that you conduct this wheat challenge on a weekend in case you have an IBS reaction.

In Chapter 3, we talk about rotating your diet so you don't eat the same foods every day, and this story helps show you why. One of Carolyn's patients avoided wheat for two weeks and then challenged by eating some simple pancakes made with whole-wheat flour. She noted that her symptoms included indigestion and heartburn, but she felt that was tolerable discomfort and not IBS-related, so she continued to eat wheat. On the third day of reintroducing wheat into her diet, she had a return of her IBS symptoms. When she only eats wheat once or twice a week she has no symptoms of IBS.

Karen gives up wheat

Karen suspected that wheat was a trigger for her IBS symptoms, which included bloating, so she decided to try the challenge by avoiding wheat and then reintroducing it into her diet.

Within a week of eliminating wheat from her diet, Karen noticed a change in the way her intestines felt — the bloating seemed to be subsiding. Heartened by this, she eliminated other gluten foods and felt a further shift in her symptoms accompanied by what seemed like her first normal bowel movements in recent memory. For two weeks, Karen was diligent in avoiding gluten products, and then she was ready to challenge the wheat. Unfortunately she did so at a dinner party, deciding to snack on the crackers offered as an appetizer. It wasn't long before she felt the gas collect in her intestines, and she found that she was holding back uncomfortable flatulence. Karen had to excuse herself several times to release the gas privately, and she eventually cut her evening short. The next morning she welcomed several gassy, mucosy bowel movements, confirming her intolerance to wheat. Karen's experience is very common, including the way she began by eliminating wheat and then removing all gluten foods. She found that she could tolerate oats, barley, and rye with no symptoms but continued her ban on wheat.

Sugar as a Trigger Food

Sugar isn't a food group, but you'd hardly know that given that the average per-person consumption of sugar in America is about 140 pounds annually. We're talking about the refined sugar that has found its way into thousands of food products to both sweeten and bulk up the product. Refined sugar is linked inextricably with special occasions, parties, and just treating yourself to a sweet. Giving up sugar can seem tremendously difficult to anyone, including people with IBS, but we encourage you to consider the effect that sugar may be having on your GI system.

Refined sugar and IBS

SIBO (small intestine bacteria overgrowth) may be a newly found cause of IBS. SIBO's role in IBS is still being researched. In the medical worlds, the current thinking is that the SIBO may be the culprit for a portion of IBS patients. For those who have SIBO, the bacteria in the small intestine set upon carbohydrates, resulting in symptoms of gas, bloating, and diarrhea.

However, according to the clinical research of Dr. Heiko Santelmann, refined sugar can also stimulate the growth of yeast in the intestines, which leads to symptoms of IBS. Candida is a yeast that is naturally present in the human body. Excessive sugar in your diet (among other causes) can cause the yeast to multiply, leading to a number of health problems, from vaginal yeast infections to severe fatigue. And these yeast, when present in abnormally high numbers, can cause strong cravings for sweet, starchy foods, thus perpetuating the problem. Chapter 18 gives you more information about yeast and how to treat it.

Why eat sugar-free?

Sugar is a simple carbohydrate found naturally in many foods, including fruits and grains. If the only sugar you consumed were in natural, whole foods, your intestines would be able to cope. But the average American diet is full of refined, nutrient-depleted foods and contains an average of 20 teaspoons of added, refined sugar every day. That's twice the amount recommended by the United States Department of Agriculture (USDA), which specifies 10 teaspoons, and four times the maximum Carolyn personally recommends to her patients.

So what's wrong with refined sugar? Many things.

- **Refined sugar compromises immune function.** Two cans of soda, which contain 24 teaspoons of sugar total, reduce the efficiency of white blood cells by 92 percent — an effect that lasts up to five hours, according to Kenneth Bock, M.D., an expert in nutritional and environmental health. Because white blood cells are an integral part of your immune system, if you happen to meet a nasty virus or bacteria within five hours of drinking a few sodas, your immune system may be unable to fight off the invader.

- **Refined sugar overworks the pancreas and adrenal glands as they struggle to keep the blood sugar levels in balance.** When you eat sugar, it's quickly absorbed into your bloodstream in the form of glucose. This speedy absorption puts your pancreas into overdrive making insulin (which carries glucose to your cells to be used for energy) to normalize blood sugar levels. But the rapid release of insulin causes a sudden drop in blood sugar. In reaction to the falling blood sugar, excess adrenal cortisone is stimulated to raise blood sugar back to normal. A constantly high intake of simple dietary sugar keeps this roller coaster going and eventually overworks or "burns out" normal pancreas and adrenal function, leading to abnormal serotonin levels in the intestines, early menopause, adult-onset diabetes, hypoglycemia, and chronic fatigue.

- **Processing sugarcane, or any whole food, strips it of most if not all of its nutritional value; the refining process of sugar removes between 83 and 98 percent of its chromium, manganese, cobalt, copper, zinc, and magnesium.** Ironically, the end product, refined sugar, is what you consume, and the nutritious residues are discarded and generally fed to cattle.

- **Because refined sugar is devoid of nutrients, the body must actually draw from its nutrient reserves to metabolize it.** When these storehouses are depleted, the body becomes unable to properly metabolize fatty acids and cholesterol, leading to higher cholesterol and triglyceride levels. Drawing on the body's nutrient reserves can also lead to chronic mineral deficits, especially in magnesium (a mineral required for more than 300 different enzyme activities) and chromium (a trace element that regulates hormones such as insulin); magnesium and chromium deficiencies put you at risk for dozens of diseases, including constipation, depression, attention deficit disorder, and asthma.

We want you to read labels to understand the hidden foods in your diet, but when it comes to sugar, you have to apply for a detective license to find the hidden sugars in foods. You probably know the "-ose's" (maltose, sucrose, glucose, and fructose), but there are dozens more names for sugar that you'd never suspect; check out Appendix D for a list of these aliases.

Taking the sugar challenge

Eliminating refined sugar for two weeks further hones your skills at reading food labels and hopefully introduces you to your kitchen to prepare food from scratch (because refined sugar is everywhere in prefab food)! For example, ketchup contains more sugar than it does tomatoes.

Actually, this is the avoidance and challenge adventure that kids love most. To help determine whether there is a dietary cause of hyperactivity, Carolyn often tells parents to have their kids do an experiment to avoid sugar for one week, then on Saturday, load up on candies and sugar treats to their hearts' content. The kids love the idea of gorging on candy, but then on Sunday they look and feel like they're totally hungover. The kids get the message, and we hope you will too. Do the experiment of avoiding sugar yourself for one or two weeks, and then eat candy all day and see how you react. You can learn a lot about your body this way. Remember that you should honestly record your symptoms in your food diary — even if you don't want to admit to them.

Of course, if you're diabetic, we don't recommend you undertake this experiment.

Sugar substitutes and IBS

Sorbitol is a sugar alcohol that's neither digested nor absorbed by the human gut. Intact, it reaches the large intestine, where it is acted upon by gut bacteria and yeast, encouraging them to overgrow. Gas, bloating, intestinal cramps, and diarrhea are the natural consequence.

Sorbitol is used as a sugar substitute in many confections — even those in the health food section. However, sorbitol causes bloating, flatulence and diarrhea — even at only 2 teaspoons consumed a day. If you have a magnifying glass when you read labels, you can sometimes spot the warning "Excess consumption can have a laxative effect." In fact, when we searched "sorbitol" online, the third result that popped up was "How Sorbitol Causes Irritable Bowel Syndrome."

Sorbitol is found naturally in prunes and pears, explaining why these fruits have a laxative effect. It's even the principle ingredient of an OTC laxative called Sorbilax. Chronic chewing of sorbitol-laced gum can cause chronic diarrhea. Similar diarrhea label warnings should be on products containing mannitol, maltitol, and xylitol.

If you decide to avoid sugar in all its forms, be aware that you're changing how you feed your intestinal yeast. Without sugar, yeast can die off in large numbers, and you may experience some symptoms as a result. Yeast can produce up to 178 different toxins that are normally released as they die. These toxins may cross the intestinal wall into the bloodstream and cause reactions that can feel like allergic reactions. When greater numbers of yeast die off, you may feel a little more tired, have a coated tongue, or even develop a skin rash.

Fructose as a Trigger Food

Fructose is a simple single sugar in the carbohydrate family. It's found in fruits; root vegetables, such as beets, sweet potatoes, parsnips, and onions; honey; cane sugar; and high fructose corn syrup. Fructose actually requires less digestion than white sugar (sucrose), which is a double sugar with equal parts of glucose and fructose.

Is fructose healthier than sugar? Many people mistakenly believe that fructose is a healthier sugar because one of its sources is fruit. The fact that it's used in many so-called "natural" foods also makes it seem benign. Although fructose is naturally present in fruit, the fructose that's added to many commercially prepared foods is even more refined than plain white sugar.

Hereditary fructose intolerance is a genetic disease caused by lack of a particular enzyme that breaks down fructose. It's a rare condition that only occurs in about 1 in 10,000 people. What we're talking about in terms of fructose as an IBS trigger is *fructose malabsorption,* commonly referred to as fructose intolerance, which occurs when absorptive cells in the intestinal lining don't accept and transport fructose into the bloodstream. The intestinal contents become supersaturated with fructose, causing gas and bloating and providing food for intestinal bacteria and yeast. Fructose malabsorption is quite common; according to www.foodintol.com, about 30 percent of the population has some level of sugar sensitivity, mostly to fructose.

Fructose and IBS

Fructose, just like its cousin, sucrose (table sugar), feeds intestinal bacteria and yeast and can cause an imbalance in the number of organisms in the intestines. Refer to the earlier section "Sugar as a Trigger Food" for an explanation of the biological problem of sugar in the gut.

Fructose from fresh fruit (sometimes referred to as *fruit sugar*) has the same effect as fructose sweeteners, but fruit can have the added effect of irritation due to the insoluble fiber in the skin of the fruit. But remember, fruit isn't just empty sugar — it also has the added benefit of vitamins, minerals, and fiber. The goal here isn't to get you to eliminate all fruit; we want you to be able to identify whatever culprit is triggering your IBS.

Prunes are well known and applauded for their laxative effect. In the last generation, prunes were a staple in many households (including ours), and we fondly remember our mother popping a prune or two to prevent constipation. Because of their laxative capabilities, prunes have suffered from a lot of negative publicity; now, they're often referred to as dried plums as a way to wipe the slate clean of the negative connotations of the word *prune*.

In addition to prunes/plums, when eaten in considerable quantities, peaches, figs, kiwi, pineapple, mango, and papaya have a laxative effect in most people. However, for someone with gut sensitivity, it may not take much to cause irritation and increased bowel movements.

Eating fructose-free

Products containing added fructose number in the thousands but can be identified by closely reading labels. Most of the fructose you encounter in foods is in the form of *high-fructose corn syrup* (HFCS) or *crystalline fructose,* which have nearly eclipsed sugar as the most consumed sweeteners in the U.S. HFCS contains 55 percent fructose and 45 percent glucose. Crystalline fructose is created by enriching corn syrup with fructose, making it 98 percent fructose.

In the past decade, researchers woke up to the fact that HFCS causes an elevation in blood lipids and should be avoided. The American Diabetic Association (ADA) used to include food products containing fructose in its recommendations because fructose is absorbed more slowly into the bloodstream than table sugar. Now, however, the ADA warns diabetics to avoid HFCS because of lipid elevation.

Eating or drinking 20 to 40 teaspoons of HFCS a day can overwhelm the body's ability to digest it so that it stays in the blood and elevates the blood sugar. That sounds like a lot of sugar, but when you realize that one can of soda contains about 10 teaspoons of sugar and that many people drink soda more than water, it's not hard to down the equivalent of a cup of sugar (48 teaspoons) a day.

Taking the fructose challenge

For a two-week period, avoid all fruit and fructose-containing products. If you've determined that dairy and/or gluten are *not* an IBS challenge for you (see the sections on each earlier in this chapter), you may choose to continue to eat them during your fructose challenge. Of course, if you reacted to foods from those avoidance experiments, keep them out of your diet, too. There's no substitute for a piece of fruit, but you can use stevia, Just Like Sugar, and maybe some honey, maple syrup, or a dash of xylitol instead of fructose as a sweetener.

Keep a diary of your symptoms before and during the challenge, and see if they improve during the two weeks you're fructose-free. When the two weeks is up and you challenge fruit, choose one that you would normally eat — don't pick a new exotic fruit you've never tried before. You want to measure your reaction to your typical foods, so this isn't the time to try out new things. Eat several pieces of fruit and see how your body reacts. If that goes well and you don't have symptoms, try a bottle of fruit juice sweetened with HFCS and assess your reaction.

Make sure that you write down all the symptoms that you notice — even if they aren't IBS-related. For example, Christine remembers avoiding fruits for two weeks and then challenging by eating strawberries, which had just come into season. Her reaction was itchy hives, which indicated an actual allergy and not a digestive intolerance.

Fiber as a Trigger Food

Dietary fiber includes those parts of edible plants that your body can't digest or absorb. You need to digest protein, fats, and carbohydrates to build and run your body, but you also need fiber that remains undigested in order to act like a broom sweeping through the colon. Fiber helps keep you regular. It also keeps colonic bacteria and yeast under control, lowers cholesterol and blood sugar, and decreases the risk of hemorrhoids and diverticulitis. Soluble fiber can actually decrease the risk and symptoms of IBS, which is why this section focuses primarily on its less-friendly sibling, insoluble fiber.

There are two types of fiber:

- ✔ **Soluble fiber** dissolves in water. It forms a gel-like substance that is best exemplified by psyllium powder in its pure form. You can take psyllium powder for either IBS-D or IBS-C. Better-tasting soluble fiber foods are peas, carrots, beans, apples, pears, citrus fruits, and barley.

- ✔ **Insoluble fiber** doesn't dissolve in water. It creates bulk that helps promote the movement of matter through your GI tract. The main insoluble fibers are whole-wheat flour, wheat bran, nuts, a variety of vegetables, and the skins of some fruits.

The amount of each type of fiber varies in different plant foods.

Insoluble fiber and IBS

Insoluble fiber can be an irritant for people with IBS because the rough edges of the fibers don't soften up in water and may irritate sensitive intestines. To help soothe fiber-triggered IBS symptoms, you may eat some form of soluble fiber with every meal to help soften the intestinal contents, or you may avoid consuming insoluble fiber altogether by peeling tomatoes and apples before eating them, for example.

In terms of insoluble fiber as a trigger of IBS symptoms, beans may cause you a cacophony of gas if you have trouble digesting them. Soaking the beans well before cooking removes the indigestible complex sugar flatus factors, cleans the beans off well, and rehydrates them to allow them to cook faster.

Nuts and seeds contain insoluble fiber that may cause some intestinal scraping and digestion issues. You can overcome this problem by grinding and blending these foods into butters and pâtés that are more soothing to the intestines. We incorporate principles for combating the IBS-triggering capabilities of fiber in the recipes in Part II, and Appendix C shows you the fiber contents (soluble and insoluble) of lots of common foods.

Journaling fiber foods

It's impossible to eliminate all fiber foods in order to perform a fiber challenge to identify whether fiber is a trigger for your IBS, so we don't ask you to do it. Instead, you should pay close attention to your food diary to help determine which of the fiber foods listed in Appendix C may be causing some intestinal upset.

The connection between fiber foods and IBS symptoms is very individual and personal. You may find that certain soluble fiber foods aren't your friends and certain insoluble fiber foods are. And a person with IBS-diarrhea may determine that his symptoms are triggered by the same type of food that causes constipation in his friend who has IBS-constipation.

Chapter 3

Transitioning to an IBS-Friendly Diet

In This Chapter

▶ Using your food diary to build your new diet

▶ Rotating foods and replacing triggers to avoid reactions

▶ Planning out a safe menu

▶ Keeping tabs on your improvement

▶ Looking at diet philosophies that may help

*F*eeling like you have to change your diet beyond recognition can be daunting, especially when so many of your favorite foods are now off limits. Although you may have to make some food compromises, don't feel like you have nothing left to eat. This chapter makes easing into a good diet effortless. It does come with some restrictions, such as avoiding food additives, synthetic sweeteners, MSG, caffeine, and alcohol, but we also suggest plenty of friendly replacements for you to try. Appendix B offers additional sensible trigger food substitutes. Just like dating, you may have to try out a few before finding the perfect mate.

Changing your diet is a long-term plan and not an overnight quick fix. Go easy on yourself as you experiment with new ways of cooking and eating. Ease into the adjustments and remember that big changes like these take time, commitment, planning, and patience. You won't wake up in the morning after reading this book and have everything in place. But you will wake up with a new sense that you have more control over your IBS than you thought. If your commitment falls by the wayside for a bit, that's okay — just hop back on the wagon and continue your journey towards a healthier diet.

Eating for your type: The blood type diet

In the 1970's, Naturopath Peter D'Adamo, ND, came up with the theory that a person's blood type influenced what kind of diet she should eat. Here are some of this diet's highlights; check out Chapter 5 for more information:

✔ O blood types need high amounts of animal protein and fish in their diets. They have problems digesting dairy and wheat and may struggle with grains in general. They can eat meat, fish, and olive oil freely and eggs, nuts, seeds, certain vegetables (such as spinach, sweet potatoes, and turnips) and fruits in moderation.

✔ People with an A blood type can thrive on a plant-based vegetarian diet but have difficulty digesting red meat and dairy. Their recommended foods are nuts, seeds, beans, cereals, pasta, rice, fruits, and vegetables.

✔ Those who have B blood types can eat a varied diet, including grains, dairy, animal protein, vegetables, and fruits. They don't usually digest nuts and seeds well and should limit their carbs.

✔ AB blood types can eat a combination of the foods recommended for blood groups A and B. Their best bet is a primarily vegetarian diet with occasional meat, fish, and dairy products.

Tracking Your Transition with a Food Diary

Eating has evolved into a task most people do while focusing on something else — chowing down on a TV dinner while engrossed in the tube, or draining a latte during a skim of the morning paper. But what if you bring the attention back to what you're eating and how it affects your body? If you suffer from frequent burping, heartburn, fatigue, headaches, or if your stools are loose or hard, grab your food diary and do some detective work to see which foods may be causing those reactions.

Chapter 2 gives you more detailed instructions for creating a *food diary*, which is basically any sort of note-taking system you use to record everything you eat, when you eat it, and what if any symptoms and/or emotions you notice in conjunction with that eating. A food diary is an important part of the diet transition process for a few reasons:

✔ **It helps you keep track of what you eat.** You may be surprised by the number of snacks or sips that you indulge in throughout the day that may not quite adhere to your transition plan. If it goes in your mouth, it goes in your food diary, including grabbing a few French fries from the bottom of the bag or finishing off the milkshake your daughter left behind.

✔ **It helps you keep track of how you feel both physically and emotionally after you eat certain foods.** When a pizza is staring at you from your kitchen counter, you can easily forget the fact that the pizza you had four weeks ago sent you straight to the bathroom or messed with your streak of successive bowel movements, making you feel embarrassed and guilty. When you write what you've eaten and how you felt physically and emotionally, you have it there in your own writing and can reinforce why you want to transition away from those foods. Of course, you have to actually refer to your food diary and heed your own warnings!

✔ **It helps you monitor your results over time.** You may notice that wheat made you feel bloated and gassy when you first introduced it back into your diet four months ago. When you try another introduction, you may notice that you feel gassy but not bloated. It's a great way to see that you're making progress through this process.

If you feel like you don't have time to sit down and write in a food diary, use the memo function of your cellphone. Depending on your phone, you may be able to download the information into your computer and even blog it if you want!

Some of our IBS clients have a degree of sensitivity to all five trigger foods covered Chapter 2, and as a result, they've chosen to avoid them all for a period of one to three months. Using food substitution lists like the one in Appendix B, these clients have been able to enjoy a varied and healthy diet while healing their intestines.

Eating for your constitution: The Ayurvedic doshas

In Ayurvedic Medicine, the three *doshas or constitutions* (Vata, Pitta, and Kapha) are identified according to details about body type. According to this ancient medical tradition, eating foods that correspond to your dosha balances your body and improves your health. The following list gives you the highlights of each constitution's recommended diet; flip to Chapter 5 for more details about doshas.

✔ **Vata:** Vatas should avoid sugar, alcohol, and drugs, as well as and cold, raw, bitter, pungent, or astringent food and drinks, as well as raw foods. Recommended foods are those in the sweet (but not sugary), salty,

and sour categories, along with warming spices and cooked foods.

✔ **Pitta:** Pittas respond best to regular meals of cooling foods like oatmeal, basmati rice, sweet fruits, cottage cheese, and mint tea. They should avoid spicy, sour, salty, and pungent foods and focus on sweet, bitter and astringent foods. Raw is better than cooked, with a minimal amount of oil.

✔ **Kapha:** The best foods for Kaphas are astringent, bitter, and pungent; less desirable options include sweet, sour, and salty foods. Food should be cooked with a small amount of oil.

Rotating Your Way to Health

We mention in Chapter 2 that most nutritionists recommend a three-day rotation for people with food allergies or sensitivities. Some food groups create more sensitivity as they build up in your system, so you should only eat them every few days; within 72 hours, most foods have cleared the digestive tract, and if you don't eat the same food within that time you most likely won't accumulate an allergy load.

Dairy and wheat are two examples of foods likely to cause such sensitivity. You may be able to eat yogurt once a week, but make sure it's plain, organic, and low-fat (if you have problems digesting fat). Rotate wheat into your diet once or twice a week so you don't build up a reaction to it or feed yeast and bacteria in your gut. On the off days, try another grains like quinoa, rice, or any of the other grain products in Chapter 12 that break down into glucose at a slower rate than wheat and therefore don't feed yeast as readily.

Here's an example of a three-day rotation using different grains and dairy substitutes each day; these combinations are random, so you can mix and match the components however you want:

- ✔ **Day 1:** Grain: Rice cereal for breakfast and rice pasta in a main meal. Dairy substitute: Rice milk

- ✔ **Day 2:** Grain: Millet puffed cereal for breakfast and cooked millet as part of a main meal. Dairy substitute: Almond milk

- ✔ **Day 3:** Grain: Oatmeal cereal for breakfast and quinoa as part of a main meal. Dairy substitute: Soy milk or hemp milk

When you eat a rotation-only food, write the date on the food box or in your food diary so you don't forget and eat it again too soon.

Use the rotation rationale for your whole diet and try not to eat the same thing every day or even two days in a row. That way, you have much less chance of building up a sensitivity to it even if it's not especially prone to causing problems.

Substituting Trigger Foods

The concept of food substitution is actually the basis of a good IBS diet. This book assumes that certain foods in your current diet have something to do with your IBS symptoms and that you therefore need to get them out of your kitchen and replace them with foods that are IBS-friendly. (We're not talking about substituting plain potato chips for your sour cream potato chips but rather substituting something like baked rice crackers for potato chips.)

Go through your food diary and notice what foods have left you feeling full of IBS. No matter what you've been eating that's been aggravating your IBS, you can find healthier options; we list many in Appendix B. Granted, the IBS-friendly substitutions may not be as creamy, crunchy, rich, or sugary as your current faves, but they can help fend off feelings of deprivation as you make this diet transition. The more friendly foods you substitute into your diet, the more likely you'll feel relief from some of your symptoms.

Table 3-1 uses a food chart to show you how you can transition your diet. We're making a lot of assumptions in this section about your diet, so just look upon this table as a vast generalization about the diets that most Americans are eating. The substitution lists in Appendix B are more extensive, but here we want to give you a broad overview of your diet at a glance.

Table 3-1	Glancing at the IBS Transition Diet
Present Diet	*Transition Diet*
Processed cold cuts, hot dogs	Antibiotic-free meat
Fried fish, farm-raised fish	Wild salmon, shellfish
Pork	Free-range chicken, grass-fed lamb and beef
Canned beans with sugar, tofu	Soaked beans, lentils, canned organic beans, tempeh
Sugar, molasses, candy, chocolate, maple syrup, honey	Stevia, xylitol, Just Like Sugar
Milk, cheese, cream, coffee creamer	Nut milks (rice, almond, hazelnut), yogurt, soy cheese, rice cheese
Butter	Ghee
Fruit, fruit juices	Vegetables
Coffee, black tea, soda	Grain coffee, organic herbal teas, green tea
Diet drinks, alcohol	Mineral, spring, or filtered water
Hydrogenated oils	Organic butter, coconut oil
Light olive oil, lard	Extra-virgin olive oil, coconut oil
Genetically modified corn oil, canola oil, vegetable oil	Sesame oil, extra-virgin olive oil
Products made with refined white flour	100 percent sprouted-grain breads (such as Essene bread, Ezekiel bread, and manna), gluten- and yeast-free bread, miracle noodles

Here's the lowdown on why we recommend these swaps:

- ✔ Processed cold cuts and hot dogs are full of fat and additives. Replacing them with antibiotic-free meat (ideally grass-fed beef and lamb and free-range chicken) helps prevent yeast overgrowth and antibiotic resistance (see Chapter 18). (We shy away from pork because it may contain parasites if not cooked properly.) On the fish front, farm-raised fish absorb the antibiotics, colorings, and chemicals used in their hatcheries. Wild salmon doesn't have this problem, and it has less mercury than other fish.

- ✔ Commercial canned beans are often sweetened and have many additives. Indulge in organic kidney, pinto, black, garbanzo, and adzuki beans when the only other ingredients are water and maybe some seaweed. Tofu is a non-fermented soy product that is hard to digest, so replace it with fermented soybean tempeh.

- ✔ Stevia, xylitol, and Just Like Sugar are allowed in the IBS diet; if you're avoiding alcohol sugars like xylitol, you can stick with stevia and Just Like Sugar.

- ✔ The lactose sugar in dairy feeds bacteria and yeast in the intestines. You can substitute with nut milk and rice and soy cheese and still use plain, organic yogurt. *Remember:* A good yogurt contains little to no lactose because its bacteria have eaten it all. Butter has much less lactose than the dairy it came from but you can make it even IBS-friendlier by creating *ghee* (butter without the milk protein casein). You can find a recipe for ghee in Chapter 6.

- ✔ Fruit and especially fruit juices have loads of fruit sugar that yeast and bacteria love. If you have a yeast overgrowth (see Chapter 18), excessive fruit may cause a problem; limit yourself to two pieces of fruit a day and avoid fruit juice. Vegetable juices are your transition substitution.

- ✔ Coffee, black tea, and soda raise your blood sugar and overly stimulate the adrenal glands, which can activate your intestines. Diet drinks and alcohol are out of the running as well. "Diet" is more of a marketing slogan than it is an actual health benefit. Diet drinks have no calories, but they often contain artificial sweeteners; the most common one is *aspartame,* a chemical made up of methanol (wood alcohol) and two neurostimulatory amino acids. European studies show that aspartame can cause widespread side effects, including obesity and bowel problems. Alcohol contributes to yeast overgrowth and is damaging to the liver. The substitutions are herb teas and water flavored with essential fruit and herb oils like citrus, raspberry, and especially peppermint, which are soothing for the intestines.

Stevia comes in various flavors to naturally sweeten and flavor water at the same time.

✔ Hydrogenated oils can be irritating to the intestines and also your heart, but butter, ghee, and coconut oil are better alternatives. Light olive oil and lard aren't as healthy as extra-virgin olive oil and coconut oil. Genetically modified products consistently show digestive problems in test animals, so sub genetically modified corn and canola oil, as well as vegetable oil, with sesame oil and extra-virgin olive oil.

✔ Refined white flour products (such as bread, crackers, bagels, tortillas, pizza, cookies, cakes, muffins, pasta, pretzels, and Danish) usually contain yeast-growing sugar and bowel-irritating hydrogenated oil. 100-percent *sprouted-grain breads* (breads made from grains that have germinated) are better for IBS because the grains are not processed into flour, which breaks down quickly into glucose, and the sprouting makes them more easily digstible.

Miracle noodles may be a miracle substitution for people with IBS, especially IBS-C. The noodles are made from *glucomannan,* a water-soluble plant fiber. Medical studies confirm that their high soluble-fiber content creates bulky stool to relieve constipation; they should also be a relief to IBS-D sufferers because their fiber soothes the gut. Manufacturers claim that miracle noodles have zero carbs and calories and are gluten- and wheat-free. They're rather tasteless on their own, but they can take on the flavors of any sauce or soup.

Finding possible cheese solutions

The Specific Carbohydrate Diet (SCD) allows non-lactose dairy that you may be able to tolerate, but only you can know that for sure. The following list shows you the cheeses the SCD has deemed legal for free and occasional use, as well as those marked as always illegal. If you've avoided diary for 2 weeks, you may want to try one of the legal cheeses.

✔ **Cheeses approved for free SCD use:** Brick cheese, cheddar, Colby, dry-curd cottage cheese, Gruyère, havarti, Manchego, Provolone, and Swiss

✔ **Cheeses approved for occasional SCD use:** Asiago, blue, brie, Camembert, Edam, feta (after six months of symptom improvement), Gorgonzola, Gouda, Limburger, Monterey Jack, Muenster, Parmesan, Port du Salut, Romano, Roquefort, and Stilton

✔ **Cheeses identified as illegal for the SCD:** Chevre, cottage cheese, cream cheese, gjetost, mozzarella, Neufchâtel, primost, processed cheeses, ricotta, and Tofutti

You can read more about the SCD and its potential IBS advantages in the "Benefiting from the Specific Carbohydrate Diet (SCD)" section later in this chapter.

All a matter of tastes

Some diet theories (such as Ayurvedic and Chinese medicines — see the sidebars in this chapter) rely on certain *tastes* of foods to better balance a person's system. Here are some examples of each taste category so that you know what you're looking for when someone tells you you'd benefit from pungent food:

✔ **Astringent:** Pomegranate, beans, lentils, cherry, foods rich in *tannins* (bitter plant substances that can shrink proteins), turmeric, cruciferous vegetables such as cauliflower and cabbage, and cilantro

✔ **Bitter:** Coffee, aloe, salad greens (such as arugula and dandelion leaf), hops, lettuce, radish leaf, vinegar, many dark leafy greens, turmeric, fenugreek, and bitter gourd

✔ **Sour:** Lemon, lime, grapefruit, pear, plum, mango, many unripe fruits, yogurt, vinegar, cheese, all foods produced by fermentation, pomegranate seeds, and tamarind

✔ **Salty:** Sea salt, rock salt, kelp, salty pretzels, and pickles

✔ **Sweet:** Bread, rice, milk, butter, ghee, sweet cream, honey, raw sugar, ripe fruits, and chestnut

✔ **Pungent:** Green onion, chive, clove, parsley, coriander, peppers, onion, radish, garlic, ginger, black pepper, mustard, radish, and white daikon.

Being savvy about synthetics

Food additives come in many forms and have many useful jobs, but they're derived from chemicals that your body simply isn't meant to digest easily. Many people find this fact surprising, assuming that the government wouldn't allow manufacturers to use an additive if it were unsafe or even bad for them. But just because an additive is approved for human consumption by government agencies doesn't mean it's been approved by your unique digestive system — you may simply be someone who can't digest certain additives. We suggest watching out for and even avoiding the following kinds of food additives to reduce the impact to your gastrointestinal tract (GIT):

✔ Anti-caking agents

✔ Antioxidant preservatives

✔ Artificial sweeteners

✔ Colors

✔ Emulsifiers

✔ Food acids

- ✔ Flavors
- ✔ Flavor enhancers
- ✔ Glazing agents
- ✔ Humectants
- ✔ Preservatives
- ✔ Stabilizers
- ✔ Thickeners

Most people eat food additives every day and don't even blink an eyelash. They aren't foods, they aren't the body's normal building blocks, and they don't help metabolism. In the name of protecting freshness, additives can extend the shelf life of foods for years — you may have heard of the experiments that observe sealed jars of various foods for months or years — but you have to wonder what those foods and chemicals are really doing inside your body.

Mapping Your Weekly Meal Plan

Earlier in this chapter, we discuss rotating foods and substituting safe foods for your triggers. If you have your safe list of foods, you can start to map your weekly meal plan. (For help compiling a safe food list, head to Chapter 2.) For the first five days, build your daily menus around five of your safe proteins (one per day). See "Planning a menu first" later in this chapter for more advice on menu-building.

On the sixth day, test something that you normally don't eat and then on the seventh day try a modified fast — a detox day — that helps your body rest and even clears out any reactions from your day-six test. To make about six quarts of the detox drink, combine the following ingredients:

- ✔ 6 quarts of water
- ✔ Juice of four lemons
- ✔ ⅛ teaspoon of cayenne
- ✔ The contents of six 500 milligram ginger capsules, or 1 level teaspoon of ginger powder, or 3 inches of raw ginger run through a garlic press or juicer
- ✔ 2 tablespoons maple syrup, agave, or blackstrap molasses

If you're on medications and have other conditions besides IBS, if you're run down, have weight loss, or other medical symptoms, check with your doctor before doing a detox day. After you're clear to undertake this adventure, drink five to six quarts of the detox mixture copiously throughout the day. You may be surprised that you have fewer symptoms of IBS as you proceed through the day. We suggest that your detox day fall on a weekend in case you experience any side effects (such as headache, stomach rumbling, or feeling generally icky and like you need to stay close to the bathroom). These side effects are generally greater for longer, five-to-seven-day detox cleanses, but you may experience some effects on a one-day detox.

You can also use the drink as a morning elixir (although not five to six quarts of it) to transition into your new IBS diet — in fact, we called the drink the Morning Elixir in *IBS For Dummies* (Wiley).

Building your basic recipe list

Part II provides recipes for you to sort and sample using your safe food list as a guide, and you may have other resources as well. As you experiment with recipes, think about how you can mix and match them to create meals.

Go ahead and mark off recipes you know you absolutely can't have, but think about revisiting them in a month or two as your symptoms improve.

Planning a menu first

To get the most out of your meal planning and shopping, grab your recipe list (see the preceding section) and figure out what you can and want to eat for the next few days. Say you can eat chicken, beef, tuna, eggs, and almonds with no problems. These five protein foods will form the structural base of your diet. If you're a vegetarian, your choices are more limited, but they may include beans and grains, nuts and seeds, eggs (unless you're vegan, of course), and fermented soy. With five protein foods, you have a protein base for each of the next five days and can choose appropriate recipes from your arsenal (and add their ingredients to your shopping list if necessary).

If you know what you're planning later in the week, and have the ingredients on hand then you may be able to do some extra cooking on a day you're feeling good.

Some days and even weeks, planning a day ahead makes no sense because your symptoms are fluctuating so much. The best plan to have is to have the ingredients and foods already in your house so when you feel like you can eat, you're prepared.

Shopping for success

Whether you shop online or in co-ops, markets, supermarkets, or buying clubs, always take your trusty shopping list and your safe food list (and stick to them). You're likely getting more groceries than before you had IBS (because you're cooking more), and you may be buying for a whole IBS-free family, so the trip can get pretty harried pretty fast if you're not prepared.

If certain family members don't have a lot of patience in grocery stores or markets, drag them along on your shopping adventures. If you normally shop for people in your family who don't have IBS, ask them to shop for their own food as often as possible. That takes some of the pressure off you and it may give them the freedom to grab some snacks that you wouldn't think to buy. Just make them promise to store those foods out of your reach so they don't tempt you.

Reading food labels

Bring out the magnifying glass. Reading the labels on the food already in your house isn't enough — you can't support your IBS unless you read the labels of every food you buy to make sure you know what you're eating. Appendix D gives you a hand with this task by showing you some foods and ingredients that may be hiding triggers.

If a product that you buy regularly suddenly has a change in its packaging, check the ingredient list to see whether it's undergone an ingredient change as well.

If you have a child who has IBS, have her learn to read labels so she can be on the lookout for her own safe foods. Of course, bringing kids to the store and helping them learn about product ingredients adds some time to your shopping trip, but after a couple of these outings, the little shoppers become more invested in their own diets.

Being Patient with Results: Charting Your Numbers

Carolyn often tells her clients that a healing program barely registers in your consciousness when you only feel 49 percent better, but when you're 51 percent better, a light bulb suddenly goes on. You're finally over the great divide and are on your way to health. Keeping a food diary helps you see the progress you're making, and Figure 3-1 gives you a survey to help track the improvement in your symptoms.

Use this survey to register your symptoms on a scale of zero to ten, with zero meaning no symptoms and ten meaning they're so bad you're writing from your hospital bed. The key helps you to determine if your symptoms are viral, bacteria, fungal, or parasitic. Print 12 of these pages and use one per month. Don't peek at last month's when you complete each new form — we guarantee you'll be amazed that some of your symptoms are lessening and you didn't even notice. Doing this simple exercise helps validate what you're doing and also helps keep you on the highway to health.

Date: _____

Scoring: Enter *1* for very mild symptoms and *10* for very severe symptoms; leave blank for no symptoms

Key: V = Virus, B = Bacteria, F = Fungus/Candida, P = Parasites, T = Thyroid, L = Lyme disease

Symptom	Severity	Symptom	Severity
V-Dark circles under eyes		V-Flu like symptoms	
V-Muscle aches and pains		V-Swollen glands	
V-Shortness of breath		V-Muscle weakness and exhaustion	
V-Numbness/ tingling/burning of extremities		V-Cloudy/burning/ tearing eyes	
V-Hair loss		V-Vertigo	
V-Metallic body odor		V-Feeling of uselessness	
B-Cough/lung infection		B-Sinus trouble	
B-Sore throat		B-Bladder infection	
B-Fever		B-Craving bread/carbs	
F-Craving sugar/alcohol		F-Postnasel drip	
F-White-coated tongue		F-Symptoms worsen with damp weather	
F-Dry/burning/ metallic mouth		F-Ear pain/itching	
F-Burning urination		F-Athlete's foot/nail fungus	
F-Vaginal or penile itching/burning		F-Rashes/skin breakouts	

Figure 3-1:
Symptom survey.

Symptom	Severity	Symptom	Severity
F-Sensitivity to tobacco smoke		F-Sensitivity to chemical and perfume smells	
F-Yeasty body odor		F-Confusion/poor concentration	
P-Gas that feels stuck		P-Pain in upper abdomen	
P-Incomplete bowel movement		P-Pain in lower abdomen	
P-Ravenous hunger		P-Worse symptoms at night	
P-Swollen/sore breasts		P-Night sweats	
P-Melancholy/sense of impending doom		P-Weight loss	
F&P-Air Hunger (can't get enough air)		F&P-Allergies	
F&P-Joint pain		F&P-Constipation/ diarrhea	
F&P-Anxiety		F&P-Abdominal gas/bloating	
F&P-Weight gain		F&P-Fatigue	
F&P-Drowsiness		F&P-Puffy hands/feet	
F&P-PMS		F&P-Hot flashes	
F&P-Panic attacks		T-Hatband headache	
T-Thinning eyebrows		T-Cold hands/feet	
T-Below-normal body temperature		T-Disinterest, inability to cope	
T&P-Insomnia		T&P-Trouble waking	
L-Arthritic pains that move and radiate		L-Lack of balance	
L-Muscle spasms/ twitches		L-Numb/tingling/ burning skin	
L-Feeling spacey		L-Violent temper	
	Subtotal:		Total:

Eating for your constitution: The Chinese elements

Chinese medicine bases diet on the five element theory of body type, with a specific food taste assigned to each. The Chinese are quick to acknowledge that you need to eat a balance of all the tastes, but if you're a particular elemental type you can emphasize one taste to benefit the body. You can read more about the five elements in Chapter 5; for more on the tastes, check out the "All a matter of tastes" sidebar in this chapter.

✔ **Wood:** Sour is the predominant taste that can help balance the liver and gallbladder symptoms that Wood types may be prone to.

✔ **Fire:** Bitter helps stimulate beneficial juices in the small intestine, the most important organ for Fire types.

✔ **Earth:** Sweet is the taste that soothes the stomach, the main organ that needs to be balanced in Earth types.

✔ **Metal:** Pungent foods aid balance in a Metal's large intestine, and they have a lot of antifungal properties.

✔ **Water:** Salty foods aid the balance of water in the body for the Water type.

Considering Common Diet Solutions

The diets we surveyed to develop recipes for IBS run the gamut of meat and potatoes to Raw. We have no prejudices, and we don't make our diet advice into a religion. We simply want to give you information about the diets you may be less familiar with and our reasons for featuring them in this book.

One size shoe doesn't fit everyone, so why should one diet? Individualize your own diet by keeping a food diary and mixing and matching what works for you.

Benefiting from the Specific Carbohydrate Diet (SCD)

Carolyn had the great fortune of knowing Elaine Gottschall, SCD groundbreaker, before the latter passed away in 2005. Elaine became a hero to many people suffering bowel disorders when she discovered the nutritional research of Dr. Sidney Haas and implemented his diet to heal her young daughter of ulcerative colitis. Elaine's *Breaking The Vicious Cycle: Intestinal Health Through Diet* (Kirkton Press) is the definitive book on the SCD.

The SCD is a diet for Crohn's disease, colitis, IBS, and other intestinal conditions. The premise underlying the SCD is that certain bacteria (the ones that produce disease) and yeast overgrow to such an extent that they spread their byproducts, which become toxins in the intestines that cause irritation and are absorbed in the blood stream, disrupting the immune system.

The overgrowth also interferes with the natural balance of good bacteria in the intestines, and masses of yeast and bacteria cause abnormal food fermentation. The foods these bad guys most often go after are double sugars (fructose, sucrose, and lactose) as well as carbohydrates in grains and some starchy vegetables.

SCD belief maintains that yeast alone or bacteria alone don't cause bowel symptoms. Rather, bacteria and yeast are partners in crime, living together in groups and helping each other survive. In fact, research shows that a bacterial toxin called LPS transforms yeast into a harmful pathogen.

The SCD does not completely omit any one food group and consists of most vegetables, nuts, some fruit, lactose-free dairy, meat, fish, poultry, and eggs. The diet relies on nut meal rather than flour to make bread and cookies. Though the SCD may appear to be restrictive, you may be amazed at how healthy and tasty the SCD-friendly recipes in Part II are.

In the vast clinical experience of Dr. Ronald Hoffman (a colleague of Carolyn's), he has found that "patients with IBD often note significant improvement in their symptoms within three weeks of starting the Gottschall diet. By twelve weeks, the majority are recovering definitively."

An SCD success story

Here's an email to Carolyn from Cathy, a 39-year-old U.K. mother of three children under six, who has been on the SCD for 23 days for her ulcerative colitis. Though ulcerative colitis and IBS are different conditions, Cathy's triumph shows how the SCD can improve not only digestive symptoms but also the psychological strain that can come with bowel conditions:

I just wanted to update you on my situation as I don't want to just be in touch when the news is bad! After a grueling beginning week to the SCD diet (I got much worse and was a bit worried but stuck it out), gradually the blood stopped in week two and next the watery (10 times a day) stool stopped by the end of the week. I am now eating a good many foods on the allowed list and feeling very well. I made sure not to try anything else at the same time so I would be sure what was having an effect. I have checked that all my supplements are SCD safe, so have stayed on these. I feel really well and so happy to be eating. I just wanted to let you know how shockingly quickly things began to improve for me on the SCD. I have never had such quick results without special meds or herbal treatments — just FOOD this time! I love the foods and have made many delicious things. I know the diet states it is often a long road with bumps in the first two years but I am feeling very positive about this being the right thing for me. Thank you for all your help and advice — I will keep updating you so I can be a part of your data collecting! All the best, Cathy

Although the SCD tends to focus more on helping folks with IBD (inflammatory bowel disease) than it does those with IBS, we still want to do our small part to introduce the IBS community to the potential benefits of an SCD program.

The creators of the Web site www.pecanbread.com/ibs have designed it specifically to help readers of *IBS Cookbook For Dummies* (Wiley) find more information about the diet and its supporting research.

Eating Raw for IBS

The *Raw food movement* is the new vegetarianism with a big enzyme kick. Every food has its own digestive enzymes that help it decompose. When you eat food that still contains living enzymes, you use fewer of our own digestive enzymes to break down food into digestible bits. This shift means fewer digestive upsets, better absorption of food, and fewer undigested food bits leftover to feed yeast and bacteria.

If you take antacids, don't eat enough protein, and drink a lot of fluids with your meal, you suppress your own ability to digest foods, and no amount of Raw eating is going to make up for that. Antacids neutralize stomach acid, lack of protein makes that acid difficult to produce, and fluids dilute the acid.

Heat destroys the food's enzymes, so you kill them when you cook food above the magic temperature of 120 degrees Fahrenheit. Raw foodists also contend that applying high-temperature heat to food damages vitamins and changes protein and fats into forms that are more difficult to digest.

We're talking specifically about the Raw food movement here. You can find many forms of raw cuisine, including eating raw meat and of course sushi. We don't advocate that IBS sufferers eat raw fish because sushi presents its own digestive and parasitic challenges.

Raw is an important culinary style to explore because it relies on unprocessed food straight from the farm. Most Raw food chefs recommend organic ingredients, which we encourage you to use whenever you can. Raw food retains the rich and exotic tastes that your body craves and doesn't require heavy spices and sweeteners that can upset the digestive system or irritate the intestines. Eating Raw also allows you to focus on foods high in magnesium, such as nuts, seeds, and deep leafy green vegetables; we discuss the benefits of magnesium in Chapter 1. Plus, you may be surprised how quickly you can prepare a raw meal and how little cleanup it requires.

Some people think they can't eat Raw because raw foods trigger IBS. Nothing could be further from the truth. Raw gets a bad rap because folks with sensitive guts can also have issues with their digestive enzymes, with not chewing food properly, and with drinking too much liquid with meals. The Raw recipes in Part II use preparation techniques that emphasize soluble fiber and minimize insoluble fiber minimized. We also flag some of the salads as being for folks who know they can handle veggies well.

Nuts and seeds also have something of a bad reputation in the IBS literature because their tiny shards can irritate the gut if you don't chew them completely. Underchewing nuts and seeds causes them to miss an essential stage of digestion, which is why you may see those shards in the toilet when you have a bowel movement.

Soaking nuts and seeds (as well as lentils and legumes) helps improve your ability to absorb their minerals. Check out the Soaking Nuts and Seeds recipe in Chapter 8 for instructions on soaking nuts and seeds.

Don't let the nuts and seeds stop you from trying our Raw recipes in Part II — we blend the offending ingredients to a creamy consistency that is as soothing as it is delicious and healthy.

Getting the most out of vegetarianism

Vegetarian staples like vegetables and grains get little respect in the IBS diet world because they have all that roughage (insoluble fiber). Even the word *roughage* is like scratching your fingernails on a chalkboard to someone with a sensitive gut. Unfortunately, committed vegetarians with IBS tend to live in a world of wheat pasta and white rice, only dabbling in vegetables that are overcooked and unappetizing. Such a bland diet may keep your IBS under some control, but it's hardly healthy in the long run.

Juicing is one IBS-friendly way to enjoy a vegetarian diet. Throwing away the fiber of fruits and vegetables and drinking all the nutrient-filled juice is very healthy for the intestines and lessens the chances of irritation. Chapter 8 is all about IBS drinks and juices.

Another safe way to get your vegetables is to make a salad and then blend it into a green pudding. We can hear the blechs from here, but give it a try — you may fall in love with blended salads. If that's not going to work, you can find lots of organic green powders on the market that you shake or blend into a green smoothie.

Vegetarians can benefit from the reasoning and recipes in the Raw diet (see the preceding section) because they incorporate blended nuts and seeds (so the fiber is broken down). Nuts and seeds provide an exceptional source of protein. For example, 1 cup of almonds has the same amount of protein as 4 ounces of meat.

Looking at organic eating

Eating *organic* (choosing foods grown without chemical pesticides, insecticides, and herbicides) is becoming more popular and affordable. An organic diet assures that your intestines aren't receiving or having to digest any of those unwanted chemicals that may trigger your symptoms. U.S First Lady Michelle Obama sparked great interest when she planted an organic garden on the White House lawn in March of 2009. Not to be outdone, the next month the U.S. Department of Agriculture released plans for an organic People's Garden on the Washington Mall.

According to the Environmental Working Group (www.ewg.org), some fruits and vegetables soak up more pesticides than others:

- ✔ **Pesticide-heavy:** Only buy these fruits and veggies organic if possible: Apples, bell peppers, carrots, celery, cherries, grapes, kale, lettuce, nectarines, peaches, pears, and strawberries.

- ✔ **Lower-pesticide:** These options have fewer pesticides and toxins, but you should still try to get organic versions when you can: Asparagus, avocados, broccoli, cabbages, sweet corn, eggplants, kiwis, mangoes, onions, sweet peas, papayas, pineapples, sweet potatoes, tomatoes, and watermelons.

Chapter 4

Stocking Your Kitchen to Support Your Diet

In This Chapter

▶ Kicking your unsafe food to the curb

▶ Filling your kitchen with IBS-friendly substitutes

▶ Making your kitchen work for you

*Y*ou're sitting at home when your stomach growls to tell you that you need a meal or snack. What are the first things that come to mind?

✔ I wonder what to eat from the assortment of tasty, healthy treats in my kitchen.

✔ I wonder whether I have any applesauce left.

✔ When is the last time I went grocery shopping?

✔ I hate that I don't have choices.

✔ Did I see something move in the fridge?

✔ I'm so hungry I don't care what I grab.

Read the first bullet again and notice your thoughts. You may be mumbling "Yeah, right — who has the time?" But most people discover that the mere thought of a well-stocked kitchen is a relief. The well-planned kitchen is a good friend of a healthy colon.

Now read the final bullet again. How often do you just grab food to fill space in your stomach? How does your body feel when you're so hungry that you don't care what you eat? Feeling like you have no food choices makes the stress of IBS even worse, especially when you feel like you have no safe food in the house. And choices are important when you're dealing with IBS. When you have been relieved of the choice of when you relieve yourself, you want to increase the control and choice you have in other areas of your life.

In this chapter, we help you get your kitchen, shopping, and cooking habits in shape to support your IBS challenges. Lots of our clients report feeling fewer symptoms and IBS attacks when they take charge of their kitchens.

Getting Rid of the Junk in Your Pantry and Freezer

Before you can stock your kitchen, you have to unstock it to get rid of the things that are unhealthy for you. When you're hungry, you may be tempted to eat whatever is in front of you even if you know you'll pay tomorrow, so the solution is simply not to have bad foods in front of you (or next to you, or stashed behind the toaster).

In Chapter 1, we discuss your gastrointestinal tract's (GIT) role as the gate-keeper of every bite you eat or drink. Its defense system is all set up to do the job of keeping nasty bugs and chemicals out of your blood stream and tissues, but it can only handle so much. If you throw caution to the wind and eat foods that have 50 different ingredients, most of them fresh from a chemistry lab, what's a poor GIT to do but dump them out in a hurry or hold onto them like a failing lab experiment trying to neutralize each chemical? That's why recognizing the type of food you eat and making your kitchen a safe zone are so important.

Take a look at the food you have in your home. Some of it likely is prefabri-cated, preserved, frozen, heat-and-eat stuff that you may not really know the contents of. Survey your freezer and cupboards for prepackaged meals and check the ingredient list against your safe food list. You particularly want to keep an eye out for these kinds of foods; this list isn't a complete rundown of potential IBS landmines, but it will get you thinking along the right lines:

- **Foods with ingredients you can't pronounce:** If your brain can't digest the word enough to even pronounce it, your colon likely can't process it either, and you should get it out of the house.

- **Foods full of cream and/or sugar:** Ice cream (even the homemade stuff) and other frozen sweet desserts can be an insult to a sensitive colon. Even if you aren't lactose intolerant, the cream and sugar can loosen things up for someone with IBS-D.

- **Foods full of trans fats:** Tubs of frozen dessert topping, and the cakes you put it on, are full of trans fats, which can act as a laxative in IBS-D and disrupt cell membranes potentially causing leaky gut (which we discuss in Chapter 18). In fact, most frozen dessert toppings are just fla-vored whipped oils.

Worried about wasting food? Take a few boxes of the nonperishable stuff to your local homeless shelter or food bank.

Fast food fasting

We believe the fact that this fast food generation has a 20-percent chance of having IBS is no coincidence. A 2004 study looked at the daily diets of more than 6,000 children nationwide and found that on a typical day more than 30 percent of the children ate some kind of fast food. This diet means they ate more fat, sugar, and carbs, all of which can be IBS trigger foods.

Check your food diary to see how many times in the past two weeks you've gotten fast food. Whether you sit down or go through drive-through, it's still fast food! If you have IBS-D, fast food might also mean that you (well, your bowels) move faster after you eat it.. For the next two weeks, stay away from eating on the run. Just slowing down at dinner time may be a relief for your colon.

Stocking IBS-Safe Essentials

An IBS diagnosis (or even a suspicion that you have IBS) is a wake-up call to take more control over what you put in your mouth. If you've decided to purge your kitchen of all the foods your IBS can't tolerate (see the preceding section), you may feel like you don't have any food left. We don't want you to be feeling deprived, but as you adjust to a new way of eating, you need to have healthy choices around you. For everything that you take out of your cupboard, fridge, or freezer, we want you to have an IBS-friendly choice to replace it with, so the following sections guide you to safer alternatives to some of the foods you may have had to toss.

Putting together a list of foods your intestines can handle is the first step toward restocking your IBS-friendly kitchen. (If you haven't compiled your safe food list yet, head to Chapter 2 for guidance on setting one up.) Your next task is to make sure you have items from that list close at hand. Having safer food choices at the ready doesn't have to be a chore if you know what to look for, and the following sections give you some suggestions to start off your shopping list.

Starting with snacks

Many snack crackers, cookies, and chips contain lots of wheat and fat, which are two major IBS triggers. However, friendlier options may be easier to find than you think. Although white flour has low nutritional value, it is high in fiber and an okay replacement in snacks when your choices are limited and you're having symptoms. Try plain white flour saltine crackers to replace your whole wheat-based ones (which have the extra insoluble fiber). Coconut cookies can have a welcome binding effect in IBS-D and are a better choice than most other cookies. Check out our recipe for Coconut Currant Cookies in Chapter 13.

Chips basically come in four varieties: potato, corn, rice, and wheat. Avoid the wheat stuff and look for options such as the following in your grocery or health food store.

You don't necessarily have to replace your chips with more chips. Try subbing fruits and veggies from your safe list instead.

- ✔ **Rice cakes:** Many people think eating rice cakes is worse than eating packing foam, but you can dress these cakes up with almond butter or organic peanut butter. (And anyway, those people exaggerate.) We recommend choosing a simple rice cake with two ingredients (rice and salt), which you can get from any health food stores. Watch out for the flavored rice cakes at the supermarket. Just because they're rice cakes doesn't mean they're healthy for you — depending on the flavor, they may contain sugar, yeast, milk, buttermilk, cheese, food coloring, fructose (fruit sugar), and/or maltodextrin (a food additive).

- ✔ **Rice chips:** Rice chips are made with rice flour, corn flour, and contain sesame seeds. Check out all the Lundberg brand rice chips; our favorites are the gluten-free Fiesta Lime (which contain a small amount of buttermilk) and the gluten- and dairy-free Honey Dijon flavors.

- ✔ **Baked organic corn chips:** Guiltless Gourmet makes a line of baked corn tortilla chips. The yellow and blue corn options have simple ingredients of corn, salt, oil, and a bit of lime. The flavored options may contain cane sugar (which is unrefined, but still sugar) and autolyzed yeast, if you are avoiding yeast. We recommend choosing organic corn products to avoid any genetic modifications to the ingredients and their potential harm to the gut.

- ✔ **Baked potato chips:** Baked potato chips have less fat than regular potato chips. Kettle Brand lightly salted baked potato chips have 3 grams of fat per serving and the regular version has 9 grams of fat. If you stick to the lightly salted option, the ingredients are simply potatoes, sunflower oil, and salt. As with any food, added flavors mean added and potentially triggering ingredients, so choose carefully.

- ✔ **Oat cakes:** If oats are on your list of safe foods, oat cakes are a great cracker substitute. Nairn's makes a product with simple ingredients: oats, oil, salt, and baking soda.

- ✔ **Mochi:** *Mochi* is pounded rice that's cut up and toasted. It's crunchy on the outside and chewy on the inside, so it can satisfy whatever texture you crave.

To make these chip replacements even tastier, try them with the dips in Chapter 7.

Sifting through breakfast cereals

Sugary cereals and granola are usually full of a variety of grains, sugars, and even yeast. Here are some healthier alternatives:

- ✔ Oats and oatmeal
- ✔ Rice puffs
- ✔ Millet puffs
- ✔ Kamut puffs

Looking at lunch

Frozen prefab pizzas, pastas, and other entrees are quick, easy, and even tasty, but the ingredients in most of the major brands are geared to flavor more than nutrition. The best alternative is to make your own meals, but if you just can't swing that, Organic Bistro (www.theorganicbistro.com/organic_bistro_meals.html) and Amy's Kitchen (www.amys.com) offer gluten- and dairy-free frozen meals. You may also be able to find them in your grocery store.

If canned spaghetti, ravioli, chili, and cream soups have always been more your style, try subbing them with one of the following; just remember that anything in a can or box, even if it's natural and organic, can come with a long list of added ingredients that your gut may not like, so check your labels.

- ✔ Amy's Kitchen (www.amys.com) has a wide variety of canned soups and mild chilis. Check their ingredient lists against your safe food list for some that fit for you.
- ✔ Eden Organic (www.edenfoods.com) has canned chili and rice-and-beans options whose ingredients are likely okay for your system.
- ✔ Canned wild salmon
- ✔ Low-mercury canned tuna (in water) or low-mercury tuna in pouches (without added oil)

Be sure to also check out the IBS-friendly soup recipes in Chapter 9; prep them ahead, and they can be just as convenient as the canned stuff. Salads can cause problems for some folks with IBS, but Chapter 10 offers several salad recipes that may work for you if that's your lunch of choice. For those who tend to lunch on leftover dinner, be sure to check out the following section for more replacement options.

Digging for dinner

Whether you're talking about bags of frozen fish sticks or boxes of just-add-meat meal mixes, most quick-fix dinner options just aren't IBS-friendly and have no direct, safer replacements. Having IBS tends to require you to cook more meals yourself (often especially at dinner), so we want to offer some basic guidance on putting together safe, healthy meals; head to Chapter 3 for more advice on menu planning. Your component choices for main meals follow two basic food categories:

- ✔ **Protein:** Includes lean beef, lean chicken, lean turkey, fish, nuts, seeds, and bean/grain combinations
- ✔ **Carbohydrate:** Includes vegetables, fruits, grains, and beans

Note: Grains and beans appear in both bullets because they contain both protein and carbs.

The recipes in Part II offer many choices of healthy entrees — choose the ones that are right for your safe food list.

How often have you whipped up a box of macaroni and cheese only to devour the whole thing yourself while it's still in the pot? Even the healthier versions are full of fat and calories, requiring the addition of potential triggers like milk and butter. To get your pasta fix, consider rice, kamut, and quinoa pastas.

Beefing up your baking goods

You likely do at least a little bit of actual cooking (and with IBS, you'll likely have to do a lot more), so chances are that you have some common ingredients that need replacing with safer alternatives. Baking in particular can be quite a landmine for IBS, what with all the flour, eggs, dairy, and sugar. We offer safe recipes for all sorts of baked goods in Part II; check those recipes for specific ingredient lists, but in the meantime the following list can give you a starting point for all your baking shopping.

- ✔ **Assorted flours:** Use whatever flour your recipe calls for, but coconut flour, almond flour, and rice flour are all good places to start. You may be able to buy a few cups of flour at a time out of the bulk bin at the grocery store until you determine what works for you.
- ✔ **Aluminum-free baking soda and baking powder**
- ✔ **Butter or *ghee* (casein-free butter; see the recipe in Chapter 6)**
- ✔ **Sugar substitutes (see Appendix B)**
- ✔ **Egg substitutes (see Appendix B)**
- ✔ **Milk substitutes (see Appendix B)**

- ✔ **Organic vanilla extract**
- ✔ **Sea salt**
- ✔ **Raw nuts**
- ✔ **Shredded coconut**
- ✔ **Coconut milk**
- ✔ **Raw cacao (chocolate)**

Setting Yourself Up for Success in the Kitchen

All the IBS-safe food in the world doesn't matter if you can't find it, store it, or prepare it because your kitchen isn't properly equipped. Relax — we're not talking about a bunch of fancy-schmancy equipment here, just some simple organizational and storage strategies (and, okay, a few cool gadgets) to help you get the most benefit out of your IBS-friendly food stash.

Keeping tabs on your safe foods

One challenge many IBS sufferers face when organizing their kitchens is that they share that space with other people. Ideally, you can designate special shelves in the cupboard, fridge, and freezer for your IBS foods out of the reach of little hands (or big hands, for that matter).

Give your kitchen-sharers some advance warning if you're going to rearrange the cupboards; otherwise, you may spend weeks answering, "Hey, where'd you put that again?"

If you can't get your own shelf, write your name on the packages with a permanent waterproof pen or a piece of masking tape. Safe food doesn't do you any good if it's gone when you get to it. You can also write "Don't eat the last one!" on a package you don't mind sharing from but want to keep tabs on.

If your safe cereal is also a family favorite, buy more than one box at a time, put your name on one of them, and insist that everyone else leave your box alone.

Storing food conveniently

If you buy food in bulk or in larger quantities so that you always have plenty of safe foods on hand, you need a place to put it to keep it fresh. We recommend putting storage containers on your shopping list when you first start your IBS diet so that you can take advantage of any sales on your safe foods.

The more storage capacity you have, the better, so mason jars, plastic freezer bags, and covered glass dishes are musts in your kitchen. Cooking a few meals all at once and freezing them is a way to minimize the stress associated with trying to figure out what to eat on a given day. (Flip to Chapter 14 for more on cooking and storing meals in advance.) You can even label meals for good days and bad days to leave the guess work out if you're feeling ill and have to eat. We also recommend putting the expiration day and/or the packaged date on any containers of food that you set aside.

Having handy tools at the ready

A fun part of organizing your kitchen to be IBS-friendly is that you may get to shop for new kitchen appliances (at least the small ones — you probably won't need a new fridge). Certain appliances save you time chopping and preparing food and allow you to prepare foods that you may not have tried before.

- **High-speed blender:** A high-speed blender (such as those made by Blendtec) let you grind nuts and make nut pâté, whizz up frozen desserts, and make great garlicky salad dressings in seconds without having to use a garlic press. It can take the place of multiple other appliances you may have needed to do the same job — a coffee grinder to grind nuts, a blender to mix things up, and a food processor to chop.

- **Juicer:** Fresh juices are very healing; they give you fruit's nutrients without the fiber. You can find some very good and inexpensive juicers on the market — Jack LaLanne has one for around $100.

- **Spiral slicer:** This garnishing machine turns vegetables into a pasta replacement with a few twists of the wrist, helping you easily fill your pasta craving without triggering your IBS with the real thing. Carolyn purchased hers online for about $25.

- **Chef's knife:** Vegetables are an important part of many folks' IBS diets, but chopping them can be a chore. With the right knife, however, chopping vegetables is a breeze. Shop in person for a knife that fits your hand and is easy to wield. Carolyn uses a Nakiri bocho knife, which is a Japanese-style vegetable knife with a wide, thin, straight blade. Knives with thicker blades are used to cut through bones of fish and meat.

- **Wooden cutting board:** At one point, health professionals believed that plastic cutting boards were safer than wooden ones in terms of cleanliness. However, research has shown that wooden boards are easier to clean and don't harbor bacteria the same way plastic ones do. Cutting into plastic over and over can also cause tiny bits of plastic to show up in your food.

Chapter 5

When Symptoms Strike: Soothing Your Gut on Difficult Days

In This Chapter

▶ Knowing which foods are and aren't helpful during an attack

▶ Identifying calming recipes

▶ Using non-food methods to pacify your gut

*W*hen you think of an IBS attack, you probably imagine rushing to the bathroom with urgency and frequency with IBS-D. However, IBS isn't all about diarrhea; you can also have an attack of cramping pain with both IBS-D and IBS-C. Either attack can be enough to keep you indoors for days.

Whatever causes an attack, avoiding or eating certain foods can help soothe your symptoms. In this chapter, we provide some solutions for soothing yourself with foods and other remedies.

We want to be clear here: We're not saying that if you eat some blueberries your attack is suddenly going to be cured. We simply want you to have all the tools possible to help calm your stomach, and those tools can include certain foods.

Avoiding Certain Foods During an Attack

When you have an IBS flare-up, you may be tempted to just quit eating entirely, but that's not a healthy solution. A better bet is to understand why some foods may make your attack worse, so here we guide you to some of those potential bad guys.

For example, when you have a sudden attack of diarrhea due to an infection, eating dairy or fruit can prolong the attack. *Note:* This diarrhea attack is different from chronic diarrhea, where ripe bananas and applesauce my help. The microorganisms running rampant in your intestines during an infection can wipe out the enzymes that digest sugars and instead use those sugars to make the perfect meal. This strategy of avoiding dairy and fruit can also be helpful for a non-infection attack of IBS.

Even if wheat isn't a trigger for you, you may want to avoid it during an attack because its gluten can be difficult to digest when your intestines are already irritated. And wheat breaks down into sugar so rapidly that it can quickly feed any microorganisms residing in your gut.

For an attack of either type of IBS, avoid alcohol, coffee, and soda; they can make your symptoms worse because they're all chemically irritating and (assuming you sweeten your coffee) can feed microorganisms with sugar.

So what can and should you eat? The following section details some soothing foods and drinks to keep on hand.

Focusing on Therapeutic Foods

The last thing you may feel like doing during an IBS attack is eating, but some foods can actually be helpful for your tummy during an attack. Easy soluble-fiber foods like oatmeal, rice, and bread provide safe bulk for your bowels, which means you can eat them as a therapeutic food when you need to. What this section focuses on are food remedies for both IBS-D and -C.

Here are several options to experiment with to find your soothing solution. You may be surprised by the variety of choices you have, but we want to give you as many possible comforting solutions as we can. Remember, particular food remedies may or may not work for you at any given time or place or for any and all circumstances. It's a matter of trial and error to see what suits your particular condition.

But first, a few tips:

- ✔ Pay attention to the foods in both the diarrhea and constipation sections. For example, if you have constipation but enjoy drinking pomegranate juice, a look at the diarrhea remedies reveals your pomegranate habit may aggravate your constipation.

- ✔ Keep some of the foods for your condition on hand. Just having them on standby makes you feel like you're prepared, and you know how important that feeling is when you're dealing with something as unpredictable as IBS.

✔ Eat small frequent meals so that you don't stretch your stomach and trigger the gut reflexes to dump.

✔ When you eat, chew your food well and in a slow and relaxed way. Chewing 30 to 40 times per bite can improve your digestion, making you feel full more quickly so you're satisfied by eating less and don't overeat. A sensitive bowel tolerates smaller meals better, less-rapid movement of the intestinal contents.

✔ In a pinch, just remember the acronym BRATTY. It stands for bananas, rice, apples, toast, tea, and yogurt, all foods currently recommended by doctors for soothing the symptoms of an IBS attack. Just be sure to use white bread, because it makes toast that's high in soluble fiber and can help absorb intestinal fluids, and plain, sugar-free organic yogurt, because it has beneficial bacteria for the gut that is very important in getting the intestinal flora back in balance. The BRATTY diet is palatable for both IBS-D and IBS-C because of the high content of soluble fiber.

✔ If you can, try to go for a little walk, even if it's just around the house or your office, after every meal. This habit is especially helpful for IBS-C because it can help keep things moving. It doesn't have to be a long trek; just 10 to 15 minutes is enough to get your juices flowing and your bowels moving. Make it a regular habit, and all parts of your body will benefit.

Dealing with IBS-D

Use your intuition and what you know about your personal condition to decide which of thee remedies make the most sense to try. You may find that you've already naturally gravitated to one remedy or another when faced with an IBS-D attack. You can also use the following foods to ward off attacks.

✔ Grate an apple and let it brown for two hours to allow it to begin breaking down and fermenting; this process makes the apple more digestible and puts no strain on an IBS-D gut. The pectin in apples is an excellent soluble fiber that helps absorb the excess fluid in the intestines to relieve diarrhea. (Pectin can also help treat IBS-C; check out the following section to make sure you're best utilizing pectin for your symptoms.)

✔ Apple cider vinegar is a long-standing digestive remedy with miraculous properties (and it's our personal favorite). Studies show that vinegar slows down the emptying of the stomach; this delay can be very beneficial for IBS because the stomach is less inclined to dump a whole meal into the small intestines, which can cause symptoms. Take between 1 teaspoon and 1 tablespoon in water before meals three times a day. Ease into this treatment by starting with the lower dose.

✔ Ripe bananas have the maximum amount of soluble fiber to help soak up liquid in the bowels and treat diarrhea.

✔ Blackberry and raspberry leaves are high in *tannins* (which have astringent properties that tighten tissues, making them secrete less fluid and lessen inflammation) and can serve as an aid for diarrhea. Steep 1 teaspoon of either leaf in 1 cup of boiling water for 15 minutes, strain, and drink either plain or with stevia as a sweetener.

✔ Blueberries are high in soluble fiber and contain tannins that become more concentrated when dried. You can eat the dried fruit or make a tea by steeping the berries in boiling water for 10 minutes. Blueberries also contain substances that have antibacterial properties, which is beneficial if your IBS is yeast- or bacteria-related.

✔ Carrots help ease diarrhea because of their high soluble-fiber content. They also contain significant amounts of vitamin A, an important nutrient for the health of the intestinal lining. Cook your carrots with ginger for the added benefit of settling nausea and digestive upset.

✔ Cinnamon in large doses can actually cause diarrhea, but in small amounts this powerful spice can actually help relieve it. Use ¼ to ½ teaspoon to add to the soluble fiber effects of cooked oatmeal or baked apples, or brew it as cinnamon tea.

✔ Ginger tea is an excellent remedy for nausea, diarrhea, and intestinal upset. You can sweeten with stevia, honey, or coconut milk.

✔ Whole lemon contains pectin, which is high in soluble fiber. Liquefy a (thoroughly washed) whole organic lemon (seeds, rind, and juice included) in a high-speed blender with ½ teaspoon salt and then take 1 teaspoon of this mixture three times a day. Lemon seeds have an anti-microbial effect that's especially helpful if your IBS is related to yeast or bacterial overgrowth.

✔ Mint tea and mint essential oils act as muscle relaxants to intestinal muscles to help with diarrhea and relieve gas.

✔ Papaya contains soluble fiber and enzymes that help ease diarrhea. Grate a raw green papaya and boil it in 3 cups of water for 8 to 10 minutes. Strain out the papaya pieces and drink the liquid throughout the day. Although papaya can help treat constipation as well, in this form it has a drying effect on acute diarrhea.

✔ Although raw persimmon treats constipation, cooked persimmon relieves the symptoms of diarrhea because cooking releases its tannins, which act to dry up diarrhea.

✔ Pomegranate juice acts as a powerful astringent that has a drying effect on the stool. It's available in most health food stores; mix one part juice with one part water and sip throughout the day.

Controlling IBS-C

Make sure you thoroughly wash the following fruits and vegetables before consuming. You can also use ten drops of grapefruit seed extract in a sink of clean water to eliminate bugs and parasites: Soak for ten minutes, drain, and use. They don't require rinsing after soaking.

✔ In addition to keeping the doctor away, an apple a day can help moisturize the stool. Apples are also very high in the soluble fiber called pectin, which is an excellent gentle laxative. They can absorb enough liquid from your diet to create a soft bulking fiber that helps relieve constipation. So drink a glass of water with your apple snack.

Be aware that larger amounts (such as two apples a day) can create too much moisture and intestinal gas and bloating, especially in those who have trouble digesting raw apples.

✔ Unripe bananas can help lubricate the intestines to relieve constipation.

✔ Figs contain digestive enzymes, soluble fiber, and fruit sugar, all necessary components of a gentle laxative. Figs also treat bloating and flatulence. You can soak and stew figs (as well as prunes or dates) in licorice tea to create a laxative drink.

✔ Gooseberries have a laxative effect. Soak 4 ounces of dried gooseberries in water overnight; remove the soaking water and add 1 quart of water. Bring to a boil, let stand for 30 minutes, strain off the fruit, and drink the water throughout the day.

✔ Bitter foods with high mineral content stimulate *peristalsis,* which basically means certain greens can help you go. Salad greens like arugula, lettuce (romaine in particular), and escarole are especially helpful.

If raw salads irritate your stomach, you can cook escarole and drink the liquid for its bitter properties.

✔ Kiwi, pineapple, mango, and papaya have a reputation for helping relieve indigestion and promote digestion. They're high in soluble fiber and their high fruit sugar content draws fluid into the stool to relieve constipation. Papaya also is rich in a constipation-relieving enzyme called *papain* that helps break down protein.

✔ Peaches may act as a gentle laxative. You can eat several with or without the skin, depending on your sensitivity. The fruit sugar is thought to pull water into the stool to relieve constipation.

✔ Raw persimmon can relieve constipation because their raw fruit sugar pulls water into the stool. Too much raw persimmon can eventually cause diarrhea.

✔ Snapper is a fish that Chinese medicine uses to increase the amount of moisture in the intestines and promote movement in the intestines, making it useful for constipation. Swordfish is another fish thought to lubricate the stool and treat constipation.

✔ Turnip helps relieve constipation because of its high soluble fiber content, which allows it to absorb water and create bulk to help bowel movements.

Keeping Soothing Recipes Close By

When you're feeling overwhelmed by your symptoms, simply eating can be an effort, much less taking a lot of time to seek out and prepare safe food. Part II of this book is chock-full of IBS-friendly recipes, but when your symptoms are acting up, you may not want to take the time to rifle through and pick out one that sounds good. The following list gives you a head start by describing some of this book's most soothing recipes. They won't work for everybody all the time, but they're a place to start.

Soothing teas are always a good bet whether you have IBS-C or -D. If you don't have time to brew tea, put one drop of peppermint essential oil in 32 ounces of water and sip throughout the day.

✔ **Strawberries and Cream Oatmeal (Chapter 6):** Oatmeal is high in soluble fiber; make it a little runnier to go easier on your sensitive system.

✔ **Any of the smoothies (Chapter 8):** Smoothies are a must when you're in the midst of a flare-up because they're an easy, comforting way to get the nutrients you need in a small liquid package.

✔ **Savoring Sourdough Bread (Chapter 12):** As we recommend throughout the book, sourdough bread is a great soluble side to have on hand. When you're feeling up to baking, make an extra loaf and store it sliced in a zipper bag in the freezer for days when you're feeling off your game.

✔ **Fast, Colorful Papaya Pudding (Chapter 13):** Papaya, a well-known digestive aid, can help digest foods that may be causing some irritation in your gut. Adding psyllium powder to this recipe makes it a great source of soluble fiber to soothe unsettled intestines.

✔ **Goji Berry Tapioca (Chapter 13):** If you have IBS-D, the chia seeds in this quick recipe bulk up in your intestines with safe soluble fiber. (See Chapter 13 for more on chia seeds.)

✔ **Vegan Khir Pudding (Chapter 13):** This recipe contains the healing herb cardamom, and using no-carb *miracle noodles* gives it an extra burst of soluble fiber.

Exploring Other Helpful Options

Eating or avoiding certain foods (see the sections earlier in this chapter) isn't the only way to take charge of an IBS attack. The following sections show you other methods of relieving your symptoms and maybe even preventing future flare-ups.

Snoozing away your symptoms

Sleep is a very important factor in healing IBS symptoms. If you have IBS-D, the depletion of nutrients and stress on your adrenal glands from loss of magnesium can tire you out. Those with IBS-C are often prone to irritable tiredness because of the toxins they may be reabsorbing from their large intestine; when toxins overload the liver, anger rises to the surface. You may notice that your intestines give you the most trouble when you're especially tired or run down; fatigue can make you even more sensitive to foods you think you can digest. If you're forced to pull an all-nighter, be especially careful about what you eat during the wee hours — coffee and takeout may just compound the problem. If tiredness is causing your attack, slow down and rest as much as you can.

Dealing with stress

Stress can make any disease worse, and IBS is no exception. And good stress can affect your intestines just as much as bad stress — your gut doesn't know the difference between taking an exam and standing as an attendant at your best friend's wedding.

When you feel the rumbling in your gut or the cramping in your abdomen, stop and take a deep breath. Notice what is going on in that moment. Are you rushing to get everyone and yourself ready for school and work? Are you sitting at your desk trying to finish a project? Did the mailman bring you yet another bill to pay? If you realize that stress is likely causing your attack, look for positive ways to release that stress, such as yoga, meditation, or a simple walk around the block. Deep breathing can also be incredibly relaxing, and you can do it from your chair.

Create a part of your food diary to write down your stressors so you can identify trends in what situations and activities stress you out. Then you can decide whether you want to continue them and/or how you can better deal with them.

Stressful situations aren't the time to expand your diet beyond what's on your safe food list; if stress triggers your IBS, the last thing you want to do is throw another potential trigger on top of that. Resist the urge to just grab whatever's handy or tempting. Flip to Chapter 20 for more guidance on avoiding this emotional eating.

In *IBS For Dummies* (Wiley), we introduce you to *Emotional Freedom Techniques* (EFT), a do-it-yourself stress relief technique that anybody can use. EFT is especially useful in the midst of an attack because it can have direct effects on your current symptoms. You can find out more about EFT and how to use it to relieve your symptoms on Christine's Web site (www.christinewheeler.com).

Treating with medicine

Depending on what symptoms you have, you may be prescribed any variety of medications, such as antispasmodic drugs; antidiarrheal drugs such as Lomotil or Imodium; drugs that have narcotics like codeine; laxatives; bulking agents; anti-flatulents; and antidepressants. Sometimes you get the same drug for your IBS-C that your friend is taking for IBS-D. So when you're under attack from your IBS symptoms, you may get short-term relief by taking Lomotil, Imodium, or bulking agents, but follow the guidelines, which usually tell you that they are for short-term use only.

The key word here is *short* term. In the long term, you have to address your diet and lifestyle to find what is making your symptoms worse and to make helpful changes. There's no definitive cure for IBS, but we've heard from many, many readers of *IBS For Dummies* (Wiley) who resolved their symptoms and resumed normal relationships with their bathrooms. One of our chefs told us that a client of hers claimed her IBS was cured when she read *IBS For Dummies* and took charge of her diet. Our chef said that we attained the status of rock stars in her client's eyes! We'll take a pass on the rock star status but are thrilled when our work helps and heals people.

Zelnorm: A cautionary tale about side effects

A possible result of taking any kind of medication that it can cause side effects. You may remember Zelnorm, a drug marketed for a few years as treatment for IBS-C because it manipulated the serotonin in the gut. At one point, the U.S. Food and Drug Administration demanded Zelnorm's packaging include a warning about the potential occurrence of *ischemic colitis* (bowel inflammation or injury caused by lack of blood supply to the colon), but in 2005, new label warnings only mentioned severe diarrhea and fainting. In 2007, Zelnorm was pulled from the market after several people who were taking the drug died of stroke or heart attack.

Medicating acute attacks with homeopathy and magnesium

In the previous section, we go over the failure of conventional medicine to find something to cure or even treat IBS, but that doesn't mean we're going to leave those of you suffering from acute attacks empty-handed. This section gives you several remedies that can offer at least some relief during an acute attack. (Of course, we don't expect those acute attacks to keep happening after you develop your own IBS diet — see Chapter 3 — and implement some of the advice in this book.)

Helping symptoms with homeopathic remedies

Use a qualified homeopath if you choose to explore homeopathy as a treatment for your chronic IBS symptoms.

You may not know much about *homeopathy* (treating conditions with small amounts of drugs that would produce the conditions' symptoms in a healthy person) except the use of arnica for pain and shock, but it's the best first aid for an acute IBS attack. Each remedy in Table 5-1 treats a certain set of symptoms best. Match your symptoms with a remedy or two, and then buy those remedies and keep them on hand. Because stress can contribute to IBS attacks (see "Dealing with stress" earlier in this chapter), knowing you have treatments ready to go may lessen the chances of an attack.

The dosage for acute symptoms is one dose every half hour. In the health store, you can find different *potencies* of each remedy. Choose a 6, 12, or 30 potency. If a homeopathic remedy is going to work, it should do so within four to five doses. If one remedy isn't working after five doses, try another remedy. But if you try two or three different remedies and nothing is helping — move on to other ways of helping your IBS. *Note:* The pellet forms of these remedies contain lactose, and the liquid versions have some alcohol as a preservative. Most people do just fine with either, but if you have severe lactose intolerance, use the liquid.

Anyone, infant to elderly, can take homeopathic treatments safely, and there are no interactions with any other medications or any other diseases. Still, it's smart to consult with your doctor before you begin taking any of these medications.

Table 5-1	Homeopathic Remedies for IBS	
Remedy	*GI Symptoms*	*Associated Emotions*
Argentum nitricum	Bloating, rumbling flatulence, nausea, and greenish diarrhea	Anxiety; nervousness; claustrophobia; extreme expressiveness; impulsiveness

(continued)

Table 5-1 *(continued)*

Remedy	*GI Symptoms*	*Associated Emotions*
Arsenicum album	Vomiting and diarrhea caused by eating bad meat, fruit, or vegetables; upset stomach or burning pain caused by food	Overwhelming fear of illness/death, being alone, and being closely watched; restlessness; agitation; anxiety with exaggerated weakness
Colocynthis	Cutting and cramping pains triggered by eating fruit or drinking water	Anger; indignation
Lilium tigrinum	Alternating constipation, diarrhea; possible lump in the rectum that creates the unsuccessful urge to go	Irritability; rage
Lycopodium	Bloating; gas; stomach pain; heartburn; chronic bowel problems; a ravenous appetite to the point of getting up at night to eat	Lack of confidence; worry
Magnesium phospate	Cramping of all muscle groups, including those that produce hiccups; abdominal colic	Mental exhaustion
Natrum carbonicum	Indigestion and heartburn; poor absorption of food; gas, explosive diarrhea; an empty, gnawing feeling in the stomach	Cheerfulness and considerate nature, which lead to weakness, sensitivity, and a desire to be left alone
Nux vomica	Abdominal pains; bowel symptoms accompanied by abdominal tension, which may lead to soreness in the muscles of the abdominal wall and pain from trapped gas; constipation with a largely unsuccessful urge to go; diarrhea	Irritability; aggressiveness; a hard-driving, Type-A personality

Remedy	GI Symptoms	Associated Emotions
Podophyllum	Abdominal pain and cramping accompanied by a gurgling, sinking, empty feeling and followed by watery, noxious-smelling diarrhea; alternating diarrhea and constipation; pasty yellow bowel movements containing mucus	Depression and irritability
Sulphur	Sudden morning urge to evacuate bowels; episodes of diarrhea throughout the day, alternating with constipation accompanied by offensive, odorous gas; oozing around the rectum with itching, burning, and red irritation	Strong personality; hot, fiery temperament

Making magnesium work for you

One of the really bad parts about having an IBS-C attack is the cramping pain that can cut like a knife.

Researchers are still trying to figure out what exactly causes intestinal spasms in IBS; some theories suggest that the intestines may already be in spasm from generalized tension or from lack of magnesium. In either situation, taking magnesium is going to help. We cover magnesium and its laxative properties in Chapter 1; if you have IBS-C, take two to three 200-milligram doses of magnesium citrate/magnesium chloride power or capsules throughout the day and one glass of water with each dose.

The first doses should help calm you down and begin to relax your intestines. If that amount doesn't result in more relief of your constipation, you can take more magnesium up 600 to 800 milligrams of magnesium citrate per day.

If you have IBS-D, you can easily get around the dilemma of magnesium being a laxative: Use magnesium salts in a bath or a foot bath, or spray magnesium oil on your skin, especially your abdomen. Epsom salts are magnesium sulfate and available in any drugstore in the country. Put 2 to 4 cups of Epsom salts in a moderately hot bath and relax while the magnesium penetrates your skin and relaxes your intestinal spasms. Magnesium oil is magnesium chloride highly concentrated in distilled water; put 2 ounces in a bath or 1 teaspoon directly on your skin. It's available from various online sources (such as www.globallight.net).

Defending against infections

Even if you have IBS, you can still suffer a gut infection on top of everything else, so you want to know how to recognize the difference and be able to treat an infection if you have one.

If other people around you are coming down with a stomach flu, that's a clue that your extra symptoms indicate is a newly arrived gut infection. The initial symptoms of a gut infection begin with abdominal cramping and diarrhea. These symptoms are so common in IBS that you have to judge the intensity and frequency of symptoms to know the difference. You can also have one or more of the following symptoms, which definitely indicate that something more is going on than just a bad IBS attack:

- Fever
- Nausea
- Loss of appetite
- Vomiting
- Weight loss
- Mucus or blood in the stool
- Dehydration

The following from Carolyn's e-book *Future Health Now! Encyclopedia* gives you some tips on treating a gut infection or acute attack:

- Use dietary treatment first. Antibiotic or antidiarrheal pills can be dangerous and actually prolong the illness.
- Triple your dose of *probiotics* (beneficial bacteria).
- Observe the following diet:
  - On the first day of your symptoms, drink only clear fluids such as soups, juices, and teas.
  - On day two, eat only rice, applesauce, and bananas. Three times that day, take 1 teaspoon of carob powder in some applesauce.

- For day three, you can add dry, bland foods, but nothing greasy, fried, or spicy.

- By day four, you should be able to move up to a normal diet, but do so slowly.

- Avoid dairy and citrus for at least a week.

- If your bowels loosen at any time, move back to clear fluids.

If any of the following happens, go to the nearest doctor or hospital:

✔ Any symptom of gut infection hangs on for more than five to six days.

✔ Fever and bloody diarrhea or vomiting and diarrhea occur together. Dehydration occurs when vomiting and diarrhea are present. Make sure you are drinking lots of fluids to make up for all the fluid loss associated with with vomiting and diarrhea.

Antidiarrheal pills should be used only to control diarrhea for short periods of time when absolutely necessary, such as long road trips. Antibiotics can be dangerous when used for diarrhea and should only be prescribed by a doctor. They can lead to overgrowth of bacteria and/or yeast in the intestines so be sure to take probiotics as we mention in Chapter 1 if you take an antibiotic.

Watch young children with diarrhea; they dehydrate faster. They can go without food for short periods of time but don't let them go without fluids. Warm baths can help to rehydrate.

Preventing infectious diarrhea

The nearby "Defending against infections" section presents infection as a probable cause of some cases of IBS, so we want to make sure you have some useful preventive tips and tools to help you avoid this particular kind of diarrhea attack:

✔ Don't drink the water, including in ice, fruit drinks, and milkshakes. Drink only boiled water, commercially bottled water, or mineral water (with unbroken seals). Also consider other ways you may ingest water, such as while brushing your teeth.

✔ Don't eat salads or cut fruits, except fruits you peel yourself. Eat only dry foods (which are usually safe) and freshly cooked food.

✔ Wash your hands often, using hot water and soap.

✔ Take probiotics every day to keep the good bacteria at a high level and grapefruit seed extract capsules and/or digestive hydrochloric acid tablets with every meal.

Borrowing benefits from other theories

You're an individual with your own unique symptoms and triggers, so when your symptoms strike, you may need a treatment farther off the beaten path. To help you celebrate your uniqueness, and so you won't think you have to avoid every food and trigger just because it affected someone else with IBS, we want to give you some different perspectives on healing. We give you an overview of them in Chapter 3, but this section explores how these theories can guide you to foods that may help soothe your symptoms.

Read about these theories with an open mind. Don't be alarmed if you read that a certain constitution can eat spicy food or drink coffee because it doesn't fit into the IBS picture. One man's IBS pleasure food is another man's IBS poison.

(Blood) typing your way to health

No, we aren't suggesting that you hit the keyboard of your computer to find the answers — we know that you've already drained the Internet of information about IBS. This section looks at the blood type diet and how you can use it when your intestines are under attack.

In his book *Eat Right 4 Your Type: The Individualized Diet Solution to Staying Healthy, Living Longer & Achieving Your Ideal Weight* (Putnam Adult), Dr. Peter D'Adamo describes the four blood types and the four different blood type diets. The following list gives you the highlights of each diet; if you're having trouble calming an IBS attack, find your blood type and see whether these suggestions help put your system back in harmony.

- ✔ **Blood type O:** People who are O blood types need high amounts of animal protein and fish; they can't digest dairy or wheat properly and may have problems with grains and beans in general. They can eat meat, fish, and olive oil freely and enjoy eggs, nuts, seeds, certain vegetables, and fruits in moderation.

- ✔ **Blood type A:** People with an A blood type can live a good life on a plant-based vegetarian diet that includes nuts, seeds, beans, cereals, pasta, rice, fruit, and vegetables. However, they have difficulty digesting red meat and dairy.

- ✔ **Blood type B:** B blood types can eat the most varied diet: grains, dairy, animal protein, vegetables, and fruits. They have trouble digesting nuts and seeds and they do much better only eating small amounts of carbs.

- ✔ **Blood type AB:** ABs can eat a combination of the foods recommended for blood groups A and B.

Physician, heal thyself: Carolyn's type diet story

When Carolyn first learned about the blood type diet, she was in her first year of medical practice and experimenting with a macrobiotic diet comprised of soy products, beans, grains, and vegetables. After a few weeks, she developed fluid in her lungs; even though she wasn't sick and didn't have a fever, she could feel the rasping in her chest and hear water moving around the air sacs when she listened to her breathing with a stethoscope.

Her macrobiotic doctor friend told her it was just a "healing reaction," but her husband and nurse were pretty worried about her symptoms — they thought she had pneumonia. But she thought the problem was her diet's protein deficiency. She's an O blood type, so she figured she didn't have enough protein to keep her fluids in the right places in her body! Plus, she was eating lots of soy that upset her intestines because she couldn't digest it.

She knew she couldn't get enough protein from the macrobiotic diet when she eliminated soy, so she decided it was time to eat some meat. Within 36 hours of eating organic chicken, her lungs cleared, proving her need for protein and inability to digest soy — two ideas suggested by the O blood type diet. (Check out the nearby section "(Blood) typing your way to health" for info on appropriate foods for each blood type). The information from the O type diet also helped reinforce her decision to reduce wheat and dairy, which are difficult for Os to digest. When she did that, her intestines were the happiest they had ever been.

Many years ago, Carolyn did a survey at her local health club to see whether healthy, athletic people naturally followed their blood type diet. They didn't. Then she surveyed her patient population and discovered that when people were sick and symptomatic and not following a diet appropriate for their blood type, they always benefited by making some changes.

For example, when Theresa and Pam, patients from the A and AB blood groups, came to see Carolyn with IBS symptoms, they had a lot of red meat, wheat, and dairy in their diets. Their symptoms of fatigue, headaches, and alternating constipation and diarrhea made them both feel miserable. She explained that the foods they were eating weren't being digested properly and were creating bowel toxicity (and feeding intestinal organisms that made even more toxicity). She encouraged both women to try a plant-based vegetarian diet that matched their blood type-approved food list for 3 weeks; the diet's high fiber content and their inherent ability to better digest this diet helped turn their symptoms around.

Applying Ayurvedic medicine

Ayurvedic medicine is a 5,000-year-old medical tradition of the Vedic culture in India. It centers on the three *doshas* (the energies that govern the body based on a person's body frame) or constitutions: Vata, Pitta, and Kapha. A person derives health and well-being from having balanced doshas.

We're giving you some very basic, general information about the three constitutions as examples of alternative ways to approach your IBS condition. In no way are we suggesting that you suddenly and drastically change your diet. If any of this information feels right to you, please do much more research and/ or see an Ayurvedic doctor.

The following list gives you a quick rundown of each constitution as well as some foods you should and shouldn't eat to keep your system in balance:

- ✔ **Vata:** A person with a Vata constitution is thin and cool (as in body temperature, not like the Fonz) and has dry skin. When the Vata person is out of balance, he's likely to be gassy, flatulent, constipated, and anxious. If this sounds like you, look to salt, oil, and hot and spicy foods to warm up your system and lubricate your intestines. Sour foods are also a good choice. Vatas have a cool metabolism, so cold foods put them even further out of balance, so try staying away from cold foods like beer, ice cream, and cold salads.

- ✔ **Pitta:** A person with the Pitta constitution is likely to be medium build with a well-proportioned body. The element that runs the Pitta person is fire, so Pittas often have a warm body temperature and a fiery temperament. If you have a Pitta constitution, sweet, bitter, and astringent foods are your best bets for intestinal peace; you can get into trouble and out of balance when you stoke up the fire that is already burning in your belly, especially the small intestine.

- ✔ **Kapha:** Kaphas don't have digestive issues, except a sluggish metabolism that can lead to constipation. Kaphas flourish on astringent, bitter, and pungent foods and flounder when they eat sweet, sour, and salty foods.

Finding the five elements of Chinese medicine

Chinese medicine discusses constitutions in terms of elements; the five elements of Chinese medicine are Wood, Fire, Earth, Metal, and Water. In this section, we give you a quick rundown of the elements and the foods each type can use to soothe an intestinal attack.

We know that Chinese medicine's five-element diet theory isn't an easy subject. If it seems to strike a chord with you, however, and you want to read more, we recommend Harriet Beinfield and Efrem Korngold's *Between Heaven and Earth: A Guide to Chinese Medicine* (Ballantine Books).

✔ **Wood:** A Wood type has a tendency to ward liver and gall bladder problems, possibly leading to constipation. Foods that help relieve liver and gall bladder symptoms are in the sour taste category: citrus fruit, pear, plum, mango, many unripe fruits, yogurt, vinegar, cheese, yogurt, all foods produced by fermentation, pomegranate seeds, and tamarind.

✔ **Fire:** Like a Pitta constitution in Ayurvedic medicine (see the preceding section), a Fire type can have problems with digestion and food absorption when the small intestine is out of balance. The foods that help stimulate beneficial gastric and intestinal juices are in the bitter taste category: coffee, aloe, salads, hops, lettuce, radish leaf, vinegar, many greens, turmeric, fenugreek, and bitter gourd.

✔ **Earth:** An Earth type is a worrier with a slow metabolism and relies on sweet foods to soothe the stomach. But too much sweet food coupled with the worry can make an Earth feel heavy and bloated and lead to IBS-D. To pacify your gut, look to bread, rice, milk, butter, ghee (butter without the protein casein; see the recipe in Chapter 6), sweet cream, honey, raw sugar, ripe fruits, and chestnuts.

✔ **Metal:** Metal types express their digestive symptoms in the large intestine, which can lead to dryness in the large intestine and constipation. Pungent foods help move stuff through the intestines — try green onion, chive, clove, parsley, coriander, peppers, onion, radishes, garlic, ginger, chili peppers, black pepper, mustard, radish, and white daikon.

✔ **Water:** Water types don't typically deal with digestive issues because their problem area is the kidney. They rely on salty foods to balance the fluids in their body, including sea salt, rock salt, kelp, salty pretzels, and pickles.

If your symptoms seem to sound like any of these elements, do some more research or consult with a doctor of traditional Chinese medicine.

Part II
Eating For Your Intestinal Health

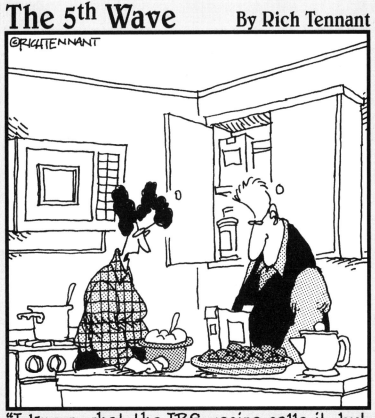

The 5th Wave   By Rich Tennant

"I know what the IBS recipe calls it, but if anyone asks, it's a seafood souffle, not an Anti-Inflammatory Bowel Souffle."

In this part . . .

We're very excited to reveal 120 delicious IBS recipes from fabulous chefs from all over North America; these folks have an interest in creating meals that support your intestinal health. From your three square meals to dessert delicacies to late-night munchies, we've collected recipes to surprise and satisfy you. We've even put some foods back on your menu that you probably thought were lost!

These recipes aren't your typical IBS fare, which is often about restricting lots of foods and adding soluble fiber (although we do advocate the latter). These recipes are eclectic and innovative as well as tasty.

Chapter 6

Beginning Your Day with Breakfast (Without the Consequences)

In This Chapter

▶ Getting serious with cereals

▶ Enjoying pancakes and breads

▶ Refusing to give up on yogurt

▶ Having your eggs and eating them too

*B*reakfast, more than any other meal, can be a touchy subject for someone with IBS. You can do the math on how many hours it's been since you last ate when you roll, lurch, or leap out of bed in the morning. If you suffer from IBS-D, lurching out of bed is designed to propel you in the direction of the bathroom as your body responds to the adrenaline surge from low blood sugar. Morning is when your blood sugar is at its lowest, which is why breakfast should be the heartiest meal of the day.

You may not want to tempt your sphincters with anything bulky, but you still need to eat something so you don't become hypoglycemic as you start your day. You can't push your adrenaline all morning to keep your blood sugar up. In fact, that action can actually overly stimulate your intestines and cause more activity than you want.

Balancing your blood sugar by eating breakfast serves many purposes. It offsets the production of adrenaline and the stimulation of your intestines. It prevents low blood sugar headaches and irritability — things we're sure you want to avoid. Breakfast done right can nourish your body without you suffering any side effects.

Especially if you have IBS-D, you can begin your day with a calming tummy tea and then a safe and soothing smoothie. Because you can enjoy our teas, smoothies, and other delicious drinks throughout the day, we feature them in Chapter 8. This chapter focuses on breakfast foods.

You don't have to limit yourself to smoothies if you have IBS-D. The following breakfast favorites served up with IBS-friendly ingredients should be safe for everyone. Just take it slow and easy, use small portions, and remember to list your food reactions as you develop your safe food list.

Factoring In Soluble Foods

You can balance any breakfast meal by eating a portion of soluble fiber food. Your best high soluble-fiber fruits are apples, bananas, mangoes, and papayas. Ideal breakfast grains include brown rice cereal, oatmeal, cornmeal or polenta, barley, quinoa, and sourdough white bread.

We aren't big on white bread, and we don't mean for you to eat the white flour and water paste that passes for bread in the grocery store. Try to find fresh, homemade sourdough white bread, or better yet, make your own! (See the recipe in Chapter 12.) The reason we favor white bread at all is because of its soluble fiber. Wheat bread and whole-wheat bread still contain the wheat bran, which is insoluble and capable of irritating your intestines. Although you also lose the vitamins and minerals from the bran by eating white bread, sometimes it's a fair trade-off to keep you from having a tummy attack.

Shoot for breakfast recipes where at least half the ingredients (or safe substitutions) are sources of soluble fiber. The soluble/insoluble fiber chart in Appendix C shows you the fiber content of many common foods — choose the ones that have at least the same amount of soluble as insoluble fiber.

Being Grateful for Grains and Cereals

If you simply want a quick breakfast out of a box or bag, you can try millet, rice, or, if you aren't too gluten-sensitive, kamut puffed cereal. They don't have much nutrition, but they have bulk, and you can dress up your dish with some fruit (like papaya, mango, or strawberries), douse it with coconut milk, and be good to go. Check out Chapter 12 for more on grains.

Then there's the old standby: What would breakfast be without good, old-fashioned oatmeal? Our grandfather told us stories of his mother making huge vats of oatmeal, pouring it into the drawers of a dresser to harden, and then cutting it out in bricks as needed!

Oatmeal is high in soluble fiber and can therefore be called an IBS health food. You can make oatmeal thick or thin; thinner is better for a sensitive stomach.

You can find different varieties of oatmeal based on their cooking times:

- ✔ **Old-fashioned:** Oat groats are called *old-fashioned oats.* They take longer to cook (around 45 minutes), are chewier, and may not be as soothing to the gut as rolled oats.

- ✔ **Steel-cut:** *Steel-cut oats* are oat groats cut into pieces but not flattened leaving them coarse and somewhat chewier than rolled oats when cooked. The coarseness may cause some intestinal irritation. Their cooking time is about 20 minutes.

- ✔ **Rolled:** *Rolled oats* are oat groats steam-heated and flattened into round, flat oats. They cook more quickly than old-fashioned oats (in about 15 minutes). In terms of stomach compatibility, they're not as coarse as groats and steel-cut oats and may be easier to digest.

- ✔ **Quick-cooking:** *Quick-cooking oats* are even flatter than rolled oats. The manufacturers probably use a laundry press on them (just kidding). Because they're flatter and more processed, you can cook them up even more rapidly than rolled oats — in about 5 minutes. They may be easier to digest because they are more processed, but they aren't as tasty as rolled oats or groats.

- ✔ **Instant:** Instant oats are the fastest cookers of all. They cook up in hot water in one to two minutes. They may be the easiest on the gut, but they have the least flavor.

Instant oatmeal in little packets is a great option when you travel. Use the coffee maker in your hotel room to heat water, pour it over your oats in a coffee cup, and stir and let sit for a few minutes for lovely oatmeal.

You may have heard that oatmeal has gluten, which can be hard on an IBS stomach. According to gluten researchers, most oatmeal contains some gluten only in the sense that it's been cross-contaminated by wheat or rye in the field, granary, or manufacturing plant. If you have celiac disease, look for gluten-free oatmeal, which guarantees noncontamination.

☙ Quick Brown Rice Protein Power Breakfast "Cereal"

Julie Beyer contributed this recipe that's quick to prepare and easy to digest, tastes great, and can hold you over for three to four hours. Julie created recipes like this one to harness the healing potential and power of organic whole foods. If you're going to warm fruit for this recipe, try using a steamer. A good tip is to keep berries in your freezer — you can quickly steam them when you're in a hurry.

Preparation time: *5 to 10 minutes*

Cooking time: *None*

Yield: *1 serving*

3 tablespoons brown rice protein powder

2 tablespoons ground flaxseed

½ teaspoon cinnamon

Pinch of sea salt

½ teaspoon stevia

1 tablespoon flaxseed oil

1 to 2 tablespoons water

1 cup fresh or warmed peaches

¼ to ½ cup coconut milk

1 teaspoon shredded coconut

Sprinkle of nut of your choice (optional)

⅛ teaspoon each cloves, nutmeg, and cinnamon, or to taste

1 to 2 teaspoons of maple or agave syrup (optional)

1 In a bowl, mix the brown rice protein powder, ground flaxseed, cinnamon, and salt.

2 Add the flaxseed oil and water to obtain a dough-like consistency. If you're steaming the peaches, you can use some of the warm water from the steamer.

3 Add the peaches, coconut milk, shredded coconut, nuts (if desired), and spices.

4 Drizzle with a small amount of maple or agave syrup if desired.

Tip: *Freshly ground flaxseed is best. Use a coffee grinder to make this healthy addition to breakfast.*

Tip: *Flaxseed oil tends to go rancid quickly. Therefore, it's best to buy only the smallest bottles and use within 3 weeks. You can buy several and preserve the extras in the freezer for up to one year.*

Per serving: *Calories 558; Fat 37.9 g (Saturated 17 g); Cholesterol 0mg; Sodium 256 mg; Carbohydrate 33 g (Fiber 9.2 g); Protein 38.1 g; Sugar 14.9 g.*

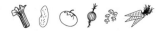

◌ *Hand-Milled Gluten-Free Breakfast Cereal*

When our contributor Laura Pole (www.eatingforalifetime.com) developed IBS, she was sensitive to dairy, gluten, corn, and soy, so she came up with this deliciously pleasing hot breakfast cereal to satisfy her desire for safe grains. As an added benefit, when you travel you can mix up a batch of the dry ingredients ahead of time, add a bit of Rapadura (unrefined cane sugar), put it in a small container, and take it on the road. You use the hotel coffee maker to brew hot water, pour it over the cereal, and let it cook for 10 minutes.

Preparation time: *10 minutes*

Cooking time: *10 to 15 minutes*

Yield: *4 servings*

¼ cup long grain brown rice

¼ cup millet

¼ cup quinoa (red or white)

¼ cup walnut or other nut pieces, ground if nut pieces are irritating

¼ cup dried blueberries

½ teaspoon cinnamon

Pinch of salt

1½ cups water

¼ cup organic whole milk or non-dairy milk (such as unsweetened Rice Dream)

Grade B maple syrup (optional)

Butter or coconut oil (optional)

1 Grind the rice, millet, and quinoa in a coffee/spice grinder or a sturdy blender.

2 Mix ground grains with the nuts, dried blueberries, cinnamon, salt, and water.

3 Bring to a boil and reduce heat to simmer. Cover and allow to simmer about 10 to 15 minutes, stirring occasionally and adding more water to create desired consistency.

4 Add the milk, syrup, and butter as desired.

Vary It! You can substitute other dried fruit such as raisins or cherries for the dried blueberries.

Tip: You can also use coconut milk for an extra creamy taste.

Per serving: Calories 211; Fat 6.5 g (Saturated 1.5 g); Cholesterol 0.7 mg; Sodium 51 mg; Carbohydrate 32.9 g (Fiber 3.3 g); Protein 5.1 g; Sugar 12 g.

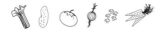

☺ *Caramelized Banana and Date "Porridge" (SCD)*

Michelle Gay (www.eatingjourney.wordpress.com) uses leftover pureed cooked cauliflower to create this breakfast treat that has the consistency of porridge. Yes, we said cauliflower. What a great way to make use of leftovers! Be sure to heat the cauliflower thoroughly because when cauliflower puree is hot, the flavor blends well with the other ingredients. When cold, it may have a distinct taste. This recipe is safe for the Specific Carbohydrate Diet (SCD); see Chapter 3 for more on the SCD.

Preparation time: *5 minutes*

Cooking time: *10 minutes*

Yield: *2 servings*

1 banana	*½ a head of cauliflower, pureed*
2 dates	*Dash of cinnamon*
1 teaspoon butter	*½ to 1 tablespoon honey (optional)*

1 Slice the banana. Pit the dates and slice them into small pieces.

2 Place the butter into a small frying pan and heat on a medium-high burner.

3 At the first sign of melting, add the banana and dates and sauté for 2 to 3 minutes, constantly turning.

4 When the banana starts turning golden, reduce the heat to medium and add the pureed cauliflower. Heat thoroughly.

5 Sprinkle cinnamon over the top and add honey if you like.

Per serving: *Calories 197; Fat 2.3 g (Saturated 1.3 g); Cholesterol 0 mg; Sodium 58 mg; Carbohydrate 45.7 g (Fiber 6.9 g) Protein 4 g; Sugar 33.1 g.*

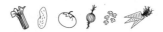

☉ Soaked Oats Porridge

This recipe is a family favorite from Shannon Leone's collection; you can find Shannon at www.rawmom.com. It's just one way you can enjoy an oatmeal breakfast, the ultimate comfort food and a universal meal that sticks to your ribs.

Tools: *High-speed blender (optional)*

Soaking time: *Overnight*

Preparation time: *5 minutes*

Yield: *1 serving*

2 cups organic oat groats

¼ cup dried figs

1 tablespoon walnuts

1 tablespoon shredded coconut

1 cup coconut juice or water to mix ingredients

4 ounces of coconut milk

Pinch of cinnamon or nutmeg (optional)

1 The night before, put the oats, figs, nuts, and shredded coconut together in a bowl and cover with water to soak overnight.

2 In the morning, carefully rinse the ingredients in fresh water to eliminate residue.

3 Put the soaked mixture in a blender or food processor with the coconut juice or water and blend until smooth.

4 Pour the coconut milk over the blended mixture and serve with a pinch of cinnamon or nutmeg (if desired).

Tip: *For all grains (whether raw, sprouted, or cooked), vegetables, fruits, dried fruit, and nuts, use 5 drops of grapefruit seed extract in the soaking water to eliminate fungi and bacteria. Sensitivity to fungi, mold, and bacteria may be a major reason why some people with an already-sensitive gut can't digest grains, vegetables, or nuts.*

Per serving: *Calories 1599; Fat 52 g (Saturated 27 g); Cholesterol 0 mg; Sodium 40 mg; Carbohydrate 237.3 g (Fiber 37.8 g); Protein 57.4 g; Sugar 19.9 g.*

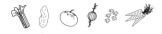

○ Strawberries and Cream Oatmeal

This dish is Carolyn's favorite breakfast; find it featured in the color section. While her quick oats are cooking, she cuts up strawberries and bananas (an IBS staple) and gets the coconut milk out of the fridge. As soon as that's done, the oatmeal is usually ready to pour. You can add different fruits and even nuts as your diet allows.

Preparation time: *2 minutes*

Cooking time: *8 minutes*

Yield: *4 servings*

1 cup quick-cooking rolled oats	5 strawberries, cut up
2 cups water	2 ounces coconut milk
1 banana, cut up	

1 Put the rolled oats and water into a pot on a cold stove.

2 Bring to a boil, turn the heat to the lowest setting, and let cook for 5 minutes.

3 Put the banana and strawberries into the bowl, add the oats, and cover with the coconut milk.

Per serving: Calories 211; Fat 5.8 g (Saturated 3.3 g); Cholesterol 0 mg; Sodium 6 mg; Carbohydrate 34.3 g (Fiber 5.3 g); Protein 7.2 g; Sugar 3.6 g.

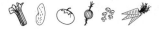

Piling On the Pancakes

If you thought your IBS meant you'd never have pancakes again, think again! Our chefs who formulate SCD recipes give you the perfect way to enjoy pancakes without wheat (actually, without any grains at all).

You can also purchase wheat-free or gluten-free pancake mixes in the health food store. They're a bit pricey but still much cheaper than any similar restaurant fare. One product that gets rave reviews is Pamela's Ultimate Baking and Pancake Mix.

☾ Cinnamon Pancakes with Ghee

Imagine pancakes that give your morning an energy boost and are worry-free. Thanks to Kendall Conrad for contributing this SCD version of a morning favorite that everyone in the family can enjoy. Kendall chose this recipe to share with us from her book *Eat Well Feel Well* (Clarkson Potter), which you can read about at her Web site www.eatwell feelwellthebook.com.

Preparation time: *10 minutes*

Cooking time: *10 minutes*

Yield: *4 servings of 4 pancakes each*

1 cup whole organic cashews	*Splash of vanilla*
½ teaspoon baking soda	*Pinch of salt*
3 eggs	*2 tablespoons of honey*
1 tablespoon Kendall's SCD Dairy Yogurt (see the recipe later in this chapter)	*1 teaspoon cinnamon*
	1 tablespoon coconut oil

1 Using a food processor, grind the cashews into a paste.

2 Add the baking soda, eggs, yogurt, vanilla, salt, honey, and cinnamon and blend well.

3 Turn the oven burner to medium-low heat and melt the coconut oil in a frying pan.

4 Pour the batter into the pan in ¼-cup pools.

5 Flip when golden.

> **Vary It!** *If you're in a hurry (or just don't want to make your own yogurt), you can substitute plain organic cow or goat yogurt.*

> **Tip:** *Drizzle extra honey and melted butter or ghee (see the following recipe) over pancakes.*

> **Per serving:** *Calories 292; Fat 21.4 g (Saturated 6.5 g); Cholesterol 160 mg; Sodium 232 mg; Carbohydrate 18.7 g (Fiber 1.4 g); Protein 11.2 g; Sugar 9.2 g.*

Gratifying Ghee

Ghee is a type of butter from which all the milk solids have been removed, which makes it safer for people who have both lactose intolerance and *casein* (milk protein) allergies. (Butter has no lactose but does contain casein.) Ghee has been used for centuries in India; it's prized by practitioners of Ayurvedic medicine (see Chapter 3).

Making ghee is a fairly simple procedure to heat the butter and separate the fat and the solids. The results are magical. Ghee looks semisolid at room temperature. You don't need to refrigerate it, and it can keep for several months. Always use a clean utensil in the ghee bottle.

Tools: *4 sheets of cheesecloth*

Preparation time: *2 minutes*

Cooking time: *10 minutes*

Yield: *About 1 pound*

1 pound unsalted butter (organic if available)

1 Melt the butter gradually over low heat in a deep pot with a thick bottom. Do not stir.

2 Continue cooking over low heat until the melted butter is a clear golden liquid. It will bubble and may foam but won't boil over if you have a deep enough pot. The milk solids will turn golden or light brown and may settle at bottom. You can skim off and discard the thick foam.

3 Remove from heat while the liquid is a clear gold. A darker color means overdone ghee.

4 Line a sieve with the 4 sheets of cheesecloth and place the sieve over a clean pot. Strain the still-hot ghee through the sieve.

5 Transfer the strained ghee into a clean jar and screw the lid on securely.

Per serving: Calories 102; Fat 11.5 g (Saturated 7.3 g); Cholesterol 31 mg; Sodium 2 mg; Carbohydrate 0 g (Fiber 0 g); Protein 0.1 g; Sugar 0 g.

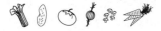

Basking in Bread

Would we eliminate the staff of life from your world? Not a chance. You can still enjoy bread that is healthy and delicious; this section gives you a couple delicious breakfast options, and Chapter 12 has the recipe for our great-with-any-meal sourdough bread.

☺ Gluten-Free Pumpkin Spice Bread

You don't have to be gluten-intolerant to enjoy this great gluten-free recipe. Personal chef, nutritional consultant, and cooking instructor Andrea Boje (`www.myfoodmyhealth.com/OurChefs/index.php?chefid=23`) provided this morning recipe that's even tastier the next day.

You can substitute 1 cup maple crystals plus ½ cup sucanat plus ½ cup brown sugar for the 2 cups of sugar. In place of gluten-free flour, you can also try ½ cup brown rice plus ½ cup quinoa flour plus ¼ cup each of sorghum, potato starch, tapioca flour, and millet flour. Cover the finished bread with plastic wrap and keep in the refrigerator for a week to 10 days. You can also freeze it for up to 3 weeks.

Tools: _Parchment paper_

Preparation time: _8 minutes_

Cooking time: _35 minutes_

Yield: _Sixteen 1-slice servings_

3 large eggs	_1 teaspoon baking powder_
2 cups sugar	_1 teaspoon baking soda_
½ cup grapeseed oil	_2 teaspoons cinnamon_
One 15-ounce can organic pumpkin	_½ teaspoon ground cloves_
2 teaspoons vanilla	_¾ teaspoon nutmeg_
2 cups gluten-free flour	_¾ teaspoon ground ginger_
1½ teaspoons xanthan gum	_1 teaspoon sea salt_

_**1**_ Heat the oven to 350 degrees.

_**2**_ Spray two loaf pans with a little olive oil, line with the parchment paper, and set aside.

_**3**_ Beat the eggs in a medium mixing bowl with a hand mixer until a little frothy. Add the sugar and continue to beat until smooth.

_**4**_ Add the oil, pumpkin, and vanilla and stir together with a spatula.

_**5**_ In a separate bowl, mix the remaining ingredients.

_**6**_ Add the dry ingredients to the wet and stir to mix.

_**7**_ Pour the batter into the prepared pans and bake for 35 minutes, turning the pans half way through. The bread is done when a toothpick or wooden skewer inserted into the middle of the loaf comes out clean. Cool on a wire rack.

Tip: _Dress it up for company with a maple cream cheese frosting._

Per serving: _Calories 248; Fat 8.4 g (Saturated 1 g); Cholesterol 40 mg; Sodium 270 mg; Carbohydrate 40.5 g (Fiber 2.1 g); Protein 3 g; Sugar 27.7 g._

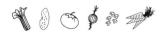

🍑 Banana Bread

Banana bread is such a comfort food, and thanks to Jenny Lass and Jodi Bager at www.grainfreegourmet.com, you can enjoy it even with your IBS restrictions. This recipe is grain-free, gluten-free, and dairy-free, but it tastes authentic and so delicious. Enjoy a slice warm from the toaster on its own or with a little butter.

Preparation time: *10 minutes*

Cooking time: *40 minutes*

Yield: *Eight 1-slice servings*

2 cups finely ground almond flour	¼ cup honey
½ teaspoon baking soda	1 large ripe banana, mashed
½ teaspoon salt	3 large eggs

1 Preheat the oven to 300 degrees and line a greased 9-x-5-inch loaf pan with parchment paper.

2 Mix the almond flour, baking soda, and salt in a bowl.

3 Combine the honey, mashed banana, and eggs and mix well.

4 Pour the wet mixture into the dry ingredients and stir until well combined.

5 Pour the batter into the prepared loaf pan and bake until a knife comes out clean when inserted, about 40 minutes. Let cool.

Per serving: Calories 232; Fat 15.9 g (Saturated 1.6 g); Cholesterol 79 mg; Sodium 251 mg; Carbohydrate 18.2 g (Fiber 1.4 g); Protein 8.6 g; Sugar 10.6 g.

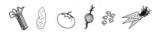

Devouring Dairy (And Dairyless) Yogurt

We love dairy, but because of dairy sensitivity, which causes some nasal mucus, we limit our intake to one serving of plain, unsweetened organic yogurt to which we add bananas, raspberries, or strawberries. Properly-made yogurt should have no lactose sugars left. The bacteria growing in the yogurt should digest all the lactose, leaving nothing for your lactose-intolerant body to deal with.

However, not all yogurts are this well made. Because some dairy lovers can't digest milk sugar or even the casein in those yogurts, the Raw food community has found ways around that specific problem with non-dairy yogurt, which recreates the taste and consistency without the side effects. You can read more about the Raw food movement in Chapter 3.

☞ *Shannon's Non-Dairy "Yogurt"*

This dairy-free yogurt replacement from Shannon Leone (www.rawmom.com) is a healthy and Raw alternative for people who are lactose intolerant or allergic to casein, or just want a change of pace. Serve it with fresh fruit that fits for you, or try it with the porridge or cereals in this chapter.

Soaking time: *1 hour*

Preparation time: *5 minutes*

Cooking time: *None*

Yield: *4 servings*

2 cups raw cashews	*½ teaspoon vanilla*
Juice of 2 lemons (about ½ cup)	*Pinch of sea salt*
3 tablespoons agave or raw honey	

1 Soak the cashews in water for 1 hour and rinse.

2 Add all ingredients into a blender or food processor and blend until smooth.

Per serving: *Calories 367; Fat 24 g (Saturated 4 g); Cholesterol 0 mg; Sodium 43 mg; Carbohydrate 33.7 g (Fiber 2.1 g) Protein 10.2 g; Sugar 17.7 g.*

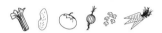

☞ Kendall's SCD Dairy Yogurt

Thanks to Kendall Conrad at www.eatwellfeelwellthebook.com for this 32-hour yogurt that makes a half-gallon of fresh, rich, Greek-style yogurt.

You need a yogurt machine for this one. You also need Yogourmet (pronounced yo-gourmet), a freeze-dried yogurt starter containing L. Bulgaricus, S. thermophilus, and L. acidophilus bacteria. One box of starter has three 10-gram packs (each pack makes 2 fresh quarts of yogurt).

Tools: *Yogurt maker*

Preparation time: *45 minutes (including cooling time)*

Incubation time: *32 hours*

Yield: *Sixteen ½-cup servings (½ gallon total)*

1 quart organic whole milk	*One 10-gram package of Yogourmet starter*
1 quart organic half and half (no careegenan)	

1 Bring milk and half and half to a simmer. Remove from stove and cover. Place in the fridge until lukewarm, about 25 to 30 minutes. When lukewarm, pour a cup of the liquid through a strainer into the inner bucket of the yogurt maker.

2 Add the contents of the starter packets and whisk 20 times in each direction. Strain the remaining milk mixture into the bucket and whisk 10 more times each way. Put the top on the bucket and place in the outer container of the yogurt maker with 1½ cups of water.

3 Plug in the machine and leave it for 24 hours. After the 24 hours has passed, leave the lid on the inner container and place it in the fridge for 8 hours more.

4 Spoon into a bowl, add honey and vanilla, and eat!

Per serving: Calories 179; Fat 8.4 g (Saturated 0.9 g); Cholesterol 49 mg; Sodium 92 mg; Carbohydrate 7.3 g (Fiber 0 g); Protein 46 g; Sugar 7.3 g.

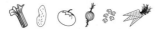

Savoring Eggcellence

First, we want to bust some misconceptions about eggs. Eggs don't count as dairy, so don't even go there. You can have eggs — the whites *and* the yolks. The story about egg yolks causing cholesterol problems is just a myth probably cooked up to sell margarine.

Eggs do have cholesterol; cholesterol is a fat, and some people are more sensitive to fat, but that doesn't translate into egg yolks triggering IBS. In summary, enjoy your eggs!

Having said all that, yes, some people don't digest eggs well. Neither of us do, and we drink powdered eggs for breakfast. Our eggs come in serving-size pouches mixed with pea powder and apple flakes. We shake the powder with water, and we're good to go.

◌ Herb Scramble

Chef and nutritionist Caroline Nation, who founded www.myfoodmyhealth.com, contributed this high protein kick-off to the day. You can enjoy it with any herbs you find tasty and healthy. For a generally nutritious scramble, try parsley, but it's also delicious with chives, dill, basil, or cilantro. Blanching the herbs for one minute keeps them bright green if that's important to you.

Preparation time: *10 minutes*

Cooking time: *5 minutes*

Yield: *4 servings*

1 bunch parsley, finely chopped

8 eggs

¼ teaspoon salt

¼ teaspoon freshly ground black pepper

1 tablespoon extra virgin olive oil

1 Bring a medium pot of water to a boil over high heat. Add the parsley (and any other herbs) and cook for 1 minute. Drain and rinse under cold water.

2 Whisk the eggs in a medium bowl. Add the parsley, salt, and several grinds of pepper and whisk to combine.

3 Warm the oil in a large nonstick or cast-iron skillet over medium heat. Pour in the eggs and stir gently and constantly until the eggs form large curds and are cooked to your preference, about 2 to 3 minutes. Serve immediately.

Per serving: Calories 149; Fat 12.6 g (Saturated 3.8 g); Cholesterol 420 mg; Sodium 178 mg; Carbohydrate 3.2 g (Fiber 1 g); Protein 6.3 g; Sugar 0.4 g.

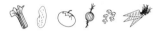

☺ Huevos Rancheros
(Eggs Country-Style)

Raman Prasad (www.scdrecipe.com/cookbook) provided us with this traditional Mexican breakfast dish from his book *Recipes for the Specific Carbohydrate Diet™* (Fair Winds Press). This dish, which is featured in the color section, translates from Spanish as "eggs country-style," because it was often served as a late-morning or early afternoon treat for farm laborers working since the crack of dawn.

The snap peas in this recipe add an unusual crunch. Anaheim chili is a mild green chili that most people with IBS may be able to tolerate. Start slowly and let your body decide. If you're on the SCD (see Chapter 3), don't worry about the Gruyère cheese — it's SCD-safe.

Preparation time: 10 minutes

Cooking time: 15 to 18 minutes

Yield: 3 servings

6 eggs	1 medium tomato, finely chopped
1 teaspoon olive oil	¼ teaspoon oregano
1 small onion, finely chopped	¼ cup fresh cilantro leaves, finely chopped
1 Anaheim chili, deseeded and finely chopped	⅛ teaspoon each salt and pepper, or to taste
9 chives, finely chopped	¼ to ½ ounce grated Gruyère cheese
10 snow peas, finely chopped	

1 Break the eggs into a bowl, mix, and set aside.

2 Heat the olive oil in a nonstick pan over medium heat. Add the onion and Anaheim chili. Sauté and allow the onion and chili to brown, 3 to 4 minutes. Add the chives and snow peas to the pan and cook together for about 1 minute.

3 Add the chopped tomato and cook until soft, 2 to 4 minutes. Sprinkle the oregano into the mixture, and add the eggs. Throw in the cilantro immediately. Add salt and pepper to taste.

4 Allow the eggs to cook for 3 to 5 minutes until they reach the desired consistency, stirring often to make sure they don't stick to the pan. Top with the grated cheese.

Per serving: Calories 165; Fat 11.8 g (Saturated 4.1 g); Cholesterol 423 mg; Sodium 226 mg; Carbohydrate 7.9 g (Fiber 1.8 g); Protein 7.6 g; Sugar 3.7 g.

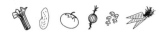

Chapter 7

Satisfying the Munchies and Your Stomach: Snacks and Appetizers

In This Chapter

▶ Whetting your taste buds with appetizers

▶ Dunking into dips and spreads

▶ Dishing out the fish snacks

Some people are convinced that snacking is the answer to IBS. Preparation time is short, so you can eat quickly if you're ravenous. The snack size is small, and the after effects are minimal; as we mention in Chapter 1, comfortable eating has to do with the sphincters in your gastrointestinal (GI) tract not being stretched to the max, allowing food to sneak in and out without you really noticing it! Now, those are magic words to someone with IBS.

You don't have to skimp on the appetizers at your next dinner party, either. The recipes we provide here let you nosh right along with your guests worry-free. But don't wait for a dinner party to prepare your favorites. Spend an afternoon in the kitchen whipping up a bunch of these "snackatizers" and put them in the freezer for another day.

Of course you can take any meal in this book and make it a small portion and achieve the desired results. However, when you want something fast and tasty or a few dishes to get the party started right, you're in the right chapter.

Choosing Soluble-Fiber Finger Foods

The following foods are your best bets for incorporating soluble fiber in your snacks and appetizers. Ideally, your munchies and starters should include at least 50 percent soluble fiber. Although this chapter's recipes don't feature all these ingredients, they're foods that you can add or substitute to raise your food-solubility factor. For a broader list, check out Appendix C for the fiber contents of lots of common foods.

- **Grains:** Barley, brown rice, cornmeal, non-wheat pasta, non-wheat flour tortillas, and quinoa
- **Vegetables:** Beets, carrots, mushrooms, parsnips, potatoes, pumpkins, rutabagas, squash, sweet potatoes, turnips, and yams
- **Fruit:** Avocado

Starting Things Off with Creative Appetizers

One man's appetizer is another woman's snack. We've called these appetizers because they kick any meal off to a great start, but don't limit yourself! They are great on their own to quiet the hungries at any time of day or night. If you're making hors d'oeuvres for a dinner party, double the recipe and keep the rest for yourself.

Asian Tempeh Kabobs

Andrea Boje (`www.myfoodmyhealth.com/OurChefs/index.php?chefid=23`) shared with us her favorite recipe for kabobs. *Tempeh* is fermented soybeans molded into a cake that you can cut up into cubes or other entertaining shapes. It's a great source of protein for people with IBS because it's fermented, which means it's easy to digest and doesn't produce gas. The key to really good tempeh is all in the simmering sauce — it gives it a rich, meaty flavor. Make extra sauce and save it in the refrigerator for quick meal prep later, or use it in preparing beef for a stir fry. Frying the tempeh first creates a crunchier texture and keeps it from falling apart.

Tools: *Garlic press (optional)*

Preparation time: *6 minutes*

Cooking time: *18 minutes*

Yield: *3 servings*

One 8¾-ounce package tempeh, cut into 1-inch cubes

3 tablespoons olive oil or high heat safflower oil

Simmering Sauce (see the following recipe)

Six 6-inch skewers

1 Heat the oil in a frying pan over medium heat. Add the tempeh and cook until browned on each side (about 2 minutes per side), turning over with tongs.

2 Pour the simmering sauce into the frying pan and simmer for about 8 minutes, turning the tempeh occasionally so that it soaks up the sauce evenly.

3 Remove from heat. Put 4 to 5 tempeh cubes onto each skewer and place on a serving dish.

4 Drizzle the remaining liquid from the pan over the skewers and serve.

Simmering Sauce

¼ cup tamari or soy sauce

2 tablespoons balsamic vinegar

2 tablespoons rice syrup, honey, or agave syrup

1 teaspoon ginger juice, or small piece of ginger, peeled and grated

1 tablespoon minced garlic, or 2 to 3 garlic cloves run through a garlic press

1 In a small bowl, mix the tamari, vinegar, rice syrup, ginger juice, and garlic until rice syrup has dissolved.

Vary It! *Add 2 teaspoons of chopped lemongrass to the sauce for a Thai influence, or add ¼ cup of pineapple or orange juice and ½ teaspoon of lemon zest to marinade for a tropical tang.*

Tip: *Having a barbeque? Make the skewers up to 2 days ahead of time and then put them on the grill for about 5 minutes to reheat.*

Per serving: *Calories 348; Fat 22.5 g (Saturated 3.7 g); Cholesterol 0 mg; Sodium 1351 mg; Carbohydrate 22.9 g (Fiber 0.3 g); Protein 18.1 g; Sugar 14.4 g.*

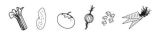

☙ Oven-Baked Yam (or Potato) UnFries

Thanks to our healing chef, Colleen Robinson (www.crimsondoorhealing.com) for this simple but delicious substitution for the universal fries. Lots of restaurants have the deep-fried version on the appetizer menu, but the baked yam version is a great alternative for IBS because it has less fat, which can be a trigger. And the UnFries have a sweet taste, so they quickly become a treat. Don't forgo the parchment paper here. It seems silly but trust us — it lets you get away with making the fries all crispy and happy with very little oil. Parsley or a French herb mix works well for the dried herb.

Tools: *Parchment paper*

Preparation time: *45 minutes*

Cooking time: *30 minutes*

Yield: *1 serving*

1 medium yam or potato, or 1 large handful new baby potatoes

¼ teaspoon sea salt

½ teaspoon dried herbs of choice

1 Preheat the oven to 350 degrees. Cover a couple of cookie sheets with parchment paper.

2 Coarsely chop the yam/potatoes into pieces roughly the same size (so they cook evenly). Soak the yam/potato pieces in a bowl of cold water for 30 minutes to pull out extra starch and make them crispier.

3 Strain out the water but do *not* leave the yams/potatoes to dry. Instead, immediately toss them with the sea salt and herbs.

4 Lightly spray the parchment paper with cooking spray and then spread the yams/ potatoes out in a single layer. Don't cram them in — they won't cook as crispily and they'll take longer.

5 Bake for about 15 minutes, flip them over with a spatula, and cook for another 15 minutes so that they're nice and soft on the inside and crisp on the outside.

Tip: If you really fall in love with this recipe, invest in a mandoline slicer to cut your yams/ potatoes up in a jiffy.

Per serving: Calories 112; Fat 0.07 g (Saturated 0.02 g); Cholesterol 0 mg; Sodium 653 mg; Carbohydrate 26.2 g (Fiber 3.9 g); Protein 2.1 g; Sugar 5.4 g.

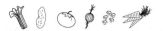

Green Chicken Egg Bake

Thanks to Michelle Gay (www.eatingjourney.wordpress.com) from Australia for this quick and easy starter for one, which is featured in the color section. Michelle is a farm girl from Oregon who is a house mom for students at an Australian university. We don't know whether she feeds her students her delicious recipes, but they would certainly benefit!

For this recipe, we recommend you use free-range chicken because they are grain-fed and free of growth hormones and antibiotics and are therefore healthier for the IBS tummy. With any chicken dish, be sure to cook whatever kind of chicken you use well. As you become more familiar with this dish, you may find that you don't need to grease the pan.

Preparation time: *15 minutes*

Cooking time: *35 minutes*

Yield: *1 serving*

4 ounces of chicken breast meat, diced

1 stalk of celery, diced

1 teaspoon olive or peanut oil

2 eggs

⅜ cup water

1 cup spinach

⅛ teaspoon each salt and pepper

¼ cup cheese, onions, peppers, bacon, or other leftovers (optional)

1 Preheat the oven to 400 degrees. Grease a loaf pan and set aside.

2 In a skillet, heat the olive or peanut oil over medium heat. Add in the celery and cook for about 1 to 2 minutes.

3 Season the chicken with salt and pepper and add it to the skillet with about ¼ cup of the water. Continue stirring until the chicken is cooked and remove from the heat.

4 In a separate bowl, whisk or beat the eggs and ⅛ cup of water with a fork. Add the spinach and any optional ingredients (if desired).

5 Place the chicken/celery mixture in the bottom of the loaf pan and cover with the egg/spinach mixture. Bake for about 20 minutes or until a knife comes out clean, meaning the egg is cooked.

Vary It! *Sprinkle the cheese on top of the dish as it bakes instead of mixing it in with the eggs.*

Tip: *If the spinach is poking out and getting burned, you can add more eggs to cover everything up.*

Per serving: *Calories 301; Fat 15.8 g (Saturated 4.1 g); Cholesterol 478 mg; Sodium 548 mg; Carbohydrate 3.2 g (Fiber 1.4 g); Protein 35.6 g; Sugar 1.6 g.*

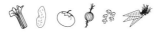

Quick 'n' Easy Quiche

Thanks to Colleen Robinson (www.crimsondoorhealing.com) for her contribution of this appetizer for the whole family. This recipe is easy to assemble, but it does take 40 minutes to cook, which gives you time to clean the kitchen! If you're looking for cheeses that are compatible with the Specific Carbohydrate Diet (SCD), you can use cheddar, havarti, brick cheese, Colby, Gruyère, or Swiss. (Check out Chapter 3 for more on the SCD.) Use soy creamer so that the creamer doesn't separate. And don't skip the hole-poking in the pie crust; it really does make a difference.

Preparation time: *10 minutes*

Cooking time: *40 minutes*

Yield: *6 servings*

3 egg whites, beaten with a fork	*1 cup mushrooms, cleaned and sliced*
⅔ cup chicken broth, preferably organic	*⅓ of a 10-ounce package frozen chopped spinach, thawed and drained*
¼ cup soy creamer	*¼ cup green onions (tops only), sliced thinly*
2 teaspoons fresh parsley, finely chopped	*9-inch frozen pie crust, unbaked*
½ teaspoon salt	
¼ cup Parmesan cheese	

1 Preheat the oven to 450 degrees.

2 In a bowl beat egg whites with the broth, soy creamer, parsley, and salt. Set aside.

3 Use a fork to poke holes in the bottom of the frozen pie crust. Bake the crust for 5 minutes and take it out of the oven.

4 Spread the spinach over the bottom of the crust and then sprinkle the green onions and mushrooms over the spinach. Pour the egg mixture over the spinach, onions, and mushrooms and sprinkle the Parmesan on top.

5 Bake for 10 minutes and then lower the heat to 325 and bake for 25 minutes more. It's done when you can stick a knife in the middle and it doesn't come out with raw egg on it.

Tip: *Clean your mushrooms by brushing them rather than washing them. Although you may be inclined to wash a fungus that grows in cool, dark, moist soil, chefs insist that washing mushrooms makes them mushy. You can buy a mushroom brush or cheat and buy a cheap, soft toothbrush; brush all the junk off them and cut the bottom bit off, and you're good to go.*

Per serving: *Calories 162; Fat 9.6 g (Saturated 3 g); Cholesterol 4 mg; Sodium 635 mg; Carbohydrate 13.1 g (Fiber 1.1 g); Protein 6.6 g; Sugar 3.2 g.*

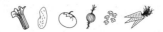

⟳ *Nori Rolls*

Chef and nutritionist Shannon Leone at www.rawmom.com provided this recipe. If you're in a rush, you can substitute avocado for the nut pâté. The nut pâté, nori, and zucchini are all IBS-friendly because of their soluble-fiber content. If you're worried about digesting the carrots, either eliminate them or shred them with a vegetable peeler. The same goes for green onions — cut them extra fine if you tend to have problems stomaching them.

Preparation time: *45 minutes*

Yield: *8 servings*

4 sheets nori

1 cup Basic Nut or Seed Pâté (see the recipe later in this chapter), or 1 cup Shannon's Quick Rice (see the recipe in Chapter 12)

1 carrot, julienned or grated

1 zucchini or cucumber, julienned

1 green onion, chopped

½ a green apple or pineapple, sliced thinly and julienned

1 Lay out one sheet of the nori at a time on a cutting board. Spread the nut pâté on the nori sheet and then place vegetables and fruit lengthwise on top of the pâté.

2 Roll the sheet into a cylinder and seal it with a wet finger. Let it stand for 30 minutes and then slice it into 6 pieces. Repeat Steps 1 and 2 for the rest of the nori sheets.

Per serving: Calories 85; Fat 5.4 g (Saturated 0.6 g); Cholesterol 0 mg; Sodium 156 mg; Carbohydrate 6.6 g (Fiber 2.7 g); Protein 3.1 g; Sugar 2.5 g.

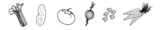

Dipping for Chips

Dips are great snack treats if you have IBS. The fact that they're in paste form means the insoluble fiber is easier to digest because it's already been broken down. With seed and nut butters, the nasty sharp bits of the nuts and seeds are ground down so that they're friendlier to sensitive stomachs.

You can try any assortment of chips available in your grocery store or health food store as edible scoops. You can also dip with cut up vegetables, or slather the goodness on pieces of flat bread or *sprouted bread* (bread made from whole grains that have sprouted or germinated).

Note that some of these dip recipes contain somewhat involved processes or unusual ingredients you may not be familiar with. We encourage you to make the leap and wander down those uncharted aisles of the grocery store — you never know what other treasures you may find.

☙ *Mango Salsa*

Raman Prasad created this cool and delicious SCD mango salsa for his book *Recipes for the Specific Carbohydrate Diet*™ (Fair Winds Press); check him out at `www.scdrecipe.com/cookbook`, and find a photo of the salsa in this book's color section. The serrano chili is optional in this dish, and leaving it out makes the salsa IBS-friendly, especially if eaten with a soluble side like quinoa or organic baked corn chips. Raman also suggests partnering it with the Herbed Tilapia with Lime in Chapter 11.

The raw onions and peppers in this dish may be setting off your IBS alarm, and if these foods have been a problem for you in the past, you're right to shy away. But if these ingredients don't specifically trigger you, consider the following: This recipe was created by a young gentleman who suffered ulcerative colitis from age 17 until he found his cure in the SCD, which allows vegetables and some spices while outlawing grains, lactose, and sucrose. If your IBS is triggered by lactose, sucrose, or grains, vegetables may not be such a problem for you, and this salsa may help you find health, not hurt.

Preparation time: *10 minutes*

Cooking time: *None*

Yield: *6 servings*

2 ripe mangoes, peeled and diced	½ yellow pepper, finely chopped
1 serrano chili, finely chopped (optional)	1 cup fresh cilantro, finely chopped
2 green onions, finely chopped	Juice of 1 lime (about 2 tablespoons), or to taste
½ red pepper, finely chopped	

1 Mix the mango pieces with the chopped chili, green onions, red and yellow bell peppers, cilantro, and lime juice in a bowl to serve as a dip or as an accompaniment to guacamole.

Tip: You also can serve Mango Salsa as a side with any of our chicken, turkey, or fish main dishes in Chapter 11 (except maybe curried shrimp). We pair it with Coconut Panko Shrimp in the color insert.

Per serving: Calories 59; Fat 0.3 g (Saturated 0.05 g); Cholesterol 0 mg; Sodium 4 mg; Carbohydrate 14.9 g (Fiber 1.9 g); Protein 0.9 g; Sugar 11.3 g.

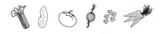

☺ Celery Root Tahini Dip

You can eat this dip on its own or with vegetables and/or crackers. *Herbs de Provence* is just a fancy name for a blend of herbs like savory, fennel, basil, thyme, and lavender. *Tahini* is a paste made of ground sesame seeds. Julie Beyer has modified many recipes such as this one to accommodate her own food sensitivities and teaches people to cook their own special, healthy meals using organic ingredients.

Tools: *Potato masher (optional)*

Preparation Time: *20 minutes*

Cooking Time: *12 minutes*

Yield: *4 servings*

1 medium celery root, skinned and chopped (about 2 cups)	*1½ teaspoons of Herbs de Provence mixture or rosemary*
2 tablespoons of olive oil or coconut oil	*2 tablespoons tahini*
½ an onion	*Juice of ½ a lemon (about ⅛ cup)*
1 to 2 cloves garlic	*⅛ teaspoon each sea salt and pepper, or to taste*
1 teaspoon turmeric	
½ to 1 teaspoon sea salt	

1 Boil the celery root for about 5 minutes or until tender and then drain it and place it in a bowl.

2 Fry the onions and garlic in the oil and then add the celery root, turmeric, sea salt, and herbs. Stir until the celery root is lightly browned.

3 Add the tahini and lemon juice. You can eat the mixture as-is at this point, mash it with a potato masher, or process it in a blender.

4 Add sea salt and pepper to taste.

Vary It! *If you don't have celery root, you can try celery as the base of this dip, although it doesn't give as rich a taste.*

Per serving: *Calories 149; Fat 11.1 g (Saturated 1.6 g); Cholesterol 0 mg; Sodium 596 mg; Carbohydrate 11.4 g (Fiber 2.6 g); Protein 2.7 g; Sugar 2 g.*

Solving the solubility problem with pea powder

Grinding nuts and seeds helps their insoluble fiber become much more digestible. However, if you still find powdered nuts and seeds slightly irritating, we have a solution for you. We both use a protein powder consisting of pea powder, whole eggs, and apple flakes, and our tummies love it. We suggest adding soluble-fiber pea powder in nut- and seed-based recipes to increase the soluble fiber content and help neutralize any possibility of irritation. One to two ounces of pea powder in a recipe can usually balance one to two cups of ground nuts or seeds.

☞ *Basic Nut or Seed Pâté*

Every Raw food chef has his favorite nut pâté, but all the recipes begin with the basic five ingredients: nuts or seeds, lemon juice, garlic, salt, and water. Juliano's Nut Cheeze is our inspiration for this nut pâté. His recipe boasts about 10 ingredients and takes a few minutes longer to prepare, but this recipe couldn't be any simpler, and it's all you need.

Twelve servings may seem like a lot, but the serving size is 2 tablespoons. It's so rich and concentrated that that's the perfect amount for a wrap or a salad dressing. For wraps, make the pâté a thicker consistency like peanut butter; for sauces (such as to pour over pasta), make it a thinner consistency. This recipe will keep in the fridge for several days because the garlic is a natural preservative.

Preparation time: *5 minutes*

Cooking time: *None*

Yield: *Twenty-four 2-tablespoon servings (3 cups total)*

2 cups of seeds or nuts (such as sunflower seeds, pumpkin seeds, almonds, macadamia nuts, or cashews)

Juice of 3 lemons (about ¾ cup)

¼ cup of water

1 heaping teaspoon of sea salt

4 cloves garlic

1 Grind the nuts or seeds in a coffee grinder or high-speed blender. If you use a coffee grinder, we recommend grinding ¼ cup at a time. Set aside the powdered mixture in a bowl.

2 Blend the lemon juice, water, salt, and garlic in a blender or food processor.

3 Add the powdered mixture to the lemon juice mixture and blend. To create the desired consistency, you may have to add another few tablespoons of water and lemon juice.

Vary It! To change the color, taste, and texture of the pâté, you can add ½ cup finely chopped or food-processed onion, or 1 teaspoon turmeric, or 1 teaspoon of powdered ginger, or ¼ cup of finely chopped fresh basil.

Tip: Add pea powder to increase the soluble fiber content. Add 1 ounce of powder and an extra ounce of water per cup of seeds. (See the nearby sidebar "Solving the solubility problem with pea powder" for more on using pea powder for digestibility.)

Tip: Take 2 ounces of the nut pâté and add 1 ounce of lemon juice and 1 ounce of water to create a wonderful mayonnaise or the basis of a Caesar-like salad dressing!

Per serving: Calories 130; Fat 10.6 g (Saturated 1.1 g); Cholesterol 0 mg; Sodium 291 mg; Carbohydrate 6.8 g (Fiber 2.5 g); Protein 4.2 g; Sugar 1 g.

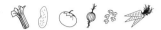

Featuring Fish

High in protein and rich in essential fatty acids, fish is a fabulous snack food and good for your brain too! Try smoked wild salmon (or any smoked fish) on a thin slice of sprouted manna bread brushed with stone ground mustard, with a side of avocado. It's a snack that takes seconds to prepare.

Every chemical and heavy metal used in the world end up in the ocean and become food for fish, and many people have justifiable concerns about some kinds of fish having high levels of mercury. Keep large game fish such as tuna, swordfish, and marlin off your snack list. For safer snacking, look to mid-sized deep-ocean fish such as cod or small tuna and smaller to mid-sized fish like tilapia, trout, and striped bass. The best fish by far is wild Alaska salmon.

Online sources of wild Alaska salmon and mercury-free or low mercury tuna are www.vitalchoice.com and www.vitacost.com/WildPlanet.

Tuna Cakes

Michelle Gay (www.eatingjourney.wordpress.com) provided us with this tasty high-protein snack that just takes moments to prepare. For this recipe, make sure you use a white albacore tuna that has been troll caught. No, we don't mean snagged by weird-looking gnomes with fishing poles. *Trolling lines* catch smaller tuna, protect dolphins, and allow fishermen to determine the size of the fish they keep. Because the level of mercury in fish is determined by the size of the fish, you want to eat the smallest fish you can. But don't go as far as eating tiny shrimp-like krill — leave those for the whales! These lovely cakes are featured in the color section.

Preparation time: *3 minutes*

Cooking time: *3 minutes*

Yield: *1 serving*

One 5-ounce can of tuna, drained

2 to 3 tablespoons almond meal

1 egg

⅛ teaspoon each salt and pepper, or to taste

1 to 2 teaspoons of olive oil, sunflower oil, or safflower oil, or ghee (see the recipe in Chapter 6)

1 In a small bowl, mix together the tuna, almond meal, egg, salt, and pepper. Set aside.

2 Heat the oil or ghee in frying pan over high heat.

3 Work the tuna mix into little cakes and drop them into the frying pan. Cook on one side for 3 to 4 minutes and then flip over and cook for 3 minutes or until crispy brown.

Tip: Believe it or not, pesto is a great addition to this tuna treat. You can find a recipe for Pesto without the Pain in Chapter 11.

Per serving: Calories 396; Fat 23.6 g (Saturated 3.1 g); Cholesterol 275 mg; Sodium 986 mg; Carbohydrate 5.4 g (Fiber 2.6 g); Protein 43.8 g; Sugar 0.4 g.

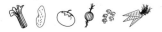

Tuna Salad, Hold the Mayo

Tuna salad is an old standard that many people with IBS miss because they can't find a replacement for the mayo. Our Down Under contributor Michelle Gay (www.eating journey.wordpress.com) found a way to make this a friendly, high-protein snack.

Preparation time: *5 minutes*

Cooking time: *8 minutes*

Yield: *1 serving*

1 hardboiled egg, diced small

¼ of an avocado

2 to 3 tablespoons of Kendall's SCD Dairy Yogurt (see the recipe in Chapter 6), or any plain yogurt

1 teaspoon curry powder (optional)

One 5-ounce can of tuna in water, drained

⅛ teaspoon each salt and pepper, or to taste

1 Place the egg and avocado in a small bowl. Add the yogurt; you may only need 2 tablespoons if your yogurt of choice isn't very thick. Add the curry powder (if desired).

2 Add the tuna, salt, and pepper and mash all together.

Vary It! *Add celery, onions, different seasonings, or apples to jazz up this tuna salad even more.*

Vary It! *Instead of yogurt, you can use our Basic Seed or Nut Pâté (see the recipe earlier in this chapter). You may have to dilute it with more water and lemon juice first to make it the right consistency.*

Per serving: *Calories 377; Fat 15.5 g (Saturated 3.9 g); Cholesterol 268 mg; Sodium 932 mg; Carbohydrate 7.8 g (Fiber 4.2 g); Protein 50.9 g; Sugar 2.6 g.*

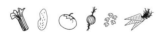

Sardine Spread

Contributing chef Caroline Nation (founder of www.myfoodmyhealth.com) recommends serving this snack on pumpernickel bread, but you may also want to try it on sprouted bread if you avoid wheat. Sardines are a good source of calcium and vitamin D, as well as omega-3 fatty acids, which are known to help reduce levels of inflammation.

Preparation time: *2 minutes*

Cooking time: *None*

Yield: *2 servings*

One 3.75-ounce tin sardines	½ teaspoon fresh lemon juice
1 teaspoon Dijon mustard	2 pieces bread of your choice
2 tablespoons finely chopped red onion	

1 Drain the sardines. In a bowl, mash the sardines and the mustard with a fork. Add the onion and lemon juice and stir to combine.

2 Spread generously on the bread to make two open-faced sandwiches.

Per serving: *Calories 102; Fat 5.4 g (Saturated 0.7 g); Cholesterol 66mg; Sodium 262 mg; Carbohydrate 1.2 g (Fiber 0.3 g); Protein 11.6 g; Sugar 0.5 g.*

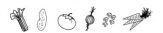

Chapter 8

Drinks for Any Time of Day or Night

In This Chapter

▶ Enjoying stomach-soothing smoothies any time of day

▶ Turning to homemade juice for some essential nutrients

▶ Going nuts for milk substitutes

▶ Checking out teas and coffees that go easy on your tummy

You've probably been told that coffee, strong tea, sodas, and alcohol aren't so great for IBS, but they aren't the only drinks in the world (although advertising can certainly make you think that). Perhaps you feel that water is your only safe liquid of choice. Au contraire! As this chapter shows, you have a wide variety of drink options to enjoy that won't set off your IBS. In fact, some of our drinks can even be called medicinal because of their healthy and healing ingredients.

Where's the Fiber?

Most of the chapters in this part give you tips on working soluble fiber into your recipes, but that's not the case here. In fact, in most of the recipes that follow, you remove all the fiber in the process of juicing or making nut milks. Even the teas are strained so that no particles of solid substance touch your tummy — just liquid. Fiber aside, though, you can use a high-speed blender to make foods more soluble — they significantly reduce food particle size, which means they shred insoluble fiber to the point of oblivion. See the nearby sidebar "The power of high-speed blending" for more on these handy machines.

The power of high-speed blending

Want to get rid of that irritating insoluble fiber as you fix your drinks? Invest in a high-speed blender. In 2008, researchers at the University of Toronto studied what happens to food when processed in a high-speed blender. They wanted to determine whether the blending process can enhance nutrient intake from whole foods. They tested high-speed blenders (specifically the Vita-Mix 5200) and found that the blenders are able to break down plant cell walls, reducing particle size and potentially increasing how quickly essential nutrients in vegetables and fruits end up in the bloodstream. You can see the microscopic details of this research at `www.vita-mix.com/household/infocenter/research.asp#`.

In terms of IBS triggers, one factor you need to watch out for in drinks is temperature. Digestion, according to Ayurvedic medicine, is the way humans cook their foods in their stomachs, absorb nutrients in their small intestines, and relieve themselves of waste through the large intestine. Starting with a warm or cool food affects how you digest it and how your intestines react to it. Flip to Chapter 3 for the skinny on the Ayurvedic *doshas* or constitutions; Vatas already have cool tendencies, so a cold drink is going to make them shiver. Pittas have more fire and sometimes needs to be cooled down, so if you have this kind of constitution, cold drinks are okay.

Soothing Your Stomach with Smoothies

A *smoothie* is defined as a blended fruit drink, but it can be so much more. A smoothie meets the needs of people who are in a rush, and in the case of IBS, it's a concentrated food source in only a few ounces.

When you consider that your stomach is only the size of your two cupped hands, you realize that you really don't need to eat too much to begin stretching the stomach, which triggers the opening of sphincters throughout the body. A few ounces of smoothie are therefore a perfect way to take in nutrients without feeling overly full.

Smoothies are also great to have any time of the day. Just make sure you sip them slowly. In fact, try chewing 'em. Swish a smoothie around in your mouth to get your salivary enzymes activated so they can help digest your smoothie before it even hits your stomach. And only drink a few ounces at a time. Then put your drink in the fridge or keep it in a thermos at work and sip it throughout the day. That way you're giving your intestines enough time to digest it and extract the goodness, ensuring you get the most nourishment possible from your smoothie.

Most people think of bananas when they hear the word *smoothie*. Bananas are high in potassium and help reduce hypertension, but you may have heard mixed stories about the benefits of bananas for the bowels. According to Carolyn's Chinese medicine teacher, unripe bananas that are still about one-third green are more lubricating for the intestines than ripe bananas and can be used to treat constipation. When they're ripe, with some brown spots forming, they can treat diarrhea. (Browning of a fruit just means the fruit is fermenting, so it's already starting to digest itself and causes less stress on a weak digestive system.)

So bananas are really like a bowel cure-all. But don't take our word for it. Try them either ripe or unripe and see how your body responds. If you've done your avoidance and challenge testing (refer to Chapter 2) and found that you can eat bananas, you're in for a smoothie treat, as the following recipes show you.

☼ Nutty Breakfast Smoothie

Michele Gay (www.eatingjourney.wordpress.com) offers this tasty and smooth way to start your day. It features the all-powerful banana as well as spinach and almond butter. We discuss the IBS benefits of bananas earlier in this section; raw spinach is high in soluble fiber when you blend it. Almond butter in its creamy state doesn't irritate the intestines.

Preparation time: *5 minutes*

Cooking time: *None*

Yield: *2 servings*

2 bananas	*1 cup water*
2 cups spinach	*1 tablespoon almond butter*

1 Cut up the bananas and spinach.

2 Put all the ingredients in a blender. Blend until smooth and enjoy.

Per serving: Calories 163; Fat 5.2 g (Saturated 1 g); Cholesterol 0 mg; Sodium 61 mg; Carbohydrate 29.7 g (Fiber 4 g); Protein 3.3 g; Sugar 14.9 g.

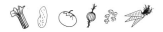

☺ Safe and Soothing Smoothie

Making a meal doesn't have to be a big deal. You don't have to turn the kitchen upside down and get out all of your pots and pans to make breakfast, but you do need breakfast. This Safe and Soothing Smoothie helps keep your blood sugar up while soothing your stomach. You can experiment with two to three of the ingredients in this recipe, and later, with the help of your food diary (outlined in Chapter 2), you can substitute different ingredients that are on your safe list.

With all the mixing and matching possibilities, you have a dozen recipes at your fingertips. We encourage you to keep it simple, though. Don't make an "everything but the kitchen sink" smoothie that can cause some intestinal distress. Stick with a few ingredients and keep a record of what your body likes and dislikes. As you experiment, you can also adjust the amount of liquid to reach your desired consistency. Check out this delicious drink in the color insert.

Tools: *High-speed blender (optional)*

Preparation time: *5 minutes*

Cooking time: *None*

Yield: *1 serving*

1 small, ripe banana

1 cup strawberries, fresh or frozen

2 tablespoons hulled hemp seeds (no soaking required)

1 to 2 tablespoons pea powder protein (such as Provide)

1 cup liquid (water, coconut juice, or half coconut juice and half coconut milk)

Natural sweetener (such as agave, stevia, or Just Like Sugar) to taste (optional)

1 Put the banana, strawberries, hemp seeds, and pea powder in a high-speed blender or a food processor. Add the liquid, making sure all the ingredients are covered, and blend well.

2 Taste the blended mixture and add sweetener to taste (if desired). Give the mixture another quick blend to incorporate any sweetener.

Tip: *Other IBS-friendly fruit includes peeled apples, apricots, peeled pears, peeled peaches, and mangoes.*

Per serving: *Calories 361; Fat 11.3 g (Saturated 1 g); Cholesterol 0 mg; Sodium 13 mg; Carbohydrate 46.7 g (Fiber 7.9 g) Protein 23 g; Sugar 22.9 g.*

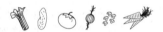

⟳ Banana and Greens Delight Smoothie

Here's another smoothie creation from Michele Gay (www.eatingjourney.wordpress.com). Like bananas, apples are a food that can swing both ways in treating IBS. Raw apples are high in pectin and fiber and can help bring fluids into the bowel and treat IBS-C. Apples in applesauce form treat IBS-D, according to the well-known BRATTY diet (bananas, rice, applesauce, toast, tea, and yogurt).

Tools: *Hand blender (optional)*

Preparation time: *5 minutes*

Cooking time: *None*

Yield: *4 servings*

1 banana, cut up	*1 pear, cored, peeled, and cut up*
2 cups baby spinach, chopped	*2 cups water*
1 apple, cored, peeled, and cut up	

1 Put all the ingredients in a blender or use a strong hand blender.

2 Blend until smooth and enjoy.

Vary It! *If you're experiencing diarrhea, use 1 cup applesauce in place of the cut-up apple.*

Per serving: *Calories 75; Fat 3 g (Saturated 0 g); Cholesterol 0 mg; Sodium 13 mg; Carbohydrate 19.3 g (Fiber 3 g); Protein 4.1 g; Sugar 12.9 g.*

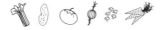

Drinking Up Your Nutrients with Juices

Everyone needs nutrition, especially people with IBS-D, who often limit themselves to white rice and white bread and can become malnourished. One of the best ways to get this nutrition is by drinking healthy juices. If you have IBS-C, juices are good for you too because they're high in antioxidants to deal with the toxins being absorbed through the large intestines along with water as you wait and wait and wait.

If you're experiencing IBS-C, prune juice and lots of water may be just what you need. Prune juice is a very gentle yet effective laxative. It contains an unpronounceable substance called *dihydrophenylisatin* (hey, we warned you it was a toughie) that's responsible for its laxative action. Water provides lubrication and bulk to help things move along and replace fluids that are continually reabsorbed through the colon.

Juices are so rich in nutrients that a couple of mouthfuls can give you a boost, especially if you chew your juice. No, don't leave chunks of juice ingredients in your drink, but *do* take a mouthful of juice and swish it around your mouth before swallowing. (You may recall that food absorption starts in your mouth, where your saliva begins to break down your food. In fact, one-third of your carbohydrate digestion process is completed in your mouth before it hits your stomach.)

Some nutritionists say that drinking juices isn't a good way to get nutrition because the contents of your glass pass too quickly through your system. We don't know if that's been studied, but Christine actually stopped drinking juices and smoothies for a while, heeding their advice, only to find that she was missing the benefits. She went back to her drinks, realizing that she felt better when she had them and really was getting nourishment from them.

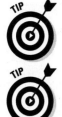

If you don't know whether you're absorbing a food or drink, just do a quick survey of the contents of your toilet bowl. You'll see the color of the juice you just drank or some bits of food that you thought you chewed and digested. If that happens, eat more slowly, chew more thoroughly, and add digestive enzymes, which we cover in Chapter 1.

Chop up your vegetables and fruits somewhat before putting them in a juicer. Doing so causes less wear and tear on your appliance.

Juicer or nut milk bag: That is the question

If you want to make your own juice at home, you have two choices for juicing: a juicer and a blender/nut milk bag combo. Just about any juicer will do the trick (unless you want a juice press where you crush out your juice and no metal blades tear up your ingredients). Nut milk bags, however, are just a bit more complex.

Nut milk bags first started as a way to strain the fiber from nuts in the making of nut milk. Then one fine day a brilliant mom decided that she could strain a vegetable drink in the very same way. All you have to do to juice the nut milk bag way is cut up some vegetables and fruits that you'd normally feed through your juicer, add a cup of water, blend thoroughly, and then pour the contents through a nut milk bag. Voilà! You have your juice.

The great part about using a nut bag versus a juicer is that you only have to rinse out the nut milk bag and not all the parts of a juicer. Cleanup is therefore a breeze!

☽ Lovely Bones Juice

Angela Elliott, author of the e-book *A Diva's Guide to Juices and Cocktails* (www.she-zencuisine.com) has found a way for you to get your calcium and magnesium in a tasty glass of juice. Apples are high in soluble fiber, ginger is a digestive aid, and lemon is good for the liver — all in all, a very IBS-friendly drink. Check out the glass of Lovely Bones Juice in the color section.

Tools: *Nut milk bag (optional)*

Preparation time: *5 minutes*

Cooking time: *None*

Yield: *2 servings*

2 apples, quartered	*Juice of ¼ of a lemon (about ¹⁄₁₆ cup)*
5 kale leaves	*1 inch ginger*
1 handful parsley (about ½ cup)	*1 celery stalk*

1 Juice all the ingredients; alternately, you can chop them up, combine them in a blender, and strain the mixture through a nut milk bag (see the nearby sidebar "Juicer or nut milk bag: That is the question" for more on this method).

2 Pour into glasses and drink up.

Per serving: Calories 125; Fat 0.7 g (Saturated 0.1 g); Cholesterol 0 mg; Sodium 42 mg; Carbohydrate 31.1 g (Fiber 5.9 g); Protein 2.2 g; Sugar 19.6 g.

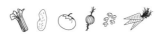

⏱ Ginger Love!

Thanks to Angela Elliott for this recipe from her e-book *A Diva's Guide to Juices and Cocktails* (www.she-zencuisine.com); it's great because we love ginger! Ginger is a true friend to people with IBS. Not only does it soothe the digestive system but it can also help alleviate the uncomfortable gas that plagues many people. Ginger has some anti-inflammatory compounds called *gingerols* that are powerful enough to work on arthritis and can soothe an inflamed colon.

Tools: *Nut milk bag (optional)*

Preparation time: *5 minutes*

Cooking time: *None*

Yield: *2 servings*

¼ inch ginger

2 apples, quartered

Juice of ½ a lemon (about ⅛ cup)

1 Run ginger and then the quartered apples through a juicer, or chop them, blend them, and strain them through a nut milk bag.

2 Mix in the lemon juice and serve.

Per serving: *Calories 101; Fat 0.3 g (Saturated 0.05 g); Cholesterol 0 mg; Sodium 3 mg; Carbohydrate 26.7 g (Fiber 4.5 g); Sodium 19.2 g; Protein 0.6 g; Sugar 16.5 g.*

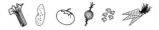

⏱ Pick Me Up

This recipe, also from Angela Elliott's *A Diva's Guide to Juices and Cocktails* (www.she-zencuisine.com), focuses on apples, which are rich in antioxidants. For people with IBS, apples are a mainstay and help with both ends of the IBS spectrum. Take them raw but peeled for IBS-C. Sauce them up into applesauce or bake them in the oven for IBS-D, again removing the peel, which has too much insoluble fiber. Cilantro gives this juice a distinct flavor that most people love. You can use just the juice of the lemons, or you can peel off the outer skin (leaving the white rind) and run the lemons through a juicer.

Tools: *Nut milk bag (optional)*

Preparation time: *5 minutes*

Cooking time: *None*

Yield: *3 servings*

1 bunch cilantro (about 12 ounces)

3 apples, cored and quartered

1 medium cucumber, cut lengthwise

8 to 10 celery stalks

Juice of 3 lemons (about ¾ cup)

1 Juice the cilantro, apple, cucumber, and celery, or chop them, blend them, and strain them through a nut milk bag.

2 Mix in the lemon juice and serve.

Vary It! *If you don't like the flavor of cilantro, try swapping out the cilantro bunch for 6 ounces of parsley or 4 to 6 ounces of mint.*

Per serving: *Calories 139; Fat 0.6 g (Saturated 0.1 g); Cholesterol 0 mg; Sodium 90 mg; Carbohydrate 36 g (Fiber 6.8 g); Protein 2.1 g; Sugar 23.7 g.*

Examining Milk Substitutes

Lactose intolerance can be absolutely intolerable. Many people have been raised on milk, that staple of meals and bedtime treats, yet your headaches, rashes, fatigue, indigestion, diarrhea, or constipation may be coming from milk. Never fear. You can easily substitute homemade nut milk (or seed milk) for store-bought milk. We share some terrific milk-replacement options for you in this section. Although store-bought milk-replacement options exist, the following homemade recipes allow you to control all the ingredients and the amount of added sugars.

Organic nuts may be more expensive, but they're free of pesticides, which is a real health bonus.

The recipes in this section (and others throughout the book) call for soaked nuts or seeds, so we've also included easy soaking instructions here.

☽ Soaking Nuts and Seeds

Soaking nuts and seeds helps remove enzyme blockers called *phytates* that block the absorption of minerals. It also begins the process of sprouting, which releases even more nutrients that are meant for the developing plant but end up in your mouth. Plus, wet nuts and seeds are easier to blend without grinding first, increasing the chances that you'll pulverize any IBS-irritating shards.

Soaking time: *At least 4 hours for seeds and 8 hours for nuts, or overnight*

Preparation time: *5 minutes*

Cooking time: *None*

Yield: *1 cup*

1 cup nuts or seeds of your choice	*Water (enough to cover nuts/seeds)*
¼ teaspoon of sea salt	

1 Rinse the nuts or seeds three times in a fine colander and set aside.

2 Combine the salt and water in a bowl or other soaking container and add the nuts/seeds. Soak seeds for at least 4 hours and nuts for at least 8 hours. Discard the soaking liquid and rinse the nuts/seeds thoroughly with fresh water.

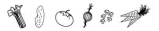

☽ Cashew Milk

This recipe from Angela Elliott's e-book, *A Diva's Guide to Juices and Cocktails,* is a simple twist on our Essential Nut Milk recipe (presented later in this chapter). Thick and creamy cashew milk is as rich as whole milk. Like the other nut milks, it removes all nut fiber and provides no dairy irritants like lactose and casein, so it's very IBS-friendly.

Tools: *Nut milk bag*

Preparation time: *5 minutes*

Cooking time: *None*

Yield: *3 servings*

1 cup raw cashews, soaked (see Soaking Nuts and Seeds earlier in this chapter)	*10 honey dates, soaked for 1 hour*
	2 cups water

1 Combine the cashews and honey dates in a blender with 1 cup of the water and blend on high until a thick cream forms. Slowly add the rest of the water and blend on high for 2 minutes.

2 Strain the mixture through a nut milk bag and collect the milk in a bowl.

Per serving: Calories 428; Fat 16.1 g (Saturated 2.7 g); Cholesterol 0 mg; Sodium 5 mg; Carbohydrate 72 g (Fiber 6.7 g); Protein 8.1 g; Sugar 55.8 g.

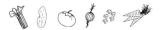

☾ Silky Chai Nut Milk

If you're feeling ill and need nutrients, this milk from Shannon Leone (www.rawmom.com) can be a great, soothing drink. Although raw nuts can be difficult to digest, you can enjoy them quite safely in milk form. *Chai* is a well-known digestive tea from India. The herbs you add make it that way. In this recipe, Shannon uses nutmeg, cinnamon, and cardamom, but you can experiment with fennel and even a touch of ginger if you want to.

Tools: *Nut milk bag*

Preparation time: *5 minutes*

Cooking time: *None*

Yield: *6 servings*

2 cups raw almonds, soaked (see Soaking Nuts and Seeds earlier in this chapter)

5 to 6 cups pure water

1 teaspoon vanilla extract

2 tablespoons raw honey or agave or 6 pitted dates (optional)

1 teaspoon nutmeg, or to taste

1½ teaspoon cinnamon, or to taste

½ teaspoon cardamom, or to taste

1 Add the soaked almonds and water to the blender and blend until the mixture is liquefied.

2 Over a large bowl, strain the mixture through a nut milk bag.

3 Pour the milk back into the blender, add the rest of the ingredients, and lightly blend to incorporate everything.

Vary It! *For a special treat, add 1 or 2 frozen or fresh ripe bananas.*

Vary It! *If you want chocolate milk, substitute 2 tablespoons raw cacao powder (if it's a food on your list, of course) for the chai spices. You can also use carob powder if chocolate isn't for you.*

Vary It! *Not an almond fan? Try making this recipe with soaked sesame seeds or pecans instead.*

Per serving: Calories 301; Fat 23.7 g (Saturated 2 g); Cholesterol 0 mg; Sodium 1 mg; Carbohydrate 16.8 g (Fiber 6.3 g); Sugar 7.9 g; Protein 10.1 g.

☺ *Essential Nut Milk*

Carolyn's work as medical director of www.yeastconnection.com and co-author of *The Yeast Connection and Women's Health* (Square One Publishers) led to including this recipe from that Web site and from *The Yeast Connection Cookbook* (Professional Books/Future Health). And we're reprinting it here because it's a simple, IBS-friendly way to substitute for dairy. Nuts don't have lactose or the dairy protein *casein,* the ingredients that typically cause adverse reactions. The nuts are safe because you're eliminating the fiber by pulverizing it. This yummy nut milk, which is featured in the color section, keeps in the refrigerator for 4 or 5 days if stored in a jar with a lid.

Tools: *Cheesecloth or cloth coffee filter*

Preparation time: *10 minutes*

Cooking time: *None*

Yield: *2 servings*

½ cup shelled raw almonds, soaked (see Soaking Nuts and Seeds earlier in this chapter)	*2 cups water*
	1 ripe banana or 1 teaspoon pure maple syrup or honey (optional)

1 Add 1 cup of the water and the banana, maple syrup, honey, or (if desired). Blend again for 1 to 2 minutes to form a smooth cream. With the blender running, add the second cup of water slowly and blend for 2 minutes.

2 Place the strainer over a large bowl and line it with cheesecloth or a cloth coffee filter. Pour the milk slowly into the strainer and allow it to filter through, using a spatula to increase the flow if desired. Pull the edges of the cheesecloth together to form something like a ball and then squeeze to extract another half cup of nut milk.

Vary It! *You can use several other nuts and seeds, including macadamia nuts, sesame seeds, sunflower seeds, pecans, walnuts, Brazil nuts, or cashews to make this recipe. If using seeds, be sure to soak them before grinding them in your blender.*

Tip: *If you don't want flecks of brown in your nut milk, you can blanch the almonds by placing them in 1 cup boiling water. Let them stand until the water has cooled slightly and then peel off the nut skins. Be sure to dry the nuts before grinding them.*

Tip: *If you're using a high-speed blender, you don't have to grind your nuts and seeds first. Just cover them with 1 cup water and blend them into a paste. Then add the second cup of water to liquefy.*

Per serving: Calories 210; Fat 17.7 g (Saturated 1.3 g); Cholesterol 0 mg; Sodium 0.5 mg; Carbohydrate 8.9 g (Fiber 4.4 g); Protein 7.6 g; Sugar 2.4 g.

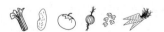

Tasting Tea and Coffee that Won't Upset Your Tummy

Tea and coffee may be the bad guys on some level, but you can still have decaffeinated green tea, lots of herbal teas, and grain/herbal coffee. So wipe that pout from your lips and wrap them around a good cup o' joe (or tea)!

Getting more than taste from tea

We grew up in a tea-drinking household, so the soothing comfort of tea is no secret to us. That's what many folks with IBS love about tea: its ability to soothe certain symptoms. Whether you use loose leaves or teabags, you can just add hot water for a taste of comfort.

Laxative herbs have a mixed reputation. Using senna tea alone can have an irritating effect on the intestines and cause cramping as it forces stool through the intestines. Cascara can be even more forceful in its action.

Gentler teas include Yogi Tea's Get Regular tea, which is mostly organic and made up of 16 herbs (840 milligrams of senna and 1,160 milligrams of the 15 other herbs). Senna contains *anthraquinone* compounds that stimulate the intestines, promoting them to expel their contents. The formula is balanced with warming, gas-reducing ingredients such as anise, cardamom, and ginger that can help alleviate gas and reduce any harsh effects of senna. The Get Regular tea also features peppermint to help speed digestion; licorice to soothe and coat the bowels, allowing for easier bowel movements; Triphala, a blend of three herbal berries (amla, bibhitaki, and haritaki), to tone and rejuvenate the eliminative functions; and yellow dock and dandelion to help the liver release more bile, assisting in promoting bowel movement through your system. Other herbal ingredients include black pepper, clove bud, celery seed, coriander seed, and stevia.

Traditional Medicinals' Organic Smooth Move is made up of eight herbs (1,080 milligrams of senna and 920 milligrams of the other seven herbs). Similar ingredients are senna, licorice root, sweet orange peel, and ginger. Smooth Move also uses bitter fennel fruit, cinnamon bark, and coriander fruit.

We like the fact that both of these teas are essentially organic. Get Regular is probably more favored because it has less senna and more healing herbs. However, people with IBS may not do so well with so many different herbs. So, once again, you must experiment to see how products react in your body.

Herbs for the teapot

Herbs are age-old healers and helpers for all sorts of ills, including the gut variety. When foods make you feel worse, brew up some of these herbs and maybe grab a hot water bottle to sit and soothe your tummy.

✔ Peppermint is most known for its ability to soothe intestinal spasms and cramps.

✔ Ginger is an anti-inflammatory that also treats nausea.

✔ Chamomile creates a general calming tea for the nerves and the intestines.

✔ Fennel is an antispasmodic that can relieve gas and bloating.

❁ A Fine Pot of Tea

Tea made the old fashioned way — the way our mother loved it — involves warming a teapot with a swish of boiling water and using a tea ball filled with loose leaves. We suggest you boil the water the old-fashioned way too — in a kettle or a pot on the stove. Don't settle for microwaved water or water poured through a coffee maker. Boiling water really lets the tea flavor fly and releases the tea's healing abilities. This herb tea has no irritants and is actually medicinal, making it perfect for IBS. Pick your favorite soothing herb, dried or fresh, and get ready to enjoy it. (See the nearby "Herbs for the teapot" sidebar for ideas and info on the medicinal properties of some common herbs.)

Tools: *Teapot, tea strainer*

Preparation time: *2 minutes*

Brewing time: *10 minutes*

Yield: *4 servings*

4 teaspoons dried peppermint, or 12 teaspoons fresh peppermint

4 cups hot water

1 teaspoon honey, or to taste

1 Warm up a teapot and add your desired herbs.

2 Pour the water into the pot. Cover the opening immediately so steam won't escape, taking the flavor and healing with it.

3 Steep the herbs for 10 minutes and strain the tea through a fine-meshed tea strainer into a cup. Add the honey to taste.

Per serving: *Calories 24; Fat 0.04 g (Saturated 0 g); Cholesterol 0 mg; Sodium 1 mg; Carbohydrate 6.3 g (Fiber 3 g); Protein 0.2 g; Sugar 5.7 g.*

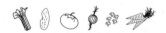

Catching up with coffee

Unfortunately for coffee lovers, the coffee bean itself, not just the caffeine, is what aggravates IBS-D — both irritate the gastrointestinal tract. That means switching to decaf coffee is not likely to help your IBS-D, so finding a hot drink alternative is the best idea. This section discusses a few coffee substitutes you may want to try; if you're not tied to that coffee feeling, check out the preceding section on tea for more hot beverage options.

Coffee substitutes have come a long way from Postum and roasted chicory, which used to be the only choices. Nowadays Nestlé makes a product called Caro made of roasted barley, malted barley, chicory, and rye. (**Note:** The barley and rye make it a gluten product.)

The newest coffee substitute is a product with the unlikely name Teeccino. It's ground and ready to brew, just like coffee, and according to reviews on the subject, it *tastes* just like coffee too. Teeccino comes in both regular and organic lines in single-serving pouches, 8.5-ounce cans, and 5-pound bags. Its ingredients include barley, so it's not gluten free. It also contains roasted carob, chicory root, figs, dates, and almonds. The organic Maya line adds roasted ramon nuts from Guatemala to the mix. Teeccino comes in a range of flavors: Original, Mocha, Almond Amaretto, Vanilla Nut, Hazelnut, Chocolate Mint, Java, Maya Chai, Maya Caffe, and Maya Mocha. Our first choice for IBS sufferers is the Maya Chai with its cinnamon, cloves, and ginger.

If regular coffee is on your list of safe beverages, but you're missing the creaminess of adding milk or cream because those aren't friendly foods for you, try adding nut milk. Christine was surprised by how tasty adding almond milk to her coffee turned out to be. You can even kick things up a notch and heat the nut milk to make yourself a latte that rivals the sugary syrup-flavored version you can get at the local coffee shop. To make your own nut milk, head to the earlier "Examining Milk Substitutes" section to peruse the recipes there.

Enjoying a Lively Lemonade

Water, lemons, and sugar are the traditional ingredients for lemonade, but we have a sweet twist for you. Lemon in the morning is a common pick-me-up for a lot of people, and it also should be one for those with IBS. It clears the palate, wakes up the brain with its pungency, and stimulates the liver just enough to get your bile flowing and jumpstart its detoxification pathways — all great things for someone with IBS.

Lemonade

Everyone needs water, and taking it in the form of lemonade makes it much more fun. Lemons are astringent, which means they help detoxify the body and although they may taste acidic, they turn alkaline and help neutralize toxins in the body.

According to its manufacturer, Just Like Sugar looks like sugar, tastes like sugar, cooks like sugar, bakes like sugar and dissolves instantly in any type of drink, hot or cold. It's made of chicory root with some added vitamin C and calcium; it's not sugar, so it doesn't elevate your blood sugar or stimulate the growth of intestinal yeast or bacteria. However, the chicory in Just Like Sugar may be irritating to some stomachs. The other natural sweetener we recommend is *stevia.* You can find so many forms and brands of stevia that you may have to experiment before you find one you really like. Because stevia is 200 times sweeter than sugar, you can use far less of it in a recipe than you would sugar or Just Like Sugar. But with either one, you have to be the judge.

Preparation time: *15 minutes*

Cooking time: *None*

Yield: *6 servings*

Juice of 6 lemons (about 1½ cups)

6 cups cold water

1 cup Just Like Sugar, or ½ to 1 teaspoon stevia

1 In a large pitcher, mix the lemon juice, water, and Just Like Sugar or stevia.

2 Stir lemonade well and serve over ice, with a lemon slice or two to garnish.

Vary It: *Use 10 to 12 limes in place of the lemons to make limeade.*

Per serving: *Calories 6; Fat 0 g (Saturated 0 g); Cholesterol 0 mg; Sodium 0.3 mg; Carbohydrate 3.5 g (Fiber 0.2 g); Protein 0.2 g; Sugar 1 g.*

Chapter 9

Settling Your Stomach with Stellar Soups

Soups are so much more than an appetizer. They're comfort foods that can be a meal in themselves. A hot soup on a cold day can warm you both physically and emotionally, and a cold soup on a blazing hot day can cool you down instantly. Soups are also a good cause for cleaning out your fridge, because you can put all of your leftovers and slightly wilted vegetables in a pot and cook them up into something tasty.

You may not necessarily want to cook and eat a hearty entrée for lunch and supper, so soups make the perfect light meal. Soup is especially convenient if you cook lots of it and freeze it in zippered freezer bags, BPA-free plastic containers, or freezer-safe mason jars. Just sit the frozen soup container on the counter when you leave for work, and it'll be ready to heat up in a few minutes when you get home all tired and hungry. Preparing foods like this ahead of time prevents the inevitable snacking on foods that don't sit well in your tummy.

Many soups are great sources of protein, vegetables, and soluble fiber all in one pot. The fact that you're cooking and simmering your soup for a long time means that you're making your vegetables even friendlier to digestion. Remember that the longer you cook your soup, the less soup you end up with, but what good is having a lot of soup if you can't digest it easily?

Bisphenol-A (BPA) is a chemical used in the manufacture of plastic. It's a hormone disruptor and therefore poses a potential danger to your health.

Finding Soluble Fiber in Soup

Cooking soups helps break down plant cell walls, eliminating some of the insoluble fiber and making soups IBS-friendlier. You can pump up the digestibility factor by adding a soluble side of safe bread.

The more soluble foods you eat at a meal, the more likely your gut will behave.

Most of the soup recipes in this chapter focus on lentils, as well as vegetables that are high in soluble fiber (think beets, carrots, mushrooms, parsnips, potatoes, rutabagas, squash, sweet potatoes, turnips, and yams). But soups are also the type of food that you want to sop up with some safe grain products. Your soluble grain choices include brown rice cereal, oatmeal, cornmeal or polenta, barley, quinoa, sourdough bread, *sprouted bread* (bread made from whole grains that have sprouted or germinated), and pita or flax bread.

Taking Stock

Broths (also known as stocks) are an essential staple to have on hand. Like juices, stocks provide great nutrition in just a few sips. They're the basis for building many other soups, but they can be satisfying all alone. Stocks are basically well-flavored liquid with no other ingredients, so they're especially handy if you have an IBS flare-up. Because you control the ingredients, homemade stocks are better than the store-bought varieties that often sneak in MSG, hydrolyzed yeast, and artificial colorings and flavorings. Be sure to keep some in your freezer at all times.

Chicken Stock

Chef and author Victoria Amory at `www.victoriaamory.com` suggests saving cooked chicken carcasses in plastic bags in your freezer and making this broth after you've collected two or three of 'em. Just make sure they have some meat left on them and include drippings if you want a good chicken flavor. You can use any vegetables that are on your food list, except for broccoli and potatoes because they'll make the broth cloudy, and broccoli can overwhelm the flavor. Chicken broth is the official meal for people starting off on the Specific Carbohydrate Diet (SCD). According to the SCD, chicken broth is almost guaranteed to soothe your gut and begin the healing process. You can store the stock in the fridge for up to 2 days, or in the freezer for up to 2 months. We suggest making several batches at a time and freezing containers of 1 or 2 cups each for future use.

Preparation time: *15 minutes*

Cooking time: *3 hours*

Yield: *Eight 1-cup servings*

2 onions, skin on, roughly chopped

1 leek, cleaned and sliced

1 turnip, peeled and roughly chopped

4 carrots, chopped

4 stalks celery, chopped

2 cooked chicken carcasses

1 sprig marjoram

1 sprig thyme

1 sprig rosemary

4 fresh bay leaves

10 peppercorns

Cold water (enough to cover the bones — about 10 cups)

1 Put all the ingredients in a large pot and add enough water to cover the chicken bones.

2 Bring the mixture to a boil. Reduce the heat and simmer over low heat for 2 to 3 hours, adding more water if the water level falls below the bones. While the stock simmers, use a spoon to remove the foam that collects on the surface.

3 Strain the stock once through a sieve. Then strain the stock a second time through a finer mesh sieve, kitchen towel, or muslin cloth.

4 Pour the stock into containers to cool, removing the fat that rises to the top.

Vary It! *If black peppercorns are one of your trigger foods, leave them out or substitute white peppercorns, which are less harsh on the intestines.*

Per serving: *Calories 106; Fat 2.1 g (Saturated 0.8 g); Cholesterol 16 mg; Sodium 81 mg; Carbohydrate 20.7 g (Fiber 2.1 g); Protein 1.8 g; Sugar 12.2 g.*

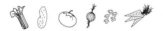

Beef Stock

The bones from ham, veal, and beef are the key to making this stock, which also comes from chef Victoria Amory (www.victoriaamory.com). You can mix them all for a rich and flavorful broth that's good for making soups and sauces that won't irritate your gut and avoids all the additives and ingredients from commercially made broths. As with the chicken stock (see the preceding recipe), any vegetables except for broccoli and potato will lend this stock a fine flavor. You can add more water during the cooking process as the stock evaporates so that you end up with 8 cups in the end.

Preparation time: *15 minutes*

Cooking time: *3 hours*

Yield: *Eight 1-cup servings*

2 onions, skin on, roughly chopped	2 tablespoons tomato paste
1 leek, washed and chopped	4 cloves garlic, peeled
1 turnip, peeled and chopped	8 stems parsley
4 carrots, peeled and chopped	8 black peppercorns
1 cup mushroom stems, chopped	Cold water (enough to cover the bones — about 10 to 12 cups)
4 stalks celery, chopped	
1-pound mix of veal, beef, or pork bones	

1 Put all the ingredients in a large pot and add enough water to cover the bones. Bring to a boil, reduce the heat, and simmer over low heat for 2 to 3 hours, adding more water if the water level falls below the bones. While the stock simmers, remove the foam that collects on the surface with a spoon.

2 Strain the stock once through a sieve. Strain it a second time through a finer mesh sieve, kitchen towel, or muslin cloth.

3 Pour the soup into containers to cool, removing any fat that rises to the top and then covering and storing them.

Tip: *Throw in the skins of the onions to give the broth a wonderful golden color.*

Vary It! *You can use white peppercorns if black peppercorns are a trigger for you, or leave the peppercorns out altogether.*

Per serving: *Calories 124; Fat 9 g (Saturated 2.4 g); Cholesterol 37 mg; Sodium 255 mg; Carbohydrate 10.3 g (Fiber 2.4 g); Protein 11.6 g; Sugar 4.7 g.*

Shellfish Stock

Victory Amory at www.victoriaamory.com suggests saving the heads of shrimp or lobsters in the freezer until you collect enough to make this tasty stock (that'd be about 24 shrimp heads or 4 lobster heads and carcasses as well). A broth without any solid ingredients is an IBS-safe meal and can also be the base of a great fish soup. You can whip up this stock in less than 30 minutes; refrigerate it for up to 2 days or freeze it for up to a month.

Preparation time: *5 minutes*

Cooking time: *20 minutes*

Yield: *Eight 1-cup servings*

2 pounds mixed seafood shells, such as shrimp and lobster

1 onion, peel on, quartered

10 whole black peppercorns

1 lemon, halved

1 bay leaf

Cold water (enough to cover the ingredients by at least 1 inch — at least 10 cups)

1 In a large stockpot, combine the shrimp and or lobster shells, onion, black peppercorns, lemon, and bay leaf. Cover the ingredients by at least 1 inch with cold water and bring everything to a boil.

2 Reduce the heat to low and simmer for about 20 minutes. Strain the stock through a fine mesh strainer or tea towel. Pour the stock into 1 cup containers to cool and then cover and store them.

Vary It! *If black peppercorns are one of your trigger foods, leave them out or substitute white peppercorns — they aren't as harsh on the intestines.*

Per serving: *Calories 78; Fat 0.03 g (Saturated 0 g); Cholesterol 18 mg; Sodium 81 mg; Carbohydrate 2 g (Fiber 0.4 g); Protein 17.2 g; Sugar 0.8 g.*

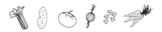

☉ Vegetable Stock

We can't think of a better way to use up the vegetables inevitably lurking in the crisper than this yummy vegetable stock! This recipe, provided by chef Victoria Amory (www.victoriaamory.com), is another staple that can be a flavorful base for soups and sauces. As with the three other stocks in this chapter, it can be a meal in itself if your IBS is acting up because it's devoid of solids and contains no synthetic flavorings or colorings. Asparagus ends, broccoli stems, cauliflowers, carrots, pea shells, and mushroom stems all make a sensational broth. You can also use leeks, scallions, turnips, and artichokes. Refrain from using potatoes and broccoli florets though, because they'll cloud the broth and give too strong a broccoli taste. Even the stems that we list below may be too much for some. You can store this stock in the fridge for 2 days or freeze it for up to 6 months.

Preparation time: *15 minutes*

Cooking time: *60 minutes*

Yield: *Eight 1-cup servings*

⅔ pound each chopped mushrooms, chopped asparagus, and chopped broccoli stems

1 onion

10 black peppercorns

1 bay leaf

Cold water (enough to cover the vegetables — about 10 cups)

1 In a large stockpot, combine the vegetables, onion, and black peppercorns. Fill the pot with cold water to cover the veggies and bring it all to a boil. Add the bay leaf. Reduce the heat and simmer for about 50 minutes.

2 Strain through a fine mesh sieve, kitchen towel, or muslin cloth. Pour into containers to cool, removing any fat that rises to the top.

Vary It! *You can substitute white peppercorns if black peppercorns are one of your trigger foods, or leave the peppercorns out completely.*

Per serving: *Calories 2; Fat 0.1 g (Saturated 0.03 g); Cholesterol 0.2 mg; Sodium 6 g; Carbohydrate 1.8g (Fiber 0.2 g); Protein 0.9 g; Sugar 0.3 g.*

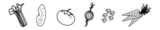

Serving Up Hot, Healthy, and Healing Soups

Hot soups, like hot drinks, are more appealing when you're chilled, during the winter, or when you don't have time to prepare a big meal. Don't get us wrong, our soups can double for a meal in themselves. They are especially welcome when you've managed to freeze some soup and cut the preparation time down to minutes.

Easily digestible soups typically have longer cooking times to help break down all the ingredients. Many of the following soups are filling; they stick to your ribs but not your intestines.

 If you like chunky soup, chop up your veggies. If you prefer a smoother soup, grate vegetables such as potatoes, beets, and carrots. And if you want a creamy soup but don't want to add the milk or cream, use a hand blender (also known as an *immersion blender*) and blend your ingredients to a creamy consistency.

Quinoa Soup with Miso

Thanks to chef Ela Guidon (`www.myfoodmyhealth.com/OurChefs/index.php?chefid=17`) for reminding us of the many uses of quinoa and providing this dairy-free recipe. Perfect any time, this delicious integration of miso and quinoa is a great use for any leftover quinoa from last night's gluten-free dinner. Quinoa is high in soluble fiber, making it a suitable grain for IBS. Miso is a fermented soybean; the fermentation process actually predigests the miso to some extent, so your gut has to do less work.

Preparation time: *5 minutes*

Cooking time: *30 minutes*

Yield: *Four 1-cup servings*

2 tablespoons olive oil

½ cup diced onion

2 garlic cloves, finely diced

2 carrots, sliced and cut in half moons

2 celery stalks, sliced

2 medium red potatoes, cut in quarter moons with skin

1 zucchini, cut in quarter moons

1 teaspoon salt

3 cups chicken stock

2 cups water

1 cup cooked quinoa

½ teaspoon dry basil

¼ teaspoon dry oregano

3 tablespoons white miso paste

1 In a medium-sized pot, heat the olive oil and sauté the onion until it's translucent. Add the garlic, carrots, and celery and cook all that together for 5 minutes.

2 Add the potatoes, zucchini, salt, chicken stock, and water. Bring everything to a boil and then simmer for 15 minutes. Meanwhile, cook the quinoa per package directions.

3 Add the cooked quinoa, basil, and oregano to the medium-sized pot and simmer for 5 minutes. Turn off the heat. Add the white miso paste and stir until dissolved.

Per serving: *Calories 301; Fat 10.6 g (Saturated 1.7 g); Cholesterol 6 mg; Sodium 1122 mg; Carbohydrate 42.5 g (Fiber 5.6 g); Protein 10.7 g; Sugar 16 g.*

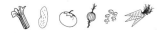

↻ Red Lentil and Coconut Soup

This luxurious gluten- and dairy-free soup is from chef Andrea Boje (www.myfoodmy health.com/OurChefs/index.php?chefid=23). Red lentils are low in fat and high in protein and fiber. Also, the addition of coconut milk gives this recipe a rich, tropical flavor, as well as a little sweetness. Your body will thank you for eating this soup because coconut milk contains immune-boosting and easy-to-digest fatty acids called *lauric acids,* which help soothe and even heal the GI tract. For even more nutrients, you can add other vegetables, such as broccoli stalks.

If they're on your food list, you can garnish your soup with a dollop of sour cream, crème fraîche, or Greek yogurt. This soup also tastes great when served with warm pieces of fresh whole-grain bread. You can keep this soup in the fridge for a week, or in the freezer to enjoy later. To reheat, warm the soup in a pot over low heat for 5 to 10 minutes, stirring occasionally. If the soup has thickened, add a little more vegetable stock or coconut milk.

Preparation time: *20 minutes*

Cooking time: *30 minutes*

Yield: *Six 1¼-cup servings*

2 tablespoons olive oil	One 14-ounce can coconut milk
1 onion, chopped	4 cloves garlic
2 carrots, chopped	½ teaspoon salt
1¾ cups red lentils, rinsed	2 teaspoons lemon juice
4 cups vegetable stock	1½ tablespoons white miso paste

1 In large soup pot, heat the olive oil over medium-low heat. Add the onion and carrot and sauté until the onions are soft, about 2 minutes. Add the lentils, stock, coconut milk, garlic, and salt to the pot. Stir and bring to a boil.

2 When the liquid is boiling, stir it some more. Reduce the heat to minimum, cover the pot, and cook for 30 minutes. Remove the pot from the heat after the lentils are completely soft.

3 Pour half of the soup into a blender and blend until smooth. Return the soup to the pot, add the lemon juice, white miso paste, and any additional desired seasonings and stir to mix. If the soup gets too thick, add additional vegetable stock.

4 Pour into bowls and serve.

Vary It! Some alternative seasonings you can use in Step 3 include 3 teaspoons grated ginger, 2 teaspoons ginger juice, and 2 teaspoons cumin or curry powder.

Tip: If you're worried about too much fat from the coconut milk stimulating your intestines, try low-fat coconut milk.

Tip: If you don't want a chunky soup, make sure to capture all the bits of vegetables you've thrown in, including the garlic cloves, when you blend the soup in Step 2.

Per serving: Calories 407; Fat 17.1 g (Saturated 8.9 g); Cholesterol 0 mg; Sodium 875 mg; Carbohydrate 44.7 g (Fiber 18.3 g); Protein 17.4 g; Sugar 6.3 g.

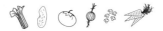

Blanching tomatoes

Some people with sensitivities to tomatoes have trouble digesting the skins, which is why blanching and skinning tomatoes can be helpful. Thanks to Colleen Robinson (`www.crimsondoor healing.com`) for demystifying the art of blanching tomatoes. It's easier than you think, and it makes tomatoes easier for IBS sufferers to digest. Blanching and skinning takes about 20 minutes to prep and another 1 to 2 minutes per batch for the actual cooking. Here's the process:

1. **Get a big pot of water boiling on the stove.**

2. **While it's boiling, rinse your tomatoes, flip them over, and cut a small, shallow *X* on the bottom.**

3. **Fill your sink half full with very cold water.**

4. **Put a few tomatoes at a time in the boiling water.**

After about a minute, the skin starts to look wrinkled and/or peel away from the cut you made in Step 2.

5. **Take the tomatoes out of the pot (using tongs or a slotted spoon) and put them in the sink of cold water.**

6. **Repeat Steps 2 through 5 until you've blanched all your tomatoes.**

7. **When the tomatoes are cool enough to touch, remove the skin by pulling it away from the *X*.**

To deseed your blanched, skinned tomatoes, cut them in half. (For the small, oval Roma tomatoes, cut top to bottom and for most other tomatoes, cut side to side.) You can squish the halves to get the seeds out or scoop them out with your fingers.

Pasta e Fagioli (Yummy Italian Pasta and Bean Soup)

Pasta e Fagioli is one of our healing chef Colleen Robinson's favorite nurturing recipes; check her out at www.crimsondoorhealing.com. This thick, hearty soup of rice and beans, which is featured in the color section, seems meaty even though it's meat-free. The white rice cooks down to create a nice soluble fiber element, and pinto beans are also high in soluble fiber. See the "Blanching tomatoes" sidebar in this chapter for instructions on blanching the skins off tomatoes.

Tools: *Potato masher*

Preparation time: *5 minutes*

Cooking time: *30 minutes*

Yield: *Four 1-cup servings*

One 15-ounce can pinto beans, rinsed well	*2 cups blanched tomatoes*
2 cups water	*Two 32-ounce containers chicken broth*
⅓ cup white rice	*¼ cup chopped fresh parsley*
1 tablespoon olive oil	*1 teaspoon dried basil*
¼ cup chopped celery	*¼ teaspoon ground black pepper*
½ cup chopped onion	*1½ cups dried short pasta (such as shells, macaroni, or fusilli)*
2 cloves garlic, minced	

1 Take ¾ of the can of pinto beans and put it in a medium-sized bowl. Mash the beans with a potato masher.

2 Boil the water on high heat in a medium saucepan. Add the white rice and stir. Cover the saucepan and lower the heat to just below medium, keeping the water at a slow boil (it should still be bubbling, but it shouldn't be making the lid jump up and down).

3 Heat the olive oil in a large pot over medium heat until a drop of water flicked from your fingers sizzles in it. Add the celery, onion, and garlic and stir off and on for 3 to 5 minutes, or until the onion softens and turns translucent.

4 Add the tomatoes, pinto beans (mashed and not mashed), chicken broth, parsley, basil, and black pepper and bring to a boil over high heat, stirring occasionally. After a minute or so, lower the heat to about halfway between medium and low and simmer for at least 10 minutes.

5 Add the pasta, raise the heat just a little bit, and boil slowly for 8 to 12 minutes, or until the pasta is cooked.

Vary It! To make this recipe vegetarian, substitute vegetable broth for the chicken broth.

Tip: Want to make the celery a little friendlier to your digestive system? Chop off the bottom and top and then cut the celery in half, but don't try to hack through all the fibers on the outside. You'll be able to peel off the really stringy bits quite quickly and easily.

Per serving: Calories 526; Fat 10.5 g (Saturated 2.4 g); Cholesterol 5 mg; Sodium 3519 mg; Carbohydrate 71.6 g (Fiber 8.6 g); Protein 36 g; Sugar 7.1 g.

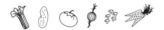

☞ Lentil Soup from the Source

This recipe comes from chef Michelle Gay (www.eatingjourney.wordpress.com). Lentils are a great source of protein often chosen by vegetarians. They've got none of the fat that's in meat protein, a fact that hikes up the digestibility factor for some people with IBS.

Preparation time: *20 minutes*

Cooking time: *40 minutes*

Yield: *Four 1-cup servings*

2 teaspoons butter

1 carrot, chopped

½ of a medium yellow onion, chopped

½ of a capsicum (a type of red pepper)

4½ cups water

1½ to 2 cups raw pumpkin, de-skinned and chopped into small chunks

Two 15-ounce cans cooked lentils, drained and rinsed, or 12 ounces of dry lentils, rinsed well but not soaked

3 to 4 cups fresh spinach

1 In a large saucepan, add the butter and sauté the carrot, onion, and capsicum for a few minutes. Add in the water and pumpkin and boil the vegetables until they're soft. If you're using dry lentils, add them here to let them cook for about 30 minutes.

2 If you're using canned lentils, add them and the fresh spinach.

3 Take ⅓ of the mixture out of the pan and blend it down with a blender, hand blender, or food processor. Add the blended-down portion back into the saucepan, stir, and serve.

Vary It! *If you're not quite up to facing a hot pepper in your lentil soup, just use ⅛ to ¼ teaspoon cayenne pepper instead. Cayenne pepper is an excellent herb for balancing the flow of stomach juices and eliminating gas. It can also help stop internal bleeding. Before you use any hot pepper products, note that at least one study has shown that people with IBS have increased nerve fibers that react with a substance in chili peppers. Use your judgment as to whether chilis, capsicum, or cayenne are safe for you to eat.*

Vary It! *You can replace the water with vegetable stock to add a different flavor and the nutrients that come from a good vegetable stock.*

Per serving: Calories 212; Fat 3.1 g (Saturated 1.3g); Cholesterol 5 mg; Sodium 396 mg; Carbohydrates 35 g (Fiber 7.6 g); Protein 13.7g; Sugar 2.5 g.

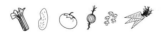

Borscht (Beet Soup)

Borscht. People can't seem to spell it right, but they can eat it happily! This recipe from our healing chef Colleen Robinson at www.crimsondoorhealing.com, calls for chicken broth, but you can easily swap that for vegetable broth if you want to make this a vegetarian dish. Beets are good for the liver and high enough in soluble fiber to pass through your intestines without a glitch. All the other vegetables are easy to digest in their well-cooked state. Think about doubling the recipe to have lots of leftovers. For instructions on blanching tomatoes, check out the "Blanching tomatoes" sidebar in this chapter.

Preparation time: *10 minutes*

Cooking time: *45 minutes*

Yield: *Eight 1-cup servings*

Two 32-ounce containers chicken broth	5 medium beets, grated
2 medium potatoes, chopped into small squares or grated	1 tomato, blanched and chopped coarsely
1 tablespoon olive oil	1 tablespoon fresh parsley, or 1 tablespoon dried parsley
1 small onion, chopped	1 teaspoon dried dill, or 1 tablespoon fresh dill
⅓ cup red or green cabbage, grated or chopped	1 bay leaf (optional)
2 carrots, grated	1 teaspoon lemon juice

1 In a large pot, bring the chicken broth to a boil and then add the potatoes. Boil for 3 minutes if the potatoes are grated and 5 minutes if the potatoes are in chunks.

2 Put the olive oil in a medium pot, toss in the onion, and cook over medium-low heat until the onion is a little translucent (about 2 to 5 minutes), stirring occasionally.

3 After the 3 or 5 minutes from Step 1 have passed, add the cabbage to the first pot and boil for another 5 minutes.

4 When the onion in the second pot is clear, add the carrots and stir occasionally for 2 to 3 minutes.

5 Put the grated beets into the pot with the carrots and onions and cook for a minute. Then add the tomato and stir-fry for another minute. Add the parsley, dill, and bay leaf (if desired) and stir for another minute.

6 Throw everything into the pot with the chicken broth, add the lemon juice, and simmer for about 30 minutes.

7 Serve when the vegetables are tender (making sure to remove any bay leaf).

Tip: *Do you like your soup chunky? Leave it as is. If you want your soup smooth, puree it right in the pot with a hand blender. Craving a creamy soup? In a bowl, mix a 12-ounce package of soft tofu with a cup of the broth, puree it with a hand blender, and add it to the broth after it has simmered for 20 minutes. And if you want a sharper taste in your soup, grate the onion (big chunks of onion become sweet when you cook them).*

Tip: *If you're going to grate the veggies in this recipe, using a decent food processor will save you grated knuckles and loads of time. Grate the beets first and empty them into a bowl. Repeat the process with the carrots, the potatoes, and then the cabbage. Don't bother cleaning the grater in between. If you have a little beet mixed in with the cabbage, it'll boil longer, which is great; you just don't want the cabbage to get mixed in and boil less.*

Per serving: *Calories 166; Fat 4.5 g (Saturated 1.1 g); Cholesterol 3 mg; Sodium 1627 mg; Carbohydrate 18.4 g (Fiber 3.6 g); Protein 13.3 g; Sugar 6.6 g.*

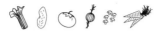

A souper food

Somewhere in history, a hungry human threw leftovers into a pot of water and invented soup, one of the cornerstones of comfort food. Soup is certainly a comforting meal for people who are ill — little to chew and easy to digest. And mom's chicken soup is always special, maybe because you know she's prepared it with love even if she just opened a can.

In 2008, a definitive study proved that chicken soup can help heal the common flu. Studies also show that people find soup more filling and satisfying. Feed the solids by themselves to a group, and folks feel less full than when they eat those same solids floating around in a tasty broth. It's all about the volume: Your mind registers a full bowl of soup as a big meal, but soup doesn't seem to make you feel too full, which is good news for people with IBS.

Orange Chicken Soup

This soup from healing chef Colleen Robinson (www.crimsondoorhealing.com) is beautiful, hearty, and delicious. The carrots and apple bring some nice sweetness to the soup without adding sugar. Cooked apple without the skin is a treatment for IBS-D, but the amount used here won't contribute to IBS-C. And of course rice is high in soluble fiber; white rice has more soluble fiber than brown rice, but the longer cooking time in a soup makes brown rice more soluble than it would be otherwise. Either kind of rice cooks and eventually dissolves, thickening the soup and balancing out the insoluble fiber in some of the vegetables.

You can use a hand blender and puree the soup right in the pot. But if you choose to scoop the hot soup into a blender or food processor, make sure you puree in quick short bursts. Otherwise, the steam can build up inside the lid and blow it off — hot, messy, dangerous, and a waste of good soup!

Tools: *Hand blender (optional)*

Preparation time: *20 minutes*

Cooking time: *60 minutes*

Yield: *Sixteen 1-cup servings*

4 quarts chicken broth	*1 apple, peeled and coarsely chopped*
¼ cup uncooked white or brown rice	*½ teaspoon cinnamon (optional)*
1 pound carrots, peeled and coarsely chopped	*½ teaspoon nutmeg (optional)*
1 small butternut or acorn squash, peeled and coarsely chopped	*1 teaspoon lemon juice*
2 medium yams/sweet potatoes, peeled and coarsely chopped	

1 In a large pot, combine the chicken broth and rice, and start simmering. Add the chopped carrots, squash, yams, and apple. Add the cinnamon and/or nutmeg (if desired).

2 Cover the pot and allow the soup to cook at a low boil (you should still see bubbles, but the lid shouldn't be jumping up and down), stirring every 10 to 15 minutes until the veggies are soft and mushy (about 20 to 60 minutes; you can start checking them with a fork after about 30 minutes).

3 Puree the soup when it's still hot or lukewarm. (Don't wait until the soup is cold to perform this step, because it'll be harder to puree that way.) Put the pureed soup back into the pot (if you used a regular blender or food processor). Stir in the lemon juice. Eat and enjoy.

Vary It! *Roasting your vegetables makes the whole process take longer, but it makes peeling the veggies a breeze. To roast the vegetables called for in this recipe, leave the yams whole and cut the squash in half. Put everything on a baking sheet and pop into a 350-degree oven for about 45 to 60 minutes, or until you can easily scoop out the insides. Then when you're boiling the soup, be careful to just boil it long enough for the rice to dissolve and the veggie flavors to mingle nicely, about 30 to 40 minutes.*

Per serving: Calories 119; Fat 2.7 g (Saturated 0.8 g) Cholesterol 3 mg; Sodium 1600 mg; Carbohydrate 12.1 g (Fiber 1.9 g); Protein 11.9 g; Sugar 4 g.

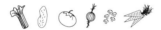

Cooling Off with Cool Soups

Sometimes a cool soup is just the sort of refreshment you need. Cool soup isn't cooked, so the vegetables are raw, but if you blend them well they become more soluble and digestible. Here are some raw soup selections that have never been near a stove.

⟡ Creamy Broccoli Soup in the Raw

Chef Angela Elliott (`www.she-zencuisine.com`) contributed this surprising creamy and cool broccoli soup that's nutritious, easy to make, and tasty while being kind to your tummy. Cashews are high in soluble fiber, and blending reduces their insoluble-fiber content. Blended broccoli may not be your first thought for a cool soup, but it's got almost as much soluble as insoluble fiber, so it's not going to irritate your IBS tummy. It's also very high in vitamins and minerals.

Soaking time: *2 hours*

Preparation time: *5 minutes*

Cooking time: *None*

Yield: *Four 1-cup servings*

1½ cups raw cashews, soaked for 2 hours

2 cups chopped broccoli

2 cups water

⅛ teaspoon each salt and black pepper, or to taste

¼ teaspoon each powdered sage, dried thyme, and garlic powder

1 Soak the raw cashews for at least 2 hours and then drain and rinse them.

2 Blend the soaked cashews, broccoli, water, and desired seasonings in a blender until smooth. Chill the soup in the fridge after blending for about 30 minutes.

3 Serve with chunks of sprouted bread (such as manna or Essene, found in the freezer section of your local health food store), Rice Mochi (pounded rice formed into flat cakes also found in your health food store's freezer), or corn chips.

Per serving: Calories 250; Fat 18.8 g (Saturated 3.3 g); Cholesterol 0 mg; Sodium 92 mg; Carbohydrate 15.8 g (Fiber 2.5 g); Protein 9.1 g; Sugar 3.3 g.

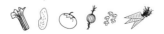

↻ *Raw Curry Spinach Soup*

Shannon Leone's Raw recipes are a tasty surprise (check out www.rawmom.com). Who knew to put creamy avocado in a curry spinach soup? Shannon did. Both avocado and spinach are high in soluble fiber, and the vegetables in the rest of the recipe offset the fat in the avocado. You can blanch and remove the skins of the bell peppers and tomatoes if you want (see the "Blanching tomatoes" sidebar in this chapter), but blending this dish chops out a lot of insoluble fiber on its own. (A food processor may give you a better blend, but the blender works too.)

Preparation time: *5 to 8 minutes*

Cooking time: *None*

Yield: *Two 1-cup servings*

1 bunch fresh spinach

¼ cup fresh dill

½ of a red bell pepper

1 small ripe tomato

½ of an avocado

¼ of a small onion (optional)

1 tablespoon Nama Shoyu (raw organic soy sauce)

2 tablespoons lemon juice

1 teaspoon curry powder

½ cup water

½ diced red or orange bell pepper

1 Combine all the ingredients in a blender or food processor.

2 Blend and enjoy.

Vary It! *If you can't find Nama Shoyu, substitute 1 teaspoon Braggs Liquid Aminos, ½ teaspoon powdered kelp, 1 teaspoon powdered dulse (both seaweeds taste salty but are low sodium and high in minerals), or ½ teaspoon Celtic sea salt.*

Per serving: *Calories 149; Fat 8.4 g (Saturated 1.2 g); Cholesterol 0 mg; Sodium 648 mg; Carbohydrate 16.2 g (Fiber 8.7 g); Protein 7.7 g; Sugar 4 g.*

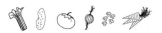

☕ *Carrot Ginger Soup*

Chef Andrea Boje (www.myfoodmyhealth.com/OurChefs/index.php?chefid=23) contributed this soup that's easy to make and has a beautiful rich orange color. The ginger is a tummy-soother, and carrot juice has all the goodness of carrots without any of the irritating fiber. You can serve it cold or at room temperature, but serving it freshly made is best. Use this dish as a first course or enjoy it for lunch with some fresh bread and grapes or cut apples. This soup will keep in the refrigerator for 5 days; avoid freezing it.

Tools: *Juicer (optional)*

Preparation time: *20 minutes*

Yield: *Four 1-cup servings*

2 pounds organic carrots, or 3 cups carrot juice

2 ripe avocados, peeled and pitted

1½ teaspoon salt

1½ teaspoons lemon juice

1 teaspoon peeled and grated ginger

Diced avocado or crème fraîche for serving

1 If using carrots, run them through a juicer to make approximately 3 cups of carrot juice.

2 Place the carrot juice, avocados, salt, lemon juice, and ginger into a blender and blend on high until smooth.

3 Taste and add more lemon, ginger, or salt if desired. Pour into bowls, top with diced avocado or crème fraîche, and serve.

Vary It! *For a sweeter taste to your soup, add 1 tablespoon agave nectar.*

Tip: *If you don't want to make your own carrot juice, Odwalla and Bolthouse Farms both make great store-bought alternatives.*

Per serving: *Calories 255; Fat 15.3 g (Saturated 2.2 g); Cholesterol 0 mg; Sodium 1035 mg; Carbohydrate 30.5 g (Fiber 13 g); Protein 4.1 g; Sugar 11.5 g.*

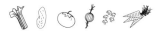

Chapter 10

Serving Up Stomach-Safe Salads

Salads may be at the bottom of your safe food list because of the potential for difficult digestion of the raw veggies. But as you progress through your own personalized IBS diet, you're likely to feel a lessening of your symptoms and be in a position to begin adding new foods to your weekly menu. And raw vegetables can be a nutritious addition.

We absolutely acknowledge that raw salads are not a good choice for people who are in the midst of regular IBS-D flare-ups and attacks, but if you've graduated to a point where your attacks are minimal, you may be ready to add a safe salad. Consider trying the salad ingredients on their own before mixing them together in a salad to check for individual reactions.

Some research shows that fiber (including that found in veggies) can be a relief for about 80 percent of people with constipation, including IBS-C. Although 20 percent find fiber irritating, the soluble and insoluble fiber in vegetables may be okay for many people with IBS-C. Tread carefully, but don't be afraid.

For an IBS sufferer, salads are all about chewing. Foods like corn may not properly digest if you don't chew them thoroughly. Let your teeth do more work and you'll digest and absorb much better as a result. An old-time cure for digestive disorders is to chew your food 40 to 50 times per bite!

If you chew long enough, you can digest a portion of the carbs in your meal with the amylase enzyme in your saliva. That action sets the stage for your stomach juices to start flowing and things to start gearing up in your gut. If you're extremely sensitive to food moving through your gut, you may cringe at that thought, assuming you're going to have a reaction to the food you're just starting to eat. However, if your stomach is presented with mush and not chunks, it has less work to do and can proceed with digestion much more calmly and smoothly.

Your constitution also plays a big role in determining how you react to salads. According to Ayurvedic practice, the Pitta constitution has enough stomach fire to digest raw salads, but the Vata constitution has very low stomach fire and therefore a difficult time digesting raw vegetables. Flip to Chapter 5 for more guidance on determining your constitution, and check out the following section to discover ways to combat the insoluble fiber in raw veggie salads.

Wash your vegetables in a sink full of water with about ten drops of grapefruit seed extract. The oil from grapefruit seeds is poisonous to parasites and bacteria and kills them on contact but it's harmless to humans. In Chapter 16, we remind you to take grapefruit seed extract capsules or tablets when you're dining out.

Sneaking Soluble Fiber into Your Salads

When you eat salads, you're consuming more plant cellulose (called *insoluble fiber,* which doesn't break down in your intestines) than the soluble fiber that's less irritating. If you want to eat salads without worry, include soluble-fiber vegetables like beets, carrots, potatoes, parsnips, squash, sweet pota-toes, turnips, or yams in your salad.

You can also balance the insoluble fiber in your salad with a side of soluble-fiber bread — store-bought manna bread or pita bread, or homemade sourdough or coconut bread (see Chapters 12 and 13 respectively for these recipes). Another simple soluble solution is to use miracle noodles as a salad ingredient. Made from *glucomannan,* a highly soluble plant fiber, these noodles are just what you need to balance the fiber in your meal without adding carbs.

Sensational Salad Recipes

We are strong advocates of organic produce for all people, but if you have IBS, we recommend getting organic greens and salad fixings whenever possible. You want to minimize the amount of non-salad stuff you get with your salad, and organic greens are free of pesticides, genetic modifications, and any "freshening" sprays or chemicals. We've had many reports of folks with IBS who were introducing salads into their diet to find that they reacted to conventional lettuce but not organic lettuce of the same sort.

You also want to keep an eye on cleanliness: Even if your greens come prewashed in a bag, somebody's hands or gloves have touched them. Just because a salad-bar worker is wearing gloves doesn't mean your salad greens are safe. People wearing gloves often perform the same tasks (making change, picking up phones, and so on) that bare-handed folks do, so don't assume gloves equal total sanitation.

French Lentil Salad

This recipe is one of Kendall Conrad's favorite salads from her book *Eat Well Feel Well* (www.eatwellfeelwellthebook.com) because it's satisfying and exotic, with lovely grapefruit and cumin flavors and the interesting combination of fresh, crunchy vegetables and sweet currants. You can serve it warm or chilled, but letting it meld for 3 to 6 hours really brings out the flavors.

This salad has a lot of ingredients but it's easy to put together. If you're worried about one or two of the ingredients not agreeing with you, just remove them. Just remember that Kendall created this dish for a family member who had severe digestive issues, so it was formulated with digestive compatibility in mind. The obvious foods you may have to be careful of are shallots and cayenne, although cayenne can be used to treat constipation and folklore credits it with stopping bleeding in the intestines. The main soluble factor in this salad is the main ingredient — lentils. Cumin, coriander, and fennel relieve gas and bloating; thyme and cilantro soothe the stomach. Garlic may help your symptoms if your IBS is being triggered by bacteria and yeast; leave it out if you know you react to it. A 2004 study showed that curry relieves abdominal pain.

Soaking time: *24 hours*

Preparation time: *About 15 minutes*

Cooking time: *None*

Yield: *7 servings*

2 tablespoons fresh thyme

½ cup (about 3 large) shallots, finely chopped

Juice of one lemon (about ¼ cup)

Juice of ½ grapefruit (about ¼ cup)

2 tablespoons ground cumin

1 tablespoon celery salt

2 teaspoons curry powder (no fillers or starches added)

1 teaspoon ground coriander

3 cloves garlic, minced

1 tablespoon freshly grated lemon zest

½ cup extra virgin olive oil

½ teaspoon cayenne pepper

2 cups cooked French green lentils

½ cup currants

1 fennel bulb, sliced very thinly with fronds removed

4 stalks of celery (about 1 cup), strings removed and finely chopped

1 cup fresh flat-leaf parsley, chopped

½ cup fresh cilantro, chopped

1 In a large mixing bowl add the thyme, shallots, lemon juice, grapefruit juice, cumin, celery salt, curry powder, coriander, garlic, lemon zest, olive oil, and cayenne pepper. Whisk ingredients together.

2 Pour the juice mixture over the lentils and add the currants, fennel, celery, parsley, and cilantro. Mix well.

Per serving: *Calories 440; Fat 19.5 g (Saturated 2.7 g); Cholesterol 0 mg; Sodium 349 mg; Carbohydrate 50.2 g (Fiber 22.5 g); Protein 18.7 g; Sugar 4.4 g.*

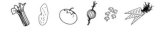

⭕ *Cauliflower Salad with Dairy-Free Dill Dressing*

Andrea Boje (www.myfoodmyhealth.com/OurChefs/index.php?chefid=23) sub-mitted this recipe that is appropriate for those whose stomachs are quite tolerant of salads. It does contain three vegetables that veer more toward insoluble fiber, but if you feel you're ready to add some peppers and onions to your diet, this recipe is a very tasty way to do it. Steaming the cauliflower makes it more digestible, as does very finely dicing and mincing the peppers and onions — you can even use a food processor and really break down the fiber that way. The dressing that goes with this recipe provides dill, an herb that's very good for digestion and soothing for the intestines.

Tools: *Steamer basket*

Preparation time: *20 minutes*

Cooking time: *3 to 5 minutes*

Yield: *4 servings*

1 large head of cauliflower

1 medium red bell pepper, finely diced

¼ cup red onion, minced

¼ teaspoon salt, or more to taste

4 grinder-turns freshly ground pepper (about ⅛ teaspoon), or more to taste

Dairy-Free Dill Dressing (enough to coat; see the following recipe)

1 Remove and discard the cauliflower stem and cut the head into small florets. Place the cauliflower in a steamer basket and steam over boiling water until slightly soft but still firm and crunchy, about 3 to 5 minutes. Remove from steam and set aside to cool.

2 Place the cooled cauliflower in the bowl of a food processor. Pulse until the cauliflower is coarsely chopped. Pour into a medium mixing bowl and cut any remaining large pieces with a knife.

3 Add the red bell pepper, red onion, salt and pepper, and enough dressing to coat. Adjust seasonings to taste. Reserve a little minced onion or bell pepper for garnishing.

Per serving: Calories 66; Fat 0.3 g (Saturated 0 g); Cholesterol 0 mg; Sodium 210 mg; Carbohydrate 13.9 g (Fiber 6.1 g); Protein 4.6 g; Sugar 6.7 g.

Dairy-Free Dill Dressing

This dressing is a great summertime recipe from chef Andrea Boje (www.myfoodmy-health.com/OurChefs/index.php?chefid=23) that accentuates the sweetness of cauliflower in the salad. If you don't heat the ingredients over 118 degrees, this dressing can complement a Raw diet (see Chapter 3).

Silken tofu is great for making creamy, dairy-free dressings. Andrea does recommend that you simmer the tofu to help with digestion, especially if you have problems digest-ing soy.

Preparation time: *20 minutes*

Cooking time: *8 minutes*

Resting time: ½ *hour to 2 hours*

Yield: *Four ⅛-cup servings (½ cup total)*

One 12-ounce package silken tofu

1 medium clove of garlic

Juice of one lemon (about ¼ cup)

4 tablespoons extra-virgin olive oil

1 tablespoon Dijon mustard

2 teaspoons sea salt

4 tablespoons fresh dill, chopped

1 Bring a small pot of water to boil. Add the silken tofu and let water come back to a boil; simmer for 3 minutes. Strain the tofu with a mesh strainer.

2 Finely chop the garlic in a food processor. Add the tofu, half of the lemon juice, and the olive oil, mustard, and sea salt. Process until smooth. Taste and add more salt and lemon juice if needed.

3 Pour into a bowl, stir in the dill, and set aside in the refrigerator for ½ an hour to 2 hours to let the flavors develop. Taste again and add more lemon juice, salt, or garlic to taste if necessary.

Per serving: Calories 194; Fat 16.1 g (Saturated 1.8 g); Cholesterol 0 mg; Sodium 1029 mg; Carbohydrate 4.6 g (Fiber 0.3 g); Protein 6.5 g; Sugar 0.4 g.

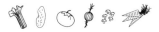

⏁ Sprouted Salad

For easy digestibility and great nutrition, try one of our favorites. The servings are small, but the sprouts are a great way to enjoy seeds packed with powerful nutrition — they're rich with enzymes and easy to digest. The ingredients in this salad are few, but you can add your favorite salad ingredients and make it your own recipe; we recommend dressing it with a tasty vinaigrette. Enjoy it with a thick slice of manna bread.

Preparation time: *About 5 minutes*

Cooking time: *None*

Yield: *7 servings*

1 cup each sunflower, broccoli, and alfalfa sprouts

1 head butternut lettuce

1 ripe avocado, halved, pitted, and peeled

1 Finely chop the sprouts and lettuce and cube the avocado.

2 Mix all the ingredients together and dress.

Per serving: Calories 140; Fat 9.4 g (Saturated 0.6 g); Cholesterol 0 mg; Sodium 4 mg; Carbohydrate 3.5 g (Fiber 2.7 g); Protein 1.6 g; Sugar 0.4 g.

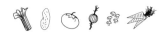

☉ *Soba Salad*

This salad from chef Caroline Nation at www.myfoodmyhealth.com is a meal in itself; check out a photo of it in the color section. It's versatile because you can easily substitute your favorite vegetables for the ones listed here. For a gluten-free salad, make sure your noodles are 100 percent buckwheat, which doesn't contain gluten. This salad is even tastier on the second day, so you may want to make it a day ahead of a planned event. (But generally speaking, we don't recommend eating the same dish two days in a row, especially if you are newly graduated into enjoying salads — see Chapter 3 for more on rotating foods.) This salad contains many raw vegetables, so it may not be for you if you're just dipping your toes into salads (which we don't recommend you do literally). Soba noodles (or substituted miracle noodles) give you a good amount of soluble fiber to balance the insoluble fiber in the raw vegetables. Remember to cut your vegetables very finely and chew them well to make them more digestible and to get the nutrients that are concentrated in raw foods.

Preparation time: *20 minutes*

Cooking time: *10 minutes*

Yield: *4 servings*

4 quarts water, salted

½ cup broccoli florets

½ cup cauliflower florets

8 ounces soba noodles

1 tablespoon toasted sesame oil

1 cup thinly sliced red cabbage

1 head green or ruby leaf lettuce, washed, drained and thinly sliced

½ cup tahini

½ cup water

2 teaspoons fresh lemon juice or brown rice vinegar

4 medium radishes, thinly sliced into rounds

2 medium carrots, shredded

1 scallion, white and green parts, thinly sliced

1 In a large pot, bring 4 quarts of salted water to a boil. Add the broccoli and blanch until barely tender, about 3 minutes. Remove with a slotted spoon and immediately plunge into a bowl of ice water or rinse under cold water to stop the cooking. Repeat the process with the cauliflower, using the same water. When cool, drain the vegetables and set aside.

2 Add the noodles to the boiling pot and cook for 6 to 8 minutes until just tender. Drain the noodles and immediately rinse under cold water. Sprinkle with the sesame oil and toss to keep the noodles from sticking.

3 Combine the cabbage and lettuce in a serving bowl. Place the noodles on top and arrange the cauliflower and broccoli around the edges.

4 Whisk the tahini, water, and lemon juice or vinegar in a small bowl until well combined. Pour the dressing over the salad and top with the radishes, carrots and scallions.

Per serving: *Calories 440; Fat 20 g (Saturated 2.8 g); Cholesterol 0 mg; Sodium 517 mg; Carbohydrate 57.4 g (Fiber 4.4 g); Protein 15.7 g; Sugar 3.3 g.*

Cobb Salad with Angie's Vinaigrette

This salad, which is featured in the color section, comes from Raman Prasad's *Recipes for the Specific Carbohydrate Diet*™ (Fair Winds Press) and fits any Specific Carbohydrate Diet (SCD) plan; see Chapter 3 for more on the SCD, and check out Raman at www.scdrecipe.com/cookbook. If your food list limits your dairy intake, replace the SCD-safe cheese with a soy cheese. Raman paired this salad with a vinaigrette recipe from a friend (included here).

Preparation time: *10 minutes*

Cooking time: *None*

Yield: *6 servings*

10 ounces spinach leaves, chopped	*10 ripe black olives, pitted and finely chopped*
3 eggs, hardboiled, peeled, and chopped into small pieces	*¼ to ½ cup grated cheddar cheese*
1 medium tomato, chopped	*¼ cup SCD-safe bacon bits (sugar-free, smoked bacon fried very crisp)*
1 to 2 avocados, stones removed and flesh scooped out of shell and sliced	*Angie's Vinaigrette (see the following recipe)*

1 Toss together the spinach, egg, tomato, and avocado in a salad bowl.

2 Sprinkle the top of the salad with the olives, cheese, and bacon bits. Toss with the dressing.

Per serving: Calories 162; Fat 11.8 g (Saturated 3.2 g); Cholesterol 113 mg; Sodium 257 mg; Carbohydrate 7.5 g (Fiber 4.2 g); Protein 7.3 g; Sugar 1.3 g.

Angie's Vinaigrette

Preparation time: *About 5 minutes*

Cooking time: *None*

Yield: *Twelve 2-tablespoon servings (1½ cups total)*

⅓ cup olive oil	*1 tablespoon honey*
2 to 4 tablespoons mock (young) balsamic vinegar	*Juice of 1 orange (about ¼ cup)*
1 tablespoon red wine vinegar	*¼ teaspoon salt and ground pepper, or to taste*
1 tablespoon ground mustard	

1 Combine all the ingredients thoroughly until they dissolve into each other.

Per serving: Calories 69; Fat 6.2 g (Saturated .8 g); Cholesterol 0.08 mg; Sodium 50 mg; Carbohydrates 3.2 g (Fiber 0.2 g); Protein 0.3 g; Sugar 2.7 g.

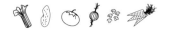

☺ Citrus Marinated Salad

Andrea Boje (www.myfoodmyhealth.com/OurChefs/index.php?chefid=23) created this refreshing summertime salad that you can enjoy on its own or on a bed of torn lettuce with canned tuna and toasted sesame oil. The longer the vegetables sit in the citrus/umeboshi vinegar marinade, the softer and more flavorful they become. Consider making the salad in large quantities because it stores in the fridge for 2 weeks.

The timing of the marinade is the key to making this recipe a safe, IBS-friendly salad. If you're comfortable with raw vegetables and want the crunch, simply pull your vegetables out of the marinade in 30 to 45 minutes. Otherwise, you can allow the marinade to do its magic for up to 3 hours. The marinade breaks down the vegetable fibers, allowing smoother digestion. You may not know umeboshi vinegar, but it's available in health food stores. It's a Japanese vinegar made from umeboshi plums and has a tart, fruity taste that's very different from apple cider vinegar but has the same ability to assist digestion. Check out this lovely salad in the color section.

Marinating time: *30 minutes to 3 hours*

Preparation time: *20 minutes*

Cooking time: *None*

Yield: *6 servings*

½ a medium green cabbage	2 tablespoons salt, divided
2 large carrots	½ a medium red cabbage
4 cups orange juice	¼ cup apple cider vinegar
Juice of 4 lemons (about 1 cup)	1 tablespoon salt
¼ cup umeboshi plum vinegar	2 tablespoons toasted sesame seeds

1 Thinly slice the green cabbage and cut the carrots into 2-inch long sticks and then cut again lengthwise to make several thin wafers. Place in a large bowl.

2 Add 2 cups of the orange juice, ½ cup of the lemon juice, and the umeboshi vinegar to the vegetables and mix the ingredients with your hands. Making sure the liquid completely covers the vegetables (weighting them down with a plate if necessary), let the mixture marinate for 1 hour or to your desired tenderness (anywhere between 30 minutes and 3 hours).

3 Thinly slice the red cabbage and place in another large bowl with the apple cider vinegar and remaining orange and lemon juice. Sprinkle with the salt and mix with your hands. Let the cabbage mixture marinate for 1 hour or to your desired tenderness (anywhere between 30 minutes and 3 hours).

4 When you're done marinating, drain both bowls of vegetables and combine them into one bowl, stirring to mix. Sprinkle with toasted sesame seeds and serve.

Vary It! *You can also add cauliflower florets to the veggies in this salad. Marinate 1 cup of chopped cauliflower florets in 1 cup of orange juice and ¼ cup of umeboshi or rice vinegar for 2 hours and then drain them and add them to the other drained vegetables.*

Tip: *You can save and reuse the vegetable marinade. Mix a little marinade with olive oil for a quick salad dressing.*

Per serving: *Calories 165; Fat 2.2 g (Saturated 0.3 g); Cholesterol 0 mg; Sodium 1733 mg; Carbohydrate 32.8 g (Fiber 4.5 g); Protein 4.2 g; Sugar 7.3 g.*

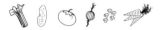

Delightful Dressings and Magnificent Mayos

Dressing up a salad is an art in itself, and here we give you some great options to choose from. We love these dressings because they are made from scratch but still deliver flavor, and you know exactly what goes in them.

In contrast, the ingredient lists of many commercial salad dressings read like a who's who of chemicals, additives, flavorings, and preservatives. In general, commercial dressings may contain starchy, wheat-based thickeners; MSG; dairy; and yeast. Fat-free or low-fat dressings often have extra sugars to create a palatable taste in the absence of the missing fat, so your "healthier" dressing may not be as beneficial as you think.

Mayonnaise is typically made with soybean oil, eggs, egg yolks, sugar, and other flavorings. Some products have less fat than the original versions, but they also contain something like twice the number of ingredients, including sulfites, which are used as a preservative but can cause headaches, heartburn, and intestinal cramps.

If you're very liberal with your condiments, be sure to use chemical-free condiments as much as possible.

☺ *Lemon Gone Wild Dressing*

Angela Elliott (www.she-zencuisine.com) shares her zesty, lemony salad dressing; she suggests you serve it on arugula, but you can also quickly open a 6-ounce package of mesclun green salad. Add a side of high soluble-fiber bread (such as sourdough white — see the recipe in Chapter 12 — or manna) and you have a meal suitable for IBS-D and IBS-C. Bottom line: Any salad will do.

Preparation time: *5 minutes*

Cooking time: *None*

Yield: *6 servings (⅔ cup total)*

¼ cup extra-virgin olive oil	¾ teaspoon salt
2 tablespoons fresh lemon juice	⅛ teaspoon freshly cracked black pepper
¾ teaspoon minced fresh garlic	¾ teaspoon fresh thyme leaves

1 Combine all the ingredients gently in a bowl to blend fully but leave the vinaigrette clear (not emulsified) for a better presentation.

> **Per serving:** *Calories 82; Fat 9 g (Saturated 1.2 g); Cholesterol 0 mg; Sodium 291 mg; Carbohydrate 0.6 g (Fiber 0.04 g); Protein 0.03 g; Sugar 0.1 g.*

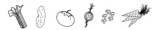

☺ *Asian Dressing*

Living on Maui, artist, writer, and chef Marilyn Jansen (www.amaryllisofhawaii.com) cooks with a Pacific Rim flair. Her Asian Dressing is best over non-wheat noodles — try thin buckwheat, rice noodles, or the no-carb miracle noodles we discuss earlier in the chapter over a bed of soft lettuce. The combination is good for IBS-C, but go light on the dressing and heavy on the soluble noodles for IBS-D.

Preparation time: *5 minutes*

Cooking time: *None*

Yield: *Eight 2-tablespoon servings (1 cup total)*

¼ cup sesame oil	¼ cup rice wine vinegar
4 tablespoons vegetable oil	2 tablespoons maple syrup
¼ cup soy sauce	1 tablespoon light miso paste (optional)

1 Whisk all ingredients vigorously to blend.

Vary It! *You can use honey instead of maple syrup to give your dressing a different sweet flavor, or if you have one on hand and not the other.*

Per serving: *Calories 140; Fat 13.8 g (Saturated 1.5 g); Cholesterol 1 mg; Sodium 413 mg; Carbohydrate 3.9 g (Fiber 0.03 g); Protein 0.2 g; Sugar 3.1 g.*

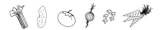

⊙ Shannon's Spicy Caesar Dressing

If you find that you're craving the zest of a Caesar salad dressing, consider this one-step IBS-friendly alternative from the kitchen of Shannon Leone (www.rawmom.com). We assure you this is IBS-friendly, especially when you read the ingredients of one of the popular commercial brands, which has about 35 ingredients including milk, cheese, cream, yeast, and flavor enhancers, any of which can act as an IBS trigger.

Preparation time: *5 minutes*

Cooking time: *None*

Yield: *15 servings (nearly 2 cups total)*

1 cup flaxseed, olive, or hemp oil

Juice of 1 to 2 lemons (about ½ cup)

⅓ cup raw tahini

1 to 2 cloves garlic

Nama Shoyu, or ½ teaspoon sea salt

1 Blend all ingredients until creamy.

Tip: *This dressing can thicken when standing, so you can add a few tablespoons of water or more lemon juice to thin.*

Per serving: *Calories 165; Fat 17 g (Saturated 1.7 g); Cholesterol 0 mg; Sodium 86 mg; Carbohydrate 2.2 g (Fiber 0.6 g); Protein 0.04 g; Sugar 0.2 g.*

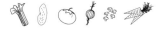

Substituting potential condiment triggers

We know how much people can be attached to their condiments. Carolyn always teased her foster son for seeming to subsist entirely on condiments. His fridge, to this day, is condiment-heavy, and he's not alone. Whether condiment use is a habit, a comfort food, or a way to mask the flavor of a healthy food, people with IBS can really miss their add-ons.

You know from reading the labels that grocery store condiments are full of sugar, wheat, and additives that may be messing with your guts. And we know that you reason that using a dash of ketchup or mayonnaise shouldn't hurt, but depending on your level of sensitivity, they may really have an ill effect.

Never fear. Here are a couple of safer condiments that you can find at most health food and grocery stores.

- ✔ If you're sensitive to the wheat and soy in soy sauce, try Braggs Liquid Aminos.

- ✔ If you're sensitive to the fat in regular mayonnaise, try nut pâté (see the recipe in Chapter 7) or Angela's Happy Mayo (which we include in this chapter)

Make sure you read the labels first and are aware that these substitutes don't taste exactly like your high-sugar condiments, but they may get the job done.

☞ Angela's Happy Mayo

Thanks to Angela Elliot (www.she-zencuisine.com) for this Raw twist on mayonnaise. It's low on fat (which makes it IBS-friendly) and high on taste, and compared to commercial mayonnaise, it's a miracle. You may even want to use it as a dressing for a salad.

Preparation time: *10 minutes*

Cooking time: *None*

Yield: *Eight 2-tablespoon servings (1 cup total)*

½ cup raw tahini	1 teaspoon sea salt
1 to 2 tablespoons fresh lemon juice	Juice of 1 orange (about ¼ cup)
2 tablespoons yacon syrup, or 6 soaked honey dates, pitted	2 tablespoons fresh dill
	1 cup water

1 Blend all the ingredients and mix with your favorite salad or spread on your favorite sandwich.

Per serving: Calories 64; Fat 3.6 g (Saturated 0.5 g); Cholesterol 0 mg; Sodium 152 mg; Carbohydrate 4.1 g (Fiber 1.8 g); Protein 1.4 g; Sugar 0.8 g.

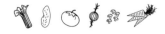

☞ Homestyle Mayonnaise

Although Carolyn remembers the days when people made mayonnaise using egg beaters, we doubt many people these days even know what an egg beater is! The mayonnaise-making job is much easier now with the use of blenders, which *emulsify* (create a suspension of the ingredients) without the elbow grease. Using a high-speed blender means you don't even have to slowly drizzle the oil into the mixture to get complete emulsification. Use a free-range or pasteurized egg to eliminate salmonella concerns, and then eat this mayo immediately or refrigerate it in a covered container for up to a week.

Preparation time: *5 minutes*

Cooking time: *None*

Yield: *Ten 2-tablespoon servings (1¼ cups total)*

1 egg	3 tablespoons lemon juice
1 teaspoon dry mustard	1 cup olive oil or safflower oil
½ teaspoon each white pepper and sea salt	1 tablespoon hot water
Pinch of cayenne pepper	

1 In a blender, combine the egg, mustard, white pepper, salt, cayenne pepper, and lemon juice and blend well.

2 With the blender still running, add the oil in a slow, steady stream and blend until all oil is emulsified. Blend in 1 tablespoon hot water at the end.

Per serving: *Calories 202; Fat 22.2 g (Saturated 3.2 g); Cholesterol 22 mg; Sodium 8 mg; Carbohydrate 0.6 g (Fiber 0.1 g); Protein 0.8 g; Sugar 0.2 g.*

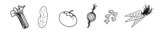

Chapter 11

Marvelous Main Dishes that Won't Torment Your Gut

Whether you're cooking and eating for one or for your whole family, we know that dinner can be a stressful time for people with IBS. You may be tired of preparing special plates for yourself while you make family favorites for everyone else that you can't enjoy.

What if you could cook one meal that the whole family can devour? In this chapter, we offer lots of IBS-friendly twists on dinner favorites as well as unique IBS recipes. Nobody needs to know they're IBS-friendly! We often hear that when people feel like they're eating typical meals, they feel better about themselves and seem to be less preoccupied about their symptoms.

The recipes in this chapter provide something for everyone, with meat, poultry, fish, and vegetarian options. You may already know that meat, poultry, and fish are high in protein; no evidence suggests that these protein foods trigger or worsen IBS. However, the company they keep can be the problem, such as the fatty skin on chicken or turkey or the marbled fat on beef. In some people with IBS, fat can increase gastric motility and lead to IBS symptoms. The fat content in fatty fish like mackerel and salmon can sometimes cause faster meal transit time. The trick is to avoid that particular part of the food or sample very little of it. Or add a side dish high in soluble fiber to help absorb the fat.

Savoring the Solubility Factor

Finding enough soluble fiber in your main dish may be easier than you think because you can work with more ingredients. Great soluble-fiber main dish ingredients include rice, pasta, barley, mushrooms, carrots, potatoes, sweet potatoes, yams, turnips, beets, squash, and pumpkin. You want at least half of your fiber to be the soluble kind. If your dish of choice isn't as high in fiber as you want, add a side of *miracle noodles* (no-carb noodles made from soluble plant fiber) or your homemade sourdough white bread (see Chapter 12 for the recipe).

To improve the solubility picture, you can reduce insoluble fiber by peeling your tomatoes and potatoes and stripping the fibrous strings from celery. When cooking and preparing your meals, the more you puree, cook, and blend your vegetables, beans, and nuts, the easier your food is to digest!

A helpful tool is the soluble/insoluble fiber chart in Appendix C. At a glance you can see the fiber content of many common foods. Choose the ones that have nearly the same amount of soluble as insoluble fiber (give or take .7 grams).

Beefing Up Your Stew for a Meaty Main Dish

If you have a sensitive gut, limit the portion size of your meat. The size of a pack of playing cards (about 3 to 4 ounces) is enough meat to satisfy your protein needs, with each ounce providing 7 grams of protein. Cooked meat freezes well, so you can make the full recipe and save some for later.

Beef has a nice hearty flavor (unlike the delicate flavor of chicken), so you want to pair it with hearty vegetables like potatoes and carrots. We forgo steak recipes in this section because they're pretty straightforward: Season the meat, heat the grill, and cook for 6 minutes on each side. Just remember to buy lean meat and pass on the ribeye — the eye is all fat.

Beef Pumpkin Stew

Here's an IBS-friendly twist on a classic beef stew; it's from chef Michelle Gay (www.eatingjourney.wordpress.com). Pumpkin is a great IBS fruit (yes, it's a fruit) that's high in soluble fiber. Cooked onions, carrots, and mushrooms are all great IBS vegetables because they are also high in soluble fiber. You can peel some of the long threads of fiber from the celery to make it more digestible. We've kept in the tomatoes; you can make them more stomach-compatible by blanching off the skins — see Chapter 9 for easy blanching instructions.

Preparation time: *20 minutes*

Cooking time: *3 to 5 hours*

Yield: *4 servings*

1 tablespoon olive oil

1 medium or ½ of a large onion, cut up

4 cloves garlic, pressed

3½ cups raw pumpkin, cut into 1-inch squares

½ of a chili pepper, diced

1 carrot, sliced

6 to 7 cups water

2 large celery stalks

3 tomatoes, chopped

6 standard-size mushrooms, sliced

3 tablespoons tomato sauce (jarred, canned, or from the Marinara Sauce recipe later in this chapter)

1 pound stew beef (top round)

½ teaspoon each salt and pepper

1½ tablespoons Italian seasoning

4 to 5 bay leaves

1 Heat the olive oil in a large saucepan over high heat. Add the onion and garlic and sauté until the onion is translucent (about 8 minutes).

2 Add in the pumpkin, chili pepper, and carrots along with 1 cup of water. Cover and steam for about 1 minute. Add the celery, tomatoes, and mushrooms. Cover and steam for about 2 minutes.

3 While the veggies are steaming, coat your meat with a liberal amount of salt and pepper and the Italian seasoning. Add the beef to the pot and cover for about 1 to 2 minutes (the meat doesn't need to cook through).

4 Add 5 to 6 cups of water and 3 tablespoons of tomato sauce. Top with the bay leaves, cover and simmer for 3 to 5 hours.

Vary It! *Because fresh pumpkins aren't always available, you can substitute butternut squash or even yams for similar results with this recipe.*

Tip: *You can add another cup or two of water in Step 4 if you want a thinner stew.*

Per serving: *Calories 261; Fat 7.9 g (Saturated 2 g); Cholesterol 52 mg; Sodium 408 mg; Carbohydrate 19.1 g (Fiber 4.3 g); Protein 30.1 g; Sugar 7.1 g.*

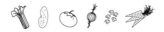

Perking Up Poultry without Ravaging Your Stomach

Some may find chicken and turkey easier to digest than beef, but crispy, fatty skin and BBQ chicken wings may trigger some symptoms of IBS-D. Luckily, you can easily remove that type of fat. All in all, chicken has the lowest fat content of any meat you may eat. The following recipes give you lots of chicken options, as well as a turkey twist on a classic.

Sabra Chicken

Chef/nutritionist Caroline Nation (www.myfoodmyhealth.com) adapted this recipe from Oded Schwartz. The marinade makes it particularly tasty, even without fat, and the sweet, tangy, salty mix of oranges and olives is particularly delicious. Make sure to dry the chicken breasts thoroughly after you remove them from the marinade to ensure even browning. This dish is a fine choice for both IBS-C and -D because chicken has very little insoluble fiber to worry about. You can easily balance potentially tricky ingredients like the olive oil and olives with a sourdough dinner roll or a soluble side (such as Basic Quinoa, Oven-Baked UnFried Rice, or Shannon's Quick "Rice" — you can find recipes for all these dishes in Chapter 12). This dish will keep in the fridge, covered, for 4 days. Take a peek at this lovely dish in the color section.

Marinating time: *2 hours*

Preparation time: *15 minutes*

Cooking time: *50 minutes*

Yield: *6 servings*

2 cups chicken stock

Zest of ½ an orange, grated or julienned

½ cup fresh orange juice

⅛ teaspoon paprika

¼ teaspoon each salt and freshly ground black pepper

Six 5-ounce chicken breasts, with skin and bones

2 tablespoons olive oil

1 medium onion, finely chopped

8 green olives, pitted

Chopped fresh mint to garnish

1 In a shallow baking dish, mix together 1 cup of the chicken stock and the zest, orange juice, and paprika with a sprinkling of salt and pepper. Add the chicken and marinate refrigerated for 2 hours, turning the chicken a couple of times to make sure it's all submerged in the marinade.

2 Remove the chicken breasts from the marinade, shake off, and pat dry thoroughly.

3 In a large skillet with sides, heat the oil over medium-high heat until your hand feels hot when held 1 inch above the pan. Add the chicken, skin side down, and cook until golden brown, about 4 minutes per side, adding more oil if the pan is too dry. Transfer the cooked chicken to a plate and set aside. Pour off all but a thin film of fat.

4 Lower the heat to medium and add the onions and the rest of the chicken stock to the skillet after a few minutes. Scrape up any brown bits and cook until the onions are translucent, about 5 minutes.

5 Return the chicken to the pan, cover, and simmer gently over low heat for another 30 minutes or until the chicken is cooked through. Transfer the chicken to a plate and tent with foil to keep hot.

6 Add the olives to the liquid, raise the heat, and cook until the sauce bubbles and thickens, about 3 to 5 minutes. Pour the sauce over the chicken. Sprinkle with the mint and serve hot.

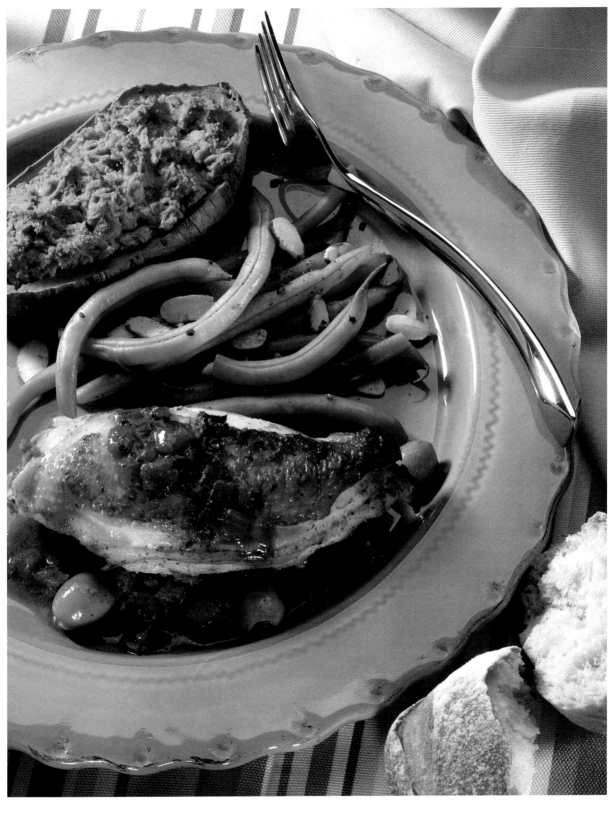

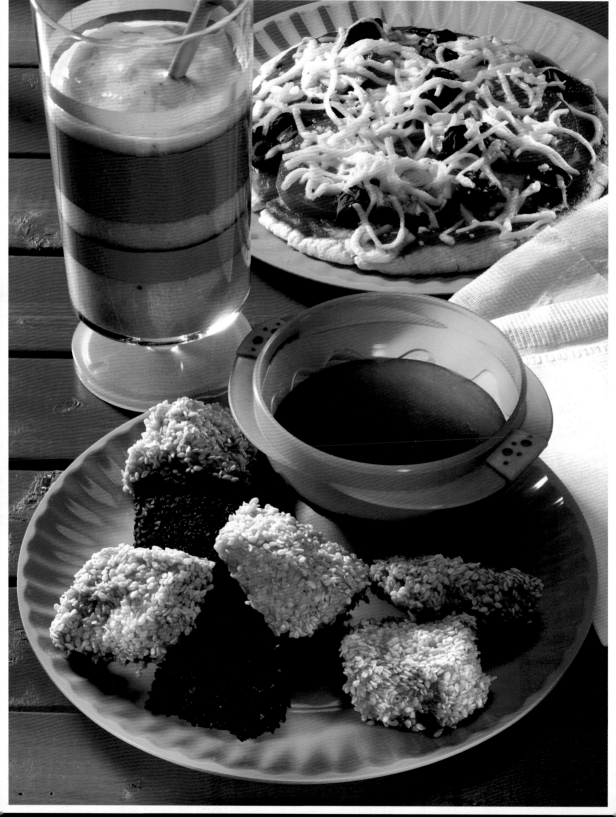

Black 'n' White Chicken Nuggets (Chapter 15), Pita Pizza (Chapter 15), and Safe and Soothing Smoothie (Chapter 9)

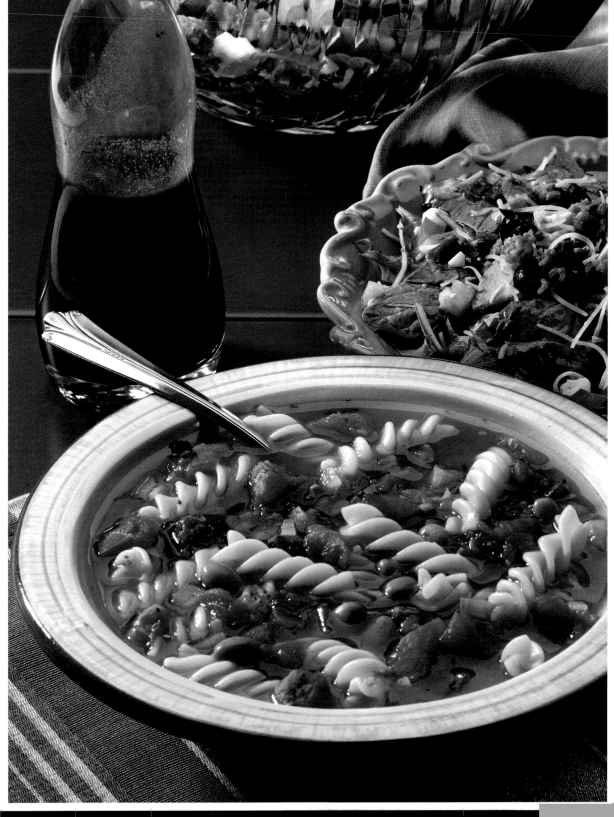

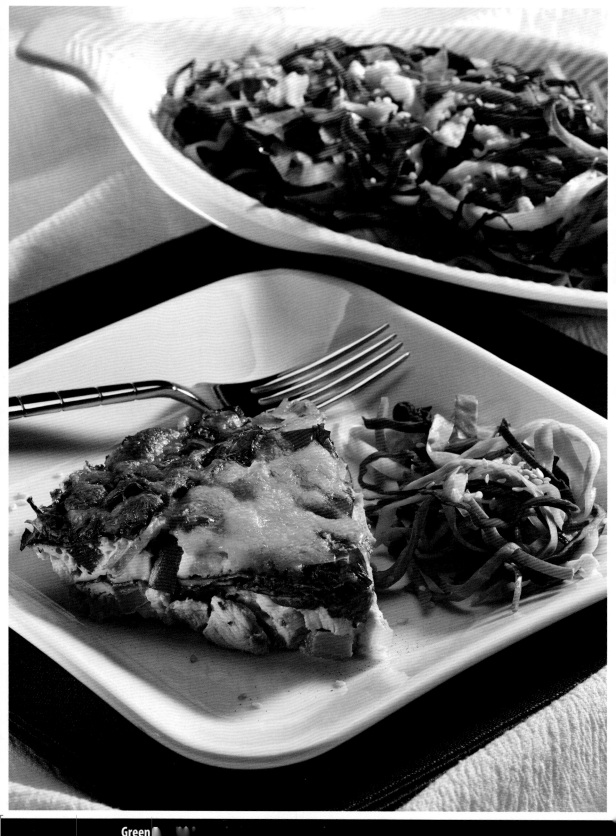

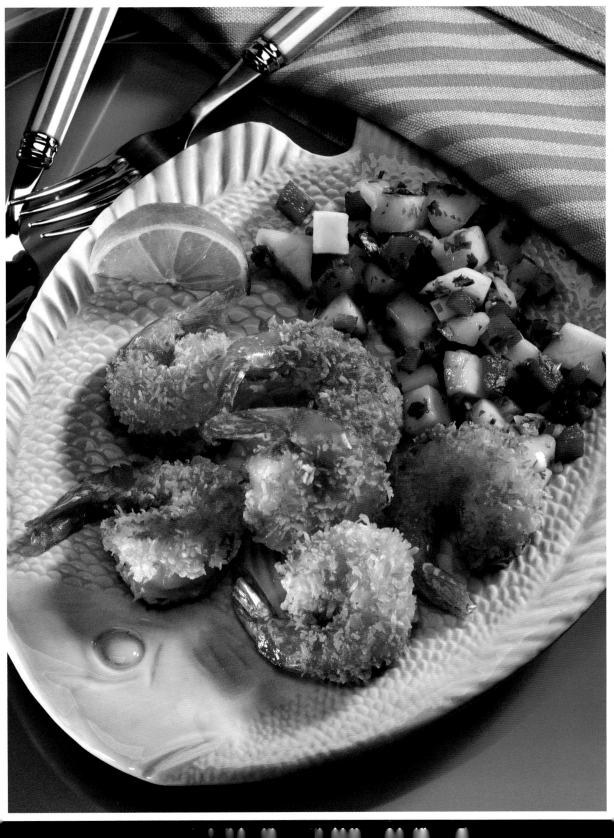

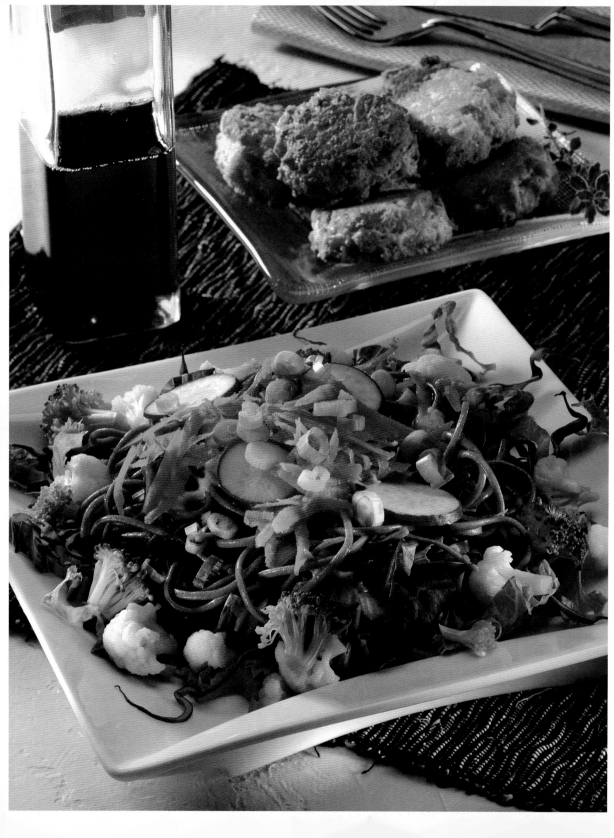

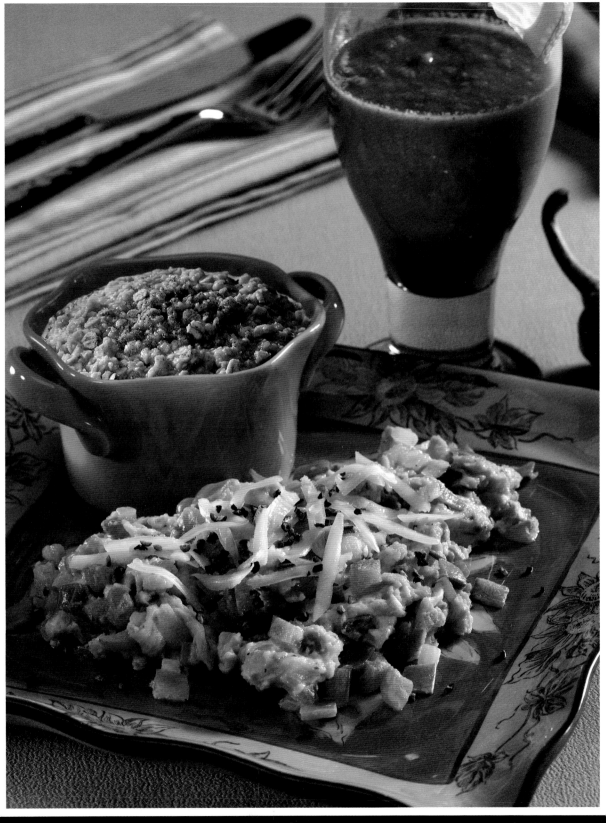

Huevos Rancheros (Chapter 6) with Strawberries and Cream Oatmeal (Chapter 6) and Lovely Bones Juice (Chapter 8)

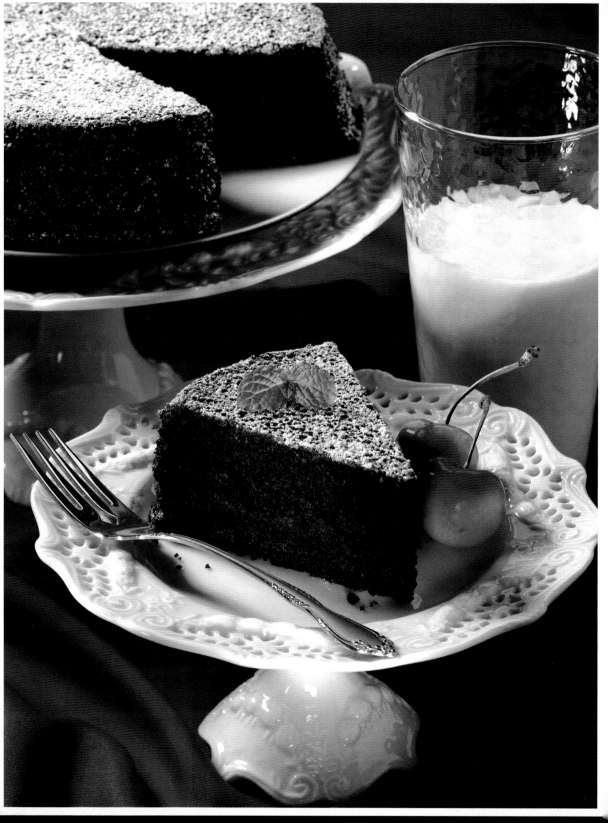

Rich and Moist Chocolate Cake (Chapter 13) and Essential Nut Milk (Chapter 8)

Vary It! *You can use vegetable stock in place of the chicken stock if that's all you have on hand.*

Per serving: Calories 315; Fat 18.1 g (Saturated 4.4 g); Cholesterol 89 mg; Sodium 301 mg; Carbohydrate 5.6 g (Fiber 0.5 g); Protein 30.2 g; Sugar 3.2 g.

Meatloaf (Turkey-Style)

Colleen Robinson (www.crimsondoorhealing.com) has adapted this family favorite for IBS sufferers by adding IBS-friendly high soluble-fiber oatmeal. Turkey has a bit more fat than chicken, but that's mainly in the skin; this recipe uses ground turkey, so the skin isn't an issue. Adding the optional tofu increases your protein intake and solubility factor. It also keeps the turkey moist, which is a bonus. For added fun, mix the ingredients with your hands; just be sure to thoroughly wash them before and after you mix.

Preparation time: 20 minutes

Cooking time: 1 hour, 30 minutes

Yield: 6 servings

2 pounds ground white-meat turkey

1 package extra-firm tofu, drained and mashed (optional)

½ cup quick-cooking rolled oats

½ cup finely chopped onions

⅓ cup finely chopped red bell pepper

1 large or 2 small eggs, gently beaten with a fork

½ teaspoon each salt, black pepper, and chili powder

1 teaspoon dried parsley, plus extra for the top

¼ cup ketchup

1 Preheat oven to 350 degrees.

2 Gently mix everything but the ketchup and cooking spray — the more you work it, the tougher the meat becomes.

3 Lightly grease a loaf pan and put the mixture into the pan, patting it down gently. Pour the ketchup on top and sprinkle with a bit more dried parsley. Bake at 325 for about 90 minutes.

Tip: *You can buy red pepper in a jar — it's more expensive, but the skin is off and it's super fast!*

Per serving: Calories 283; Fat 13.9 g (Saturated 3.8 g); Cholesterol 155 mg; Sodium 465 mg; Carbohydrate 3.4 g (Fiber 1.4 g); Protein 28.9 g; Sugar 3.4 g.

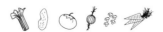

Fancy Chicken Roll-Ups

Thanks to our healing chef, Colleen Robinson (www.crimsondoorhealing.com) for this IBS-friendly version of Chicken Cordon Bleu. The low-fat chicken makes it a good option for both IBS-D and IBS-C. Asparagus is also very high in soluble fiber, but you can make it even more digestible by chopping the asparagus very finely (although you compromise the look of the dish by doing so). Soy is also high in soluble fiber.

Preparation time: *20 minutes*

Cooking time: *45 minutes*

Yield: *4 servings*

Four 5-ounce chicken breast fillets, butterflied	*1 teaspoon sea salt*
½ teaspoon butter	*1 teaspoon sage*
1 large clove garlic, minced	*1 cup chicken broth*
12 spears asparagus	*2 tablespoons flour, such as brown rice flour*
4 slices Tofutti soy cheese	

1 Preheat the oven to 350 degrees.

2 Lay the chicken fillets, cut side up, on a cutting board, dot them with butter, and sprinkle the garlic onto one side of each fillet.

3 Wash the asparagus, get rid of the ends and chop into pieces just a tiny bit longer than the chicken fillets breasts. Divide asparagus evenly among the fillets, placing them on top of the garlic and leaving the tips hanging out a little bit for enhanced appearance.

4 Place one piece of soy cheese over the asparagus on each fillet and then roll the chicken up, sealing edges with toothpicks soaked for 10 minutes in water (so they don't burn). Sprinkle the sea salt and sage over the top of each breast, crushing the sage with your fingers to break it up and release more of the flavor.

5 Pour the chicken broth in a roasting pan and add the fillets. Bake for 45 minutes, or until the juices run clear when you stick a knife in the middle of a fillet.

6 Remove the fillets and thicken the remaining pan juices with the flour to create a sauce to pour over the dish.

Vary It! *If you're avoiding soy, you can replace the soy cheese with rice cheese. If you're just avoiding the lactose, you can substitute one of these Specific Carbohydrate Diet (SCD) safe cheeses: cheddar, Colby, Swiss, or havarti*

Tip: *Butterflying chicken means that the breast has been split open and laid flat. You can buy chicken that is already flying or split it yourself.*

Per serving: *Calories 225; Fat 4.8 g (Saturated 0.9 g); Cholesterol 71 mg; Sodium 1208 mg; Carbohydrate 11.1 g (Fiber 1 g); Protein 33.3 g; Sugar 0.9 g.*

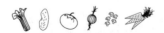

Sun-Dried and Wined Chicken

Michelle Gay in Western Australia (www.eatingjourney.wordpress.com) shared her favorite chicken recipe with us. Chicken is a safe IBS food; it has a very low fat content, and the onion, garlic, and basil in this recipe make it great for yeast-busting (see Chapter 18 for more on yeast problems). Plus, cooked onions are very high in soluble fiber, bringing the whole recipe up another notch in IBS-friendliness. Some folks feel like mushrooms shouldn't appear in a yeast-free recipe; they're high in soluble fiber, but leave them out if you prefer.

Preparation time: *15 minutes*

Cooking time: *25 minutes*

Yield: *3 servings*

3 teaspoons olive oil

2 to 3 cloves of garlic, diced

1 small onion, cut up

4 to 5 sun-dried tomatoes, diced up

4 to 6 mushrooms, sliced

Generous splash of white wine (about 3 tablespoons)

10 to 15 basil leaves

Three 5-ounce boneless, skinless chicken breasts

1 Preheat the oven to 350 degrees.

2 In a small pan, heat the oil over medium heat. Add the garlic, onion, and sun-dried tomatoes and sauté for about 3 to 4 minutes.

3 Add the mushrooms. When the mushrooms cook down to half their size (about 5 minutes), splash in white wine and cook for about 1 to 2 minutes. Turn off heat and sprinkle basil over the top of the wine mixture.

4 Measure out 3 pieces of tinfoil big enough to fully surround one chicken breast each.

5 Place one chicken breast onto each piece of foil and cover with ⅓ of the white wine mixture. Seal off the foil packets, place them on a cookie sheet, and bake them for about 20 to 25 minutes.

Vary It! *If tomato skins are irritating to your tummy and you can't find skinless sun-dried tomatoes at the store, you can substitute fresh skinless tomatoes or make your own sun-dried tomatoes. Blanch the skins off your tomatoes (you can find instructions for blanching tomatoes in Chapter 9) and then slice them into strips (discarding the seeds) and dry them in your oven on small wire cake racks (to expose the whole tomato) at 150 degrees for 10 to 15 hours. You can season with garlic powder, basil, and/or sea salt before baking if desired. A properly dried sun-dried tomato is chewy and flexible, not brittle.*

Tip: *If you don't use wine in your cooking, you can leave it out. Remember, the alcohol evaporates during cooking, leaving just the (concentrated) flavor of the wine.*

Per serving: *Calories 225; Fat 7.9 g (Saturated 1.3 g); Cholesterol 81 mg; Sodium 224 mg; Carbohydrate 7.8 g (Fiber 1.5 g); Protein 30.6 g; Sugar 3.6 g.*

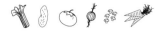

What is zest?

Zest (and we don't know why it's called that) is the outer, colorful portion of the peel of citrus fruits like limes, lemons, oranges, and tangerines. If you scrape it with your fingernail, you get an almost oily and very aromatic liquid on your finger. Zest contains aromatic oils that add a boost to certain recipes.

The trick to zesting is to scrape off the colored portion only and avoid the white *pithy* (meaning spongy, not humorous) part of the rind. Of course, that part contains bioflavonoids and is very healthy, but it's also bitter and not called for in any recipes we've heard of. You can buy a tool called a zester, or you can just use a vegetable peeler, food grater, or sharp knife to cut strips of zest (though if you go that route, you have to cut them into finer and finer strips).

Spiced Honey Chicken

This low-fat chicken dish appears in *Grain-Free Gourmet: Delicious Recipes for Healthy Living* by Jodi Bager and Jenny Lass (Whitecap Books) and became a favorite among their readers; check them out at www.grainfreegourmet.com. It may become one of your IBS favorites too; chicken is a low-fat meat, and the other ingredients shouldn't give you any trouble, although you may want to powder your almonds instead of slivering them if almonds are one of your triggers. This dish is simple to make and brings a touch of Morocco to the table. Try baking it with a head of high soluble-fiber cauliflower cut into florets to make it a one-pot meal.

Preparation time: *10 minutes*

Cooking time: *1 hour, 20 minutes*

Yield: *7 servings*

½ cup honey

2 garlic cloves, pressed

2 tablespoons plain yogurt

1 teaspoon lemon zest

1 tablespoon lemon juice

3 to 4 pounds chicken parts with bones and skin

½ teaspoon each salt and black pepper

¼ teaspoon each ground nutmeg and ground cloves

1 cup almond slivers

1 cup raisins

6 cinnamon sticks

1 Preheat the oven to 350 degrees. Place the chicken skin side up in a 10-x-15-inch casserole dish.

2 Combine the honey, garlic, yogurt, lemon rind, and lemon juice in a bowl and drizzle half of the mixture over the meat.

3 Sprinkle the meat with the salt, pepper, nutmeg, cloves, almonds, and raisins and place the cinnamon sticks evenly around the casserole dish. Pour the rest of the honey mixture over the chicken and spices.

4 Bake for 1 hour and 20 minutes, basting every 30 minutes. Check at the one hour point to test for doneness.

5 Remove from the oven and baste with the sauce before serving.

Per serving: Calories 489; Fat 14 g (Saturated 2.1 g); Cholesterol 148 mg; Sodium 341 mg; Carbohydrate 42.6 g (Fiber 2.8 g); Protein 50.4 g; Sugar 34.7 g.

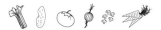

Something's Fishy: Fantastic Fish Dishes

Fish is good for your brain and for the brain in your stomach (the one that sets off your IBS), too, because of the anti-inflammatory properties of fish's omega-3 fatty acids. Fish seems to digest faster than meat or poultry, so it can be a safer food for IBS. Smaller fish are healthier for you because they eat fewer other fish and therefore ingest less mercury and fewer other toxins from increasingly polluted oceans and lakes. The best fish for your main course is wild Alaska salmon.

In *IBS For Dummies* (Wiley), we talk about *serotonin,* the feel-good neurotransmitter that's mostly found in the gut. In fact, 90 percent of the serotonin in the whole body is found in the gut, making up what is referred to as "the second brain."

Seared Salmon with Sautéed Summer Vegetables

Ela Guidon, a New York personal chef, whole-food educator, cooking instructor, and health counselor originally from Peru, contributed this quick, easy, colorful, and easy-to-digest recipe. You can find her at www.myfoodmyhealth.com/OurChefs/index.php?chefid=17.

The vegetable fiber in this recipe is made more digestible by steaming and sautéing. Cooked carrots, cucumber, and peppers have a high soluble-fiber content, more so than broccoli. To make the recipe even more IBS-friendly, you can steam the broccoli for 6 minutes, or use less broccoli and substitute more of the other vegetables. The fiber content of radish is unclear, so you can leave that vegetable out or chop it finely. You may also offset the insoluble fiber in this recipe with soluble sides such as basmati rice, millet, or sourdough white or manna bread. Make sure you pay attention to your timer so you don't overcook the salmon.

Preparation time: *10 minutes*

Cooking time: *15 to 20 minutes*

Yield: *4 servings*

3 cups broccoli florets

1 tablespoon olive oil

1 carrot, peeled and cut into ¼-inch-thick rounds

1 yellow pepper, chopped

1 red pepper, chopped

1 cucumber, peeled, seeded, and cut into 2-inch spears

1 bunch of radishes (about 5 radishes), quartered and keeping some of the greens attached

1 teaspoon lemon juice

4 basil leaves, chopped

¼ teaspoon salt

1 teaspoon coconut oil

Four 5-ounce salmon fillets

1 Steam the broccoli florets for 3 to 6 minutes and set aside.

2 In a large skillet heat the olive oil. Add the carrot and sauté for 1 to 3 minutes. Add the peppers, broccoli, cucumber, and radishes and sauté for 1 to 3 minutes. Remove to a bowl and sprinkle with lemon juice, basil, and salt.

3 Heat the coconut oil in a skillet over medium-high heat. Season the salmon with salt and then add it to the skillet searing for about 4 minutes on each side. At 8 minutes, check to make sure the salmon is cooked through. If not, cook one more minute on each side.

4 Serve the salmon on top of the sautéed vegetables.

Tip: *Squeeze more fresh lemon juice over your dish for added flavor.*

Tip: *You can serve the veggies in this recipe with any meat dish.*

Per serving: *Calories 517; Fat 31.7 g (Saturated 4.6 g); Cholesterol 109 mg; Sodium 160 mg; Carbohydrate 14.1 g (Fiber 3.9 g); Protein 43.9 g; Sugar 4.7 g.*

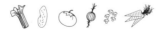

Herbed Tilapia with Lime

This recipe comes from Raman Prasad's *Recipes for the Specific Carbohydrate Diet*™ (Fair Winds Press). Visit Raman at his Web site (www.scdrecipe.com/cookbook). You can also use other kinds of white fish for this recipe, but you may need to reduce the cooking time accordingly if the fish fillets are thinner.

Tilapia is a very soft type of fish that doesn't require too much fuss; just be careful not to overcook it. It's a low-fat fish, and the seasonings in this recipe are safe for IBS, so this dish is a very IBS-friendly meal.

Preparation time: *5 minutes*

Cooking time: *15 minutes*

Yield: *2 servings*

1 tablespoon olive oil

⅛ teaspoon each thyme and dried basil

¼ teaspoon salt

Two 6-ounce tilapia fillets

Juice of ½ a lime (about ⅛ cup)

1 Heat the olive oil over medium heat in a stovetop pan.

2 Sprinkle the thyme, basil, and salt equally on both sides of the fillets. Add the fillets to the pan and cook for 5 to 7 minutes on each side, or until cooked through.

3 Place on serving plates, sprinkle the lime juice over the fillets, and serve.

Tip: *Mango Salsa makes a great side for this recipe — see the recipe in Chapter 7.*

Per serving: *Calories 228; Fat 9.7 g (Saturated 2.2 g); Cholesterol 86 mg; Sodium 380 mg; Carbohydrate 6.5 g (Fiber 0.2 g); Protein 34.4 g; Sugar 0.2 g.*

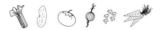

Panko: Fancy flake or basic crumb?

Although panko has been elevated to exotic status and prices in food circles, it's basically just crumbed stale bread. But panko is said to be lighter, crispier, and crunchier than Western bread crumbs, with a coarser grind and more surface area to absorb spices and seasonings. Panko's other purported powers include a lacy, airy layering of breading; a surface that doesn't absorb grease as easily; and the ability to create a great crusty topping under the broiler. You can find panko in most foodie stores and even some supermarkets, and the nearby recipe for Coconut Panko Shrimp shows you how to make your own flakes.

Coconut Panko Shrimp

Marilyn Jansen is an artist, writer, and chef Carolyn sees every Saturday morning at the farmer's market in Kahului, Maui. She contributed this recipe from her book *Amaryllis of Hawaii Loves to Cook: Recipes for Life* (Amaryllisofhawaii). You can find Marilyn at www.amaryllisofhawaii.com.

Shrimp is IBS-friendly, the eggs are fiber free, and the fat in the yolk is balanced by the healing properties of coconut, so this recipe, which is featured in the color section, shouldn't give your stomach any trouble. To make it even more of an IBS delight, make your own panko flakes from sourdough white bread. You can also add extra coconut flakes for IBS-D.

Preparation time: *20 minutes*

Cooking time: *8 minutes*

Yield: *4 servings*

2 pounds large or jumbo shrimp, tail on and deveined

½ cup rough or fine panko flakes (see the following recipe or use store-bought)

One 4-ounce bag sweetened coconut flakes

4 eggs, lightly beaten

1 cup coconut oil

1 Butterfly the shrimp and set aside in a bowl. Combine the panko flakes and coconut flakes in a bowl and put the eggs in a separate bowl.

2 Dip the shrimp into the egg and then panko/coconut mixture and place on a platter. When all the shrimp are dressed and ready to go, heat the coconut oil in a skillet over medium-high heat.

3 Add several shrimp to the skillet, leaving room to turn them when one side is golden brown. Cook for about 2 minutes on each side; remove and drain thoroughly on several layers of paper towel. Repeat for the rest of the shrimp.

Per serving: Calories 950; Fat 71.6 g (Saturated 61.8 g); Cholesterol 654 mg; Sodium 759 mg; Carbohydrate 23.9 g (Fiber 3.2 g); Protein 56.5 g; Sugar 11.3 g.

Panko

Preparation time: *5 minutes*

Cooking time: *20 minutes to 1 hour*

Yield: *3 cups*

1 loaf of day-old French or sourdough white bread

1 Preheat the oven to 150 degrees. Remove the bread crusts and rub or flake the bread into crumbs by rubbing it between your hands or using a cheese grater; you should get about 3 cups of crumbs.

2 Spread the crumbs onto baking sheets and dry in the oven for about an hour or until crunchy but not browned at all — start checking after 20 minutes. Store panko in plastic zippered bags in the fridge or glass jars inside or outside the fridge.

Tip: *To test whether your oil is hot enough for frying, place one coated shrimp into the hot oil to see whether the oil bubbles and sizzles.*

Tip: *If you're making your own panko, don't use a knife or food processor to flake; your crumbs will either be too big or completely powdered.*

Per cup: Calories 272; Fat 1.8 g (Saturated 0.4 g); Cholesterol 0 mg; Sodium 613 mg; Carbohydrate 52.7 g (Fiber 2.6 g); Protein 11 g; Sugar 3.1 g.

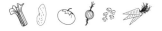

Easy Chicken Curry

A taste for curry can become addictive, but horror stories of gut-burning curry flood IBS forums. Thanks to our healing chef Colleen Robinson at www.crimsondoorhealing.com, we may have a solution to your curry needs. This recipe contains mostly soluble ingredients like onion, raisins, and potatoes that are easier to digest when they're all cooked. Cumin, cinnamon, and cardamom are spices known to help treat IBS, and good yogurt is lactose-free and soothing to the gut. The addition of some mild curry is enough to give you the taste but not the torture. Enjoy!

Preparation time: *10 minutes*

Cooking time: *25 minutes*

Yield: *4 servings*

½ tablespoon olive oil

1 to 1½ pounds white-meat chicken breast, cut into chunks

1 medium onion (optional)

¼ cup golden raisins (optional)

1 cup cooked potatoes, chopped into about 1-inch squares

½ teaspoon each cumin, cinnamon, and cardamom

1 teaspoon mild yellow curry powder

1 cup plain yogurt (see Chapter 6 for IBS yogurt recipes)

½ teaspoon salt

¼ teaspoon pepper

1 Heat the olive oil in a large pot over medium-high heat. When the pot is hot, add the chicken and quick-fry on both sides (less than one minute on each side — you don't need to worry about cooking it through yet). Set the chicken aside.

2 Add the onions, raisins (if desired), and potatoes to the pot and cook for about 5 minutes, stirring occasionally. Lower the heat to medium and add the cumin, cinnamon, cardamom, and curry powder. Cook, stirring occasionally, for about a minute to wake up the flavors in the spices.

3 Add the quick-fried chicken and cook until cooked through (about 10 to 15 minutes depending on the chunk size — to check, cut a piece in half; if it's not pink, you're safe). Add the yogurt and lower heat to medium-low. Cook, stirring continuously, until thick — about 5 minutes. Serve over rice or miracle noodles.

Vary It! *To turn this into a shrimp curry, thaw and chunk 1 to 1½ pounds of frozen shrimp. Follow the chicken recipe (minus the chicken, of course), but use 2 teaspoons of curry powder in Step 2 and allow that mixture to simmer for 5 minutes before adding the shrimp and cooking over medium heat until the shrimp are warm. Add the yogurt and finish the recipe as you would for chicken.*

Tip: *Be careful not to boil the yogurt — it'll curdle. It doesn't affect the taste, but it does mess with the texture and appearance.*

Tip: *Some people say a curry has to have onions, but if you can't stomach them, an onion-free curry is a very different but yummy experience. Who says you have to follow the rules?*

Tip: *The safest way to thaw precooked shrimp is in the fridge, which takes a few hours or overnight. A lot of people thaw it in cold water, which is faster but not necessarily the safest way. If you decide to thaw in cold water, keep the shrimp in a sealed plastic bag to keep bacteria out and to prevent the shrimp from absorbing water and getting soggy. Submerge the sealed bag in a bowl of cold water; your shrimp should thaw in an hour or so.*

Per serving: *Calories 281; Fat 8.5 g (Saturated 2.8 g); Cholesterol 122 mg; Sodium 449 mg; Carbohydrate 11.9 g (Fiber 1.3 g); Protein 37.6 g; Sugar 3.2 g.*

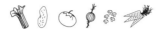

Pasta Imposters: Getting that Pasta Feeling without the Side Effects

You may think your pasta days are over if you discover you have to avoid wheat, but that's certainly not the case. You can find several non-wheat alternatives in your grocery and health food stores, such as brown rice pasta, kamut pasta, quinoa pasta, and miracle noodles; just add your favorite pesto or marinara sauce. Or you can create a whole new world of pasta with zucchini. The following recipes help you get your IBS-friendly pasta fix.

◌ Zucchini Lasagna

Chef Kendall Conrad (www.eatwellfeelwellthebook.com) finds that this dish is a great one to make with kids. You can put all of the ingredients in separate bowls and let the children assemble their own servings just how they like 'em.

Zucchini has a good soluble fiber rating for IBS, as do mushrooms and peppers. Don't be daunted by the display of cheeses in this recipe. They're all low-lactose and safe on the SCD.

Tools: *Mandoline*

Preparation time: *20 minutes*

Cooking time: *45 minutes*

Yield: *6 servings*

2 zucchinis, peeled and trimmed

1 cup farmer's cheese, crumbled

1 cup Asiago cheese, freshly grated

1 cup Monterey Jack cheese, freshly grated

1 cup Parmesan cheese, freshly grated

1 cup Classic Tomato Sauce (see the following recipe)

¼ cup of olive oil

1 Preheat the oven to 375 degrees. Using a mandoline, slice the zucchinis lengthwise into long, thin slices and set aside. Put each cheese and the tomato sauce into its own bowl.

2 Spread ½ cup of the tomato sauce in a casserole pan. Layer in some zucchini and drizzle olive oil on top. Sprinkle the cheeses on top of the zucchini (in any order you want) and repeat the process, creating several layers until all the ingredients are used, ending with the Parmesan. Top with the remaining tomato sauce.

3 Bake for 40 to 45 minutes or until bubbling on top. Let stand for 15 minutes to set the melted cheese and then slice and serve.

Vary It! *This lasagna is pretty cheesy. If you want to break some of that cheesiness up, you can also add sautéed mushrooms, sliced olives, sautéed ground beef or chicken, prosciutto, capers, and/or bell peppers (although adding meat makes the recipe non-vegetarian).*

Per serving: Calories 574; Fat 46.6 g (Saturated 23.5 g); Cholesterol 110 mg; Sodium 901 mg; Carbohydrate 5.7 g (Fiber 2.7 g); Protein 33.6 g; Sugar 1.2 g.

Classic Tomato Sauce

This great classic tomato sauce is meant for Kendall's Zucchini Lasagna, but it can also be your base for pizzas, mock pastas, and casseroles. Removing the skins from the tomatoes (see the sidebar in Chapter 9), the recipe is very IBS-friendly. You can store it in a big jar in the refrigerator for 1 week or in plastic bags in the freezer for 3 months.

Tools: *Hand blender (optional)*

Preparation time: *15 minutes*

Cooking time: *1 hour, 15 minutes*

Yield: *Twelve ½-cup servings (6 cups total)*

4 tablespoons olive oil

½ cup chopped onion

6 cloves chopped garlic

1 carrot, chopped

⅛ teaspoon each sea salt and freshly cracked pepper

Two 28-ounce cans or cartons Italian no-sugar-added whole tomatoes

1 bay leaf

2 tablespoons unsalted butter

1 big handful (about 1 cup) fresh basil

1 In a large saucepan, heat the oil over medium-high heat; add the onions and cook until they're translucent, about 5 minutes. Add the garlic and cook for one minute. Add the carrot, salt, and pepper and cook for 10 minutes, stirring occasionally to prevent burning.

2 Add the tomatoes and bay leaf and simmer for 1 hour uncovered. Remove the bay leaf and add the butter. Puree in a food processor in batches (to avoid a saucy explosion), adding basil into each batch. Or use a hand (immersion) blender if you have one handy (no pun intended).

Per serving: *Calories 87; Fat 6.6 g (Saturated 1.9 g); Cholesterol 5 mg; Sodium 218 mg; Carbohydrate 7 g (Fiber 1.7 g); Protein 1.3 g; Sugar 3.7 g.*

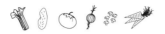

☙ Eggplant Lasagna

Michelle Gay (www.eatingjourney.wordpress.com) in Western Australia shares this hearty yet meatless lasagna recipe It does contain more insoluble fiber than soluble fiber, so it's probably more suitable for IBS-C than IBS-D. However, you can make the eggplant friendlier by peeling off the skin. The more thinly you slice the pumpkin, the better you can digest it. The marinara sauce uses skinless tomatoes, which makes it work for anyone with IBS; it's also SCD-friendly. (The sauce is great in many other dishes as well; you can even use it as a ketchup substitute.)

Roasting time: 15 minutes

Preparation time: 15 minutes

Cooking time: 25 minutes

Yield: 4 servings

1 large eggplant	2 cups Marinara Sauce (see the following recipe)
¼ of a medium pumpkin	
⅛ teaspoon each salt and pepper	7 ounces SCD-safe cheddar cheese

1 Slice the eggplant into about ¼-inch round pieces and thinly slice the pumpkin.

2 Preheat the oven to 425 degrees.

3 Place the pumpkin on tinfoil on a flat baking sheet and roast it for 15 minutes. While it's roasting, season the eggplant with salt and pepper and add it to the baking sheet after the pumpkin has roasted for about 5 minutes, so that the eggplant roasts for about 10 minutes and finishes at about the same time as the pumpkin. You can also roast them on separate sheets. Cool them down on a rack when they're done.

4 After the eggplant and pumpkin are cool, oil a baking dish and assemble the lasagna in the following order: sauce, eggplant, pumpkin, and cheese. Repeat the layering, making sure you end up with cheese on top. Bake for 20 to 25 minutes or until the cheese is melted.

Vary It! *You can use SCD-safe Colby, Swiss, or havarti cheese in place of the cheddar cheese.*

Per serving: Calories 326; Fat 18.4 g (Saturated 10.8 g); Cholesterol 52 mg; Sodium 650 mg; Carbohydrate 27.3 g (Fiber 8.4 g); Protein 17.2 g; Sugar 11.7 g.

Marinara Sauce

Preparation time: *10 minutes*

Cooking time: *3 hours*

Yield: *Eight ½-cup servings (4 cups total)*

2 teaspoons olive oil

1 small onion, diced

4 cloves garlic, pressed

4 to 6 mushrooms, chopped

1 small red pepper, diced

⅓ to ½ of a chili pepper, diced

⅓ to ½ of a zucchini, diced

2 to 3 fresh tomatoes, diced

Two 15-ounce cans skinless stewed tomatoes, juice included

2 tablespoons tomato paste

1 Heat the olive oil in a large frying pan. Add the onion and garlic and sauté for 5 minutes. You can add a tablespoon or two of water rather than more oil during this process to prevent sticking.

2 Add the mushrooms and red pepper and sauté for another 5 minutes.

3 Add the chili, zucchini, fresh tomatoes, stewed tomatoes, and tomato paste; cover and simmer on very low heat for 2 to 3 hours.

Tip: *Keep this sauce on hand to add to all kinds of dishes. Try it on turkey meatloaf (see the Meatloaf (Turkey-Style) recipe earlier in this chapter), pasta, rice, lentils, or beans.*

Tip: *Skin your own tomatoes by using the blanching technique in Chapter 9.*

Per serving: *Calories 62; Fat 1.5 g (Saturated 0.2 g); Cholesterol 0 mg; Sodium 265 mg; Carbohydrate 11.2 g (Fiber 2.1 g); Protein 2.2 g; Sugar 6.2 g.*

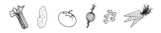

🍑 Shannon's Gourmet Zucchini Angel-Hair "Pasta"

Thanks to Shannon Leone from www.rawmom.com for this offering. It does contain a lot of raw vegetable ingredients and a fair amount of insoluble fiber, so it's best for those who know they can tolerate raw veggies well. To minimize the effects of the insoluble fiber, eat this meal with a soluble-fiber side of miracle noodles or sourdough white bread (see the recipe in Chapter 12). To minimize the fat (a common IBS trigger) in olives, use olives packed in water rather than oil. And, as always, chew well!

To make this dish, we recommend using a spiralizer or mandoline slicer. A *spiralizer* (also known as The Garnishing Machine or saladacco) may be new to you, but it's a great way to slice up zucchini pasta or any other vegetable. The thin slicing makes digestion easier. But if you don't have a spiralizer or mandoline, just grate the zucchini, or even peel it with a peeler for a flat fettuccine-type "noodle."

Tools: *Spiralizer or mandoline (optional)*

Preparation time: *15 minutes*

Cooking time: *None*

Yield: *4 servings*

1 large or 2 medium green or yellow zucchinis

12 black olives, pitted

1 cup tiny broccoli florets

4 sun-dried tomatoes, sliced

1 to 2 fresh tomatoes, finely diced

1 tablespoon balsamic vinegar

1 clove of garlic, minced

3 oyster mushrooms, sliced

¼ teaspoon each sea salt and cracked pepper, or to taste

⅛ teaspoon oregano, or to taste

1 Cut the zucchini into thin strips with a spiralizer, mandoline, grater, or vegetable peeler and set aside on a large serving platter.

2 Toss the olives, broccoli, and both kinds of tomatoes with the vinegar and garlic in a bowl. Add the olive mixture to the mushrooms, salt, pepper, and oregano.

3 Top the zucchini "pasta" with the olive-mushroom mixture and serve.

Tip: *If this recipe isn't saucy enough for you, add our Marinara Sauce (see the recipe earlier in this chapter).*

Per serving: *Calories 106; Fat 1.7 g (Saturated 0.2 g); Cholesterol 0 mg; Sodium 328 mg; Carbohydrate 17.3 g (Fiber 5.7 g); Protein 6.5 g; Sugar 6.3 g.*

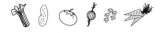

Making it a Meal: Other Hearty Main Dishes

Some dishes are just so filling that they're meals in themselves — no side dish necessary (although you can certainly add one). This section gives you recipes that'll make you forget you ever thought you could only eat rice and white bread. We also include a pizza meal that you can customize a million different ways.

Quinoa Casserole with Baked Sweet Potatoes

Preparation time: *5 minutes*

Cooking time: *60 minutes*

Yield: *4 servings*

4 sweet potatoes	½ teaspoon thyme
1 tablespoon of ghee, or coconut oil or butter (see recipe in Chapter 6)	1 cup diced zucchini
	1 cup sliced mushrooms
1 small onion, diced	1 cup frozen peas
2 chopped garlic cloves	2 cups chicken stock
1 carrot, diced	3 cups cooked quinoa
½ teaspoon turmeric	

1 Preheat the oven to 400 degrees.

2 Bake the sweet potatoes for 50 to 60 minutes. Cool, remove the skin, slice the potatoes, and set aside.

3 While the potatoes bake, heat the ghee or oil in a 12-inch sauté pan over medium heat and sauté the onions until translucent. Add the garlic and carrot and cook for 1 minute.

4 Add the turmeric, thyme, zucchini, mushrooms, peas, chicken stock, and cooked quinoa. Bring to boil and simmer for 10 minutes, stirring to prevent sticking.

5 Serve with slices of baked sweet potatoes and sprinkle on more herbs if you crave more spiciness.

Per serving: Calories 404; Fat 7.6 g (Saturated 2.4 g); Cholesterol 12 mg; Sodium 305 mg; Carbohydrate 70.9 g (Fiber 10.9 g); Protein 14.3 g; Sugar 11.8 g.

☞ Creamy Vegan Stroganoff with Caramelized Onions

This stroganoff by chef Andrea Boje (www.myfoodmyhealth.com/OurChefs/index.php?chefid=23) is dairy- and gluten-free (unlike its Russian ancestor). The combination of miso and lemon juice in the "sour cream" really makes it taste like the dairy version. The brown rice fettuccine, the onions, and the tofu in the sour cream make this dish a high soluble-fiber recipe good for anyone with IBS.

Andrea recommends using Tinkyada brand Brown Rice Fettuccini (and Christine agrees). Reduce the package-direction cooking time to 8 minutes to keep the noodles al dente. The noodles will absorb some liquid from the sauce, so you want to have them a little underdone at the beginning.

Tools: *Garlic press (optional)*

Preparation time: *7 minutes*

Cooking time: *24 minutes*

Yield: *4 servings*

2 tablespoons olive oil

1 large yellow onion, sliced from root to tip in long slices

½ cup white wine

7 ounces brown rice fettuccine, cooked and drained

1 cup tofu "Sour Cream" (see the following recipe)

2 cups tempeh, cubed

Salt and pepper to taste (optional)

½ cup olive oil-fried gluten-free breadcrumbs

1 Heat the oil in a large frying pan over medium heat. Add onions and sauté until slightly brown, about 15 minutes. Add wine and continue cooking until liquid reduces a little.

2 Reduce the heat to the lowest setting and add the cooked fettuccine to the wine mixture. Toss to coat the noodles.

3 Pour 1 cup of tofu "sour cream" into the pan and stir. Add the tempeh and continue to warm over low heat, seasoning with salt and pepper to taste (if desired).

4 Pour the noodles into a serving dish and garnish with fried gluten-free bread crumbs.

"Sour Cream"

One 12-ounce package silken tofu

2 teaspoons umeboshi vinegar

2 tablespoons plus 1 teaspoon white miso

1 teaspoon salt

½ teaspoon freshly cracked pepper

2 medium garlic cloves, minced or crushed in garlic press

1 tablespoon lemon juice

2 tablespoons olive oil (optional)

1 Blend tofu, vinegar, miso, salt, pepper, garlic, and lemon juice in a blender on high until smooth. If the mixture is too thick, begin adding the olive oil a little at a time until the cream moves freely.

2 Adjust seasonings to taste.

Vary It! *For a non-vegan alternative, substitute 2 cups of chopped cooked chicken for the tempeh. The chicken is low-fat and has no fiber, so it works well for IBS. Add it to the dish at the same time you would the tempeh.*

Tip: *Use homemade panko flakes (see the recipe in Coconut Panko Shrimp earlier in this chapter) in place of the breadcrumbs; they don't need to be fried, which makes them more IBS-friendly. And you can use gluten-free bread for the panko if you want to keep the recipe gluten-free.*

Tip: *The sour cream lasts in the refrigerator for about a week and a half. The finished stroganoff will be good for 2 to 3 days; after that, the noodles continue to get mushy as they sit in the sauce. If you know ahead of time that you're going to save some of the dish for later, keep the sour cream out of that part of the dish until you're ready to reheat. Reheat in a small frying pan with a little oil or butter over low heat for 5 minutes, stirring once.*

Per serving: *Calories 239; Fat 7.1 g (Saturated 0 g); Cholesterol 0 mg; Sodium 4770 mg; Carbohydrate 17.9 g (Fiber 3.9 g); Protein 18.1 g; Sugar 0.4 g.*

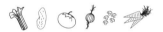

You put the knife in the coconut . . .

Living in Maui, Carolyn sees coconuts being dismembered every week at the local farmer's market. Fearless souls hold ripe coconuts in their hands and machete off the outer green rind, somehow managing to leave their hands intact. Then they slice across the top and make a hole for a straw so you can drink the liquid. After that's gone (and it takes a while because one coconut holds a lot of juice), another deft swipe with the knife splits the nut in half for you to scoop out a thin, jelly-like layer of pure white pulp. Left to dry, a *denuded* (with it's green rind removed) coconut becomes the brown, shriveled-up, dried coconut on the mainland.

If your machete is in the shop, never fear. Here's how contributing chef Angela Elliot opens about eight coconuts a day with common tools:

1. **Pick your nut, one without any soft spots, wet spots, or signs of spoilage.**

2. **Hold the coconut on its side, with the conical top toward your knife hand.**

3. **Using a large chef's knife, trim away the cone to reveal the rounded shell underneath.** This inner shell is the part you get when you buy a mature coconut that's all dried up.

4. **Set the coconut on its bottom; using the heel of your knife or, even more safely, a hammer, strike the place where the inner shell meets the thick outer rind at a 45-degree angle.** If you hit it hard enough, the shell should crack so that you can flip it back like a lid.

5. **Pour out the liquid (it should be clear or just very slightly yellowish) and scoop out the flesh.**

Vegetarian Dreamy Coconut Curry

Thanks to Angela Elliott (www.she-zencuisine.com) for this sensational, exotic concoction. Look for young coconuts at Asian grocery stores; you can also substitute four 14-ounce cans of coconut milk and 1 cup of shredded coconut. Coconut is thought to be very healing for the gut, and onions and carrots are high in soluble fiber. If you want to make the recipe even more IBS-friendly, you can substitute white basmati rice for the wild rice and use only 1 tablespoon of mild curry powder.

Preparation time: *30 minutes*

Cooking time: *45 minutes*

Yield: *6 servings*

4 Thai young coconuts, water (6⅔ cups liquid total) and meat	¼ teaspoon Celtic salt, or to taste
2 cloves of garlic	2 tablespoons yellow curry powder
2 tablespoons Thai basil	1 hot green chili pepper
Juice of ½ a lemon (about ⅛ cup)	1 fresh lemongrass stick
½ cup cilantro	¾ cup julienned carrot
3 green onions	¾ cup julienned Asian cabbage
	½ cup soaked and drained wild rice

1 In a blender, blend everything except the lemongrass stick, julienned vegetables, and rice. Transfer the blended curry to a double boiler, add the lemongrass stick, and gently warm. Cover and cook for 30 minutes.

2 Remove the lemongrass stick and check the consistency of the curry. Add water or coconut juice as necessary to thin it out. Add the julienned veggies and rice; the curry should still be warm and ready to serve.

Tip: *A double boiler (a pot of boiling water with a bowl or another pot on top) helps you control the heat in the top pot, but it isn't necessary here. If you don't want to mess with a double boiler, just use a regular pot over low heat.*

Per serving: *Calories 668; Fat 56.1 g (Saturated 49.3 g); Cholesterol 0 mg; Sodium 219 mg; Carbohydrate 42.1 g (Fiber 18.1 g); Protein 8.9 g; Sugar 13.9 g.*

Gourmet Pizza

You may have thought you had to give up pizza forever because of your IBS, but thanks to Jodi Bager and Jenny Lass at www.grainfreegourmet.com, pizza is back on the menu. This delectable recipe features an almond-flour pizza crust that appeared in their book, *Grain-Free Gourmet: Delicious Recipes for Healthy Living* (Whitecap Books). It's an SCD recipe, so it's safe for IBS (as well as colitis and Crohn's disease). The almond flour is much easier to digest and less irritating to the intestines in its pulverized form; the cheese is virtually lactose-free; and you can buy skinless tomato sauce or make your own blanched tomatoes (see Chapter 9) and marinara sauce (from the Marinara Sauce recipe earlier in this chapter).

This pizza takes minutes to throw together and tastes gourmet! You can eat it straight out of the oven, at room temperature on the go, or cold the next day. Toss your leftovers in your lunch bag — the whole office will be envious.

Tools: *Parchment paper*

Preparation time: *10 minutes*

Cooking time: *20 minutes*

Yield: *1 serving*

½ cup almond flour

1 tablespoon plus 1 cup grated Parmesan cheese

¼ teaspoon salt

½ teaspoon dried basil

½ teaspoon dried oregano

¼ teaspoon dried thyme (optional)

1 teaspoon olive oil, plus more for greasing the baking sheet and drizzling

1 large egg

¼ cup tomato sauce, or to taste depending on your level of tomato sensitivity

¼ to ½ cup each of mushrooms, red peppers, zucchini, and onions

1 Preheat the oven to 325 degrees. Line a cookie sheet with parchment paper and grease with olive oil.

2 Combine the almond flour, 1 tablespoon of the Parmesan, and the salt, basil, oregano, thyme (if desired), olive oil, and egg in a mixing bowl until the dough is the consistency of cookie batter.

3 Spread the dough thinly into a 6-to-8-inch circle on the cookie sheet. Top with tomato paste or sauce, spread on your pizza toppings, and sprinkle generously with parmesan cheese.

4 Drizzle olive oil over the pizza and bake for 18 to 20 minutes.

Vary It! *To get a thin-crust pizza, make the dough and flatten it with a rolling pin between two pieces of parchment paper or plastic wrap until it's the appropriate diameter.*

Vary It! *The toppings here are just suggestions; use any IBS-friendly pizza toppings of your choice.*

Tip: *Freeze the pizza dough for almost instant pizza. Flatten your prepared dough with a rolling pin between parchment paper or plastic wrap and then freeze the flattened dough, still between the parchment paper or plastic wrap, in a plastic freezer bag or sealed container to prevent freezer burn. No need to thaw before baking — just add the sauce and toppings, and bake at 325 degrees for 20 minutes.*

Per serving: *Calories 1072; Fat 81.6 g (Saturated 24 g); Cholesterol 304 mg; Sodium 2586 mg; Carbohydrate 31.1 g (Fiber 6.2 g); Protein 61.9 g; Sugar 9.3 g.*

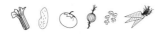

Pesto without the Pain

Thanks to Colleen Robinson (www.crismondoorhealing.com) for this creamy pesto that doesn't irritate an IBS gut. You can use it on pasta, rice, or slathered on your nut pâté wraps. Basil and parsley are high in antioxidants and vitamins, and basil and garlic are anti-microbial herbs, which can be helpful in reducing yeast or bacterial overgrowth in the intestines that may be a trigger for IBS symptoms. To make up for the insoluble fiber in garlic, basil, parsley, and almonds, pair your pesto with a high soluble-fiber pasta or rice.

Preparation time: *10 minutes*

Cooking time: *None*

Yield: *Sixteen 2-tablespoon servings (2 cups total)*

2 cloves of garlic	*⅓ cup lemon juice*
½ cup almonds	*¼ cup olive oil*
1 cup fresh basil leaves, lightly packed	*⅓ cup chicken broth*
1 cup fresh parsley, lightly packed	

1 In a food processor or blender, mix the garlic and almonds until they form a chunky paste. Add the basil and parsley and blend again. Add the lemon juice and blend again.

2 Drizzle in the olive oil slowly until you have a nice puree. Add the chicken broth and blend until it's well incorporated.

Tip: If you don't serve the whole batch at once freeze it in ice cube trays and thaw out a few cubes at a time for a fast topping over your next meal.

Tip: You can use any nut for a nutty flavor, including macadamia or walnuts.

Per serving: Calories 61; Fat 5.7 g (Saturated 0.7 g); Cholesterol 0.06 mg; Sodium 43 mg; Carbohydrate 1.8 g (Fiber 0.7 g); Protein 1.4 g; Sugar 0.4 g.

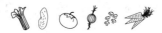

Chapter 12

Siding with Side Dishes

*O*ne definition of a side dish is a dish served with, but subordinate to, a main course. We don't think our sides are subordinate to anything, so we prefer to think of them as dishes that accompany, complete, or accentuate the entrée or main course at a meal.

Our side dishes can give you lots of variety with your meals, especially if you feel like you have limited choice in your main dishes. We've made them IBS-friendly by choosing gluten-free, dairy-free, and soluble-fiber ingredients to create them.

Sizing Up Soluble Fiber in Sides

Sides that are loaded with soluble fiber help balance the insoluble fiber in your diet. Because sides are often heavy on grains and vegetables, you can easily choose options that are at least 50 percent soluble fiber (which should be your goal).

So with a wealth of soluble fiber ingredients to choose from for your side dishes, where do you start? We know the old standby is homemade white sourdough bread (and we provide a recipe for that later in this chapter), but we want you to have many other delicious and more nutritious options available as well. The grains with the highest amount of soluble fiber are quinoa, rice, and barley. Great vegetables options include carrots, mushrooms, sweet potatoes, turnips, and yams. If you prefer a fruit side, try pumpkin or papaya (which also serves as a digestive aid for indigestion and flatulence). For more options, check out Appendix C, which gives you the fiber contents for a plethora of common foods.

Getting Familiar with Grains

If you're experimenting with the Specific Carbohydrate Diet (SCD), you're avoiding all grains and can skip this section.

Grains are the fruits or seeds of various plants, including cereal grasses. Although many foods that people think are grains are actually pseudograins or grain-like products, we include them here anyway. This section introduces you to several grains and gives you information on their basic preparations.

Contrary to what many may believe, wheat isn't the only grain on the planet. It's certainly a staple, at least in the Western world, where many people eat it three times a day, but that may be why it's become a problem for so many. Undigested wheat molecules can be absorbed through a leaky gut (see Chapter 18) into the blood and can set up a reaction in the body, creating a wheat sensitivity.

Even if you aren't avoiding wheat or gluten (contained in wheat, rye, and barley and sometimes contaminating oats) because of sensitivity, get ready to meet your new best friends: quinoa, amaranth, millet, kamut, spelt, and rice. With six choices of grains, you don't have to eat the same grain every day and run the risk of developing a sensitivity to it like many have done with wheat. The following list introduces you to quinoa, amaranth, millet, kamut, and spelt; the section "Reveling in Rice" later in this chapter gives you the lowdown on rice.

- ✔ **Quinoa:** Originally from the Andes in South America, *quinoa* (pronounced *keen*-wah) is an ancient, gluten-free substance. We have to say "substance" because it's actually a *pseudocereal* — a grainlike plant with edible seeds. Quinoa has only recently entered mainstream food production, so fewer people seem to be sensitive to it. Believe it or not, its closest relatives are beets, spinach, and tumbleweed! Quinoa has a naturally bitter coating that you rinse off before cooking; this step is especially important for those with IBS-D, because the bitter substance is somewhat laxative.

   Cooked quinoa has a fluffy, light consistency and a mild, slightly nutty flavor with a protein content registering around 16 percent. In comparison, rice has a protein content of about 7 percent. We also love the fact that quinoa is a good source of magnesium and iron.

   You can use quinoa flour along with sorghum flour, tapioca starch, and potato starch to make a gluten-free baking mix. The ratio is three parts of the quinoa flour and sorghum flour, two parts of the potato starch, and one part of the tapioca starch.

✔ **Amaranth:** *Amaranth* (known in its weed form as *pigweed*) is a beautiful plant with pretty pink blossoms. It has many purposes, but several varieties are grown in Asia and North and South America as a pseudocereal. Amaranth is a balanced protein like quinoa with a similar high protein content of 15 to 18 percent. One interesting nutrition fact is that amaranth contains twice as much calcium as milk. It's also a source of Vitamin E.

When cooked, amaranth has a tacky texture, which turns gummy if you overcook it. The flavor of amaranth flavor is sweet, nutty, and almost malt-like.

✔ **Millet:** After rice, *millet* is the second most widely used non-gluten grain (and it's a grain, not a pseudocereal or a grainlike plant). Its seeds are larger than quinoa's but smaller than rice's; it's easily digestible and one of the least-allergenic grains. It's said to be the first cereal grain used for human food and animal fodder, and it's grown around the world. The protein content is close to wheat at 11 percent. Cooked millet has a mild flavor and a heavier texture than amaranth, but it's still fluffy like rice.

✔ **Buckwheat:** *Buckwheat* is a pseudocereal with a triangular grain. It originated in Eastern Asia, and you may recognize it as the ingredient used to make Japanese soba noodles. Buckwheat is gluten-free, so it's great as a cereal, as a side dish, or in flour mixes (for things like waffles and pancakes) for those who can't tolerate gluten. It has a richer nutty flavor than other grains. Toasted buckwheat, called *kasha,* has an even stronger nutty taste. It's high in soluble fiber, much like oatmeal. Buckwheat has a higher fat content than most other grains, so store it in jars in the fridge to prevent it from spoiling.

Buckwheat helps keep blood sugar under control and has significant amounts of a flavonoid (part of the vitamin C family) called *rutin,* which can help lower cholesterol. The protein in buckwheat is only 11 percent, but it contains all the essential amino acids.

✔ **Kamut:** *Kamut* is a grain related to wheat, although it's twice the size, and also contains gluten. If you want a wheat substitute but aren't worried about the gluten, kamut may be just what you're looking for. The story goes that this grain was found, quite literally, in the Egyptian pyramids. It has the same protein content as wheat, around 11 percent. Cooked kamut's texture is chewy, and it has a nutty taste.

✔ **Spelt:** Spelt is another relative of wheat; it's a grain identified from the Bronze Age in Europe. It does contain gluten, though much less than wheat, so you want to pass on this one if you're gluten-intolerant. Spelt is more common in Europe but has made its way into American kitchens through health food stores. Its protein content is high at 17 percent. It can be used in a combination of grains but isn't usually eaten as a cooked cereal. Spelt bread is slightly sweet and has a nutty flavor.

Buy all these grains in bulk at your local health food store and store them in sealed glass containers on your shelf or kitchen counter (except buckwheat, as noted in the earlier bullet). Be sure to soak quinoa and spelt in water for four hours and overnight (respectively) and then drain and rinse before using. All the other grains need washing and rinsing as well. This step is especially important for quinoa (because of its coating; see the earlier bullet) and for millet, kamut, and spelt, which may have small stones and debris from storage.

Cook these grain products according to package directions; however, you can substitute vegetable, beef, or chicken broth for the cooking water. (Check out Chapter 9 for broth recipes.) You can also use half water and half apple juice for sweeter tasting buckwheat and amaranth. Adding fresh herbs or ginger powder to the cooking pot is another way to pump up the flavor.

◯ *Quinoa Vegetable Pilaf*

Thanks to Andrea Boje (www.myfoodmyhealth.com/OurChefs/index. php?chefid=23) for taking quinoa to the next level with this tasty side dish. If you have leftover quinoa, you can use that instead of making it from scratch; just double the amount and cut the stock/water from the recipe. Quinoa is high in soluble fiber, so it's IBS-friendly. This pilaf goes well with baked or grilled chicken, but it's so versatile, you can use it as a main dish by adding cooked cannellini beans and diced tomatoes. This dish keeps in the fridge for a week and is still tasty after being frozen.

Preparation time: *10 minutes*

Cooking time: *35 minutes*

Yield: *4 servings*

1 cup uncooked quinoa	*5 to 6 button or cremini mushrooms, sliced (optional)*
2 cups vegetable stock or water	
2 tablespoons olive oil	*¼ teaspoon each salt and pepper*
1 medium onion, finely diced	*2 teaspoons toasted sesame oil (optional)*
2 medium carrots, finely diced	*1 teaspoon toasted sesame seeds*

1 Cook quinoa according to the package directions, using stock or water, and set aside.

2 Heat the olive oil in medium frying pan over medium-high heat and sauté the onion and carrots. When the carrots have started to soften, add the mushrooms (if desired) and continue to sauté until the mushrooms are cooked.

3 Add the quinoa to the frying pan and stir until the vegetables are mixed in. Season to taste with salt and pepper and transfer to serving dish. Drizzle a little toasted sesame oil over the quinoa if desired. Top with toasted sesame seeds and serve.

*   **Tip:** *For a nuttier flavor, toast the quinoa before cooking it. Put the dry quinoa in the saucepan over low heat, stirring frequently until you can smell a nutty aroma from the pan. Add stock or water and cook.*

Tip: *Add fresh thyme to the water when cooking quinoa. You can place one or two sprigs directly into the water with the quinoa, and the small thyme leaves fall off the twigs as they cook. Remove twigs before serving.*

Tip: *Use half white quinoa and half red to make a more colorful dish. They have the same cooking time, so you can throw them in the pot together.*

Per serving: Calories 252; Fat 9.8 g (Saturated 1.3 g); Cholesterol 0 mg; Sodium 418 mg; Carbohydrate 33.4 g (Fiber 4.6 g); Protein 7.5 g; Sugar 3.5 g.

🌱 *Rainbow Vegetarian Quinoa*

Here's Shannon Leone's simple quinoa vegetable blend; you can find Shannon at www.rawmom.com. This dish only has a few ingredients, so it's less likely to set off your stomach, and the quinoa is a great soluble-fiber food. *Liquid aminos* are a low-sodium, non-fermented soybean substitute for salty, fermented soy sauce.

Preparation time: *5 minutes*

Cooking time: *15 minutes*

Yield: *4 servings*

2 cups uncooked quinoa, rinsed

4 cups water

2 cups mix of chopped carrots, peas, and corn

Dash of olive oil

Dash of Braggs Liquid Aminos, or Nama Shoyu, or miso, or pinch of salt

1 Place the quinoa in pot with the water and bring to a boil. Reduce the heat to low, cover the pot, and simmer for 15 minutes until the quinoa is fluffy.

2 Add the vegetables to the pot, turn off the heat, and let stand for 5 minutes until the vegetables are warm.

3 Lightly garnish with olive oil and Braggs Liquid Aminos, Nama Shoyu, miso, or salt.

Per serving: Calories 360; Fat 5.6 g (Saturated fat 0.8 g); Cholesterol 0 mg; Sodium 119 mg; Carbohydrate 64.4 g (Fiber 8.2); Protein 14.2 g; Sugar 46.8 g.

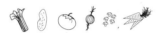

Reveling in Rice

Rice is a grain, but it's so popular that we've devoted a separate section to it. In fact, rice is eaten more than wheat on a global level. Rice comes in two main varieties: brown and white.

Brown rice is rice with its brown outer coating of bran and germ still intact. It's a staple for many people with IBS and colitis because it's hypoallergenic and high in soluble fiber, so it's a great grain to have on hand as a safe side or to balance a main meal with high amounts of insoluble fiber. Most view white rice as an important soluble-fiber food for IBS, but brown rice actually has more soluble fiber than white does (although it also has more insoluble fiber). Check out Appendix C for the actual numbers.

White rice is brown rice with the bran and germ removed. It gets a bad rap because it has been stripped of its goodness, but some people with IBS find it to be a mildly comforting food because it has no traces of rice bran to cause irritation. But we caution you against getting too friendly with white rice; like white bread, it has very few nutrients, and if you can tolerate brown rice, that's the more nutritious option.

Cook whatever rice you choose according to the package directions; for extra flavor, you can substitute chicken or vegetable stock for the water during cooking. You can cook and freeze rice in plastic containers for quick use or to throw in your survival kit (discussed in Chapter 14). If you want a more adventurous side, the following recipes give you a few interesting alternatives to straight-up rice.

If you love rice, try aromatic varieties like basmati or jasmine. They both have distinctive, nutty flavors and pleasing aromas that occur naturally in the rice. Basmati and jasmine can both be either brown or white.

☺ Oven-Baked UnFried Rice

Thanks to Colleen Robinson (www.crimsondoorhealing.com) for modifying this old favorite to feed our IBS-friendly needs by avoiding the frying pan. It calls for chestnuts, which unlike many nuts are high in soluble fiber. Rice is also high in soluble fiber, and cooking makes the vegetables easier to digest. This recipe is suitable for IBS-C and IBS-D.

Preparation time: *10 minutes*

Cooking time: *1 hour*

Yield: *5 servings*

2 cups long grain rice, uncooked

1 small onion, chopped into small pieces

1 cup chicken broth

¼ cup olive oil

¼ cup tamari, or low-sodium soy sauce

⅓ cup fresh parsley, chopped

One 8-ounce can sliced water chestnuts, rinsed and chopped

1 egg white (optional)

2 cups boiling water

1 Preheat the oven to 350 degrees.

2 Spray a small frying pan with cooking spray and quickly cook the egg white, breaking it into bits as it cooks for 1 or 2 minutes to get the look of authentic fried rice (if desired).

3 Mix all the ingredients (including the egg, if desired) into a casserole dish. Cover with tinfoil and bake for an hour.

Vary It! *Chop leftover chicken or any other meat your stomach can handle into small pieces and add it to the casserole before baking. (Of course, this addition makes the recipe non-vegetarian.)*

Per serving: *Calories 337; Fat 9.9 g (Saturated 1.5 g); Cholesterol 0.5 mg; Sodium 9 mg; Carbohydrate 53.2 g (Fiber 1.6 g); Protein 7.7 g; Sugar 1 g.*

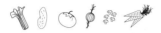

☞ *Shannon's Quick "Rice"*

This raw, vegetable-based rice alternative comes from the kitchen of Shannon Leone (www.rawmom.com). The key is to blend the ingredients until you get a rice-like texture. The blending chops through the fiber and makes your meal much easier to digest and suitable for IBS-C, which benefits from both soluble and insoluble fiber.

Preparation time: *5 minutes*

Yield: *4 servings*

1 cup parsnips, scrubbed, peeled, and chopped

1 cup chopped cauliflower

1 cup pine nuts

1 clove of garlic

1 tablespoon lemon juice

1 tablespoon Nama Shoyu (organic soy sauce)

1 to 2 tablespoons olive oil

1 tablespoon agave, or 2 dates, pitted (optional)

1 Blend all the ingredients into a food processor and process until the mixture becomes somewhat rice-like in texture.

Tip: *You can substitute the Nama Shoyu with 1 tablespoon miso, 1 teaspoon Braggs Liquid Aminos (a low-sodium soy sauce alternative), ½ teaspoon powdered kelp, 1 teaspoon powdered dulse (a seaweed; both it and kelp taste salty but are low sodium and high in minerals), or ½ teaspoon Celtic sea salt.*

Per serving: *Calories 308; Fat 28.3 g (Saturated 2.4 g); Cholesterol 0 mg; Sodium 264 mg; Carbohydrate 12.5 g (Fiber 3.6 g); Protein 6.1 g; Sugar 3.6 g.*

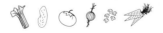

☞ Brown Rice Powder Stuffing

Thanks to Julie Beyer for this stuffing; she created it as a remedy for her own intestinal sensitivities, so you can rest assured that it's probably safer for your sensitive gut than the usual bread stuffing. Flaxseed is high in soluble fiber, and chopping and sautéing or steaming the vegetables makes them easier to digest. The addition of brown rice powder in this recipe gives you all benefits of brown rice but helps its digestibility by breaking down the fiber. Consider this brown rice stuffing as a gluten-free soluble side to go along with any of the entrees in Chapter 11.

Preparation time: *20 minutes*

Cooking time: *None*

Yield: *6 servings*

½ cup ground flaxseeds	3 celery stalks, diced
½ cup brown rice protein powder	3 apples, peeled, cored and diced
1 teaspoon sea salt	4 Swiss chard leaves, chopped
½ cup flaxseed oil	1 to 2 teaspoons nutmeg
5 tablespoons water	3 to 4 teaspoons Italian herb mixture
2 to 3 tablespoons olive or coconut oil	2 to 3 teaspoons maple syrup
1 medium onion, chopped	2 teaspoons freshly squeezed lemon juice, or to taste
2 to 3 cloves garlic	¼ teaspoon each celery salt and pepper, or to taste
½ cup pecans or walnuts, soaked (optional; see the Soaking Nuts and Seeds recipe in Chapter 8)	Fresh oregano and mint to garnish (optional)

1 Mix the ground flaxseeds, brown rice protein powder, and sea salt in a large bowl. Mix in the flaxseed oil and enough water to form a dry, doughy paste and set aside.

2 In a large skillet, heat 2 to 3 tablespoons of olive oil or coconut oil and sauté the onion, garlic, nuts (if desired), celery, and apples over medium heat until all the produce is almost tender. Add the Swiss chard and continue sautéing until all the produce is tender.

3 Add the protein powder mixture to the produce mixture and mix in the nutmeg, Italian herbs, maple syrup, lemon juice, celery salt, and pepper. Garnish with fresh oregano and mint (if desired).

Tip: *You can also lightly steam the vegetables instead of sautéing. Make sure to steam them separately because they all require different amounts of time in the steamer.*

Tip: *If nuts are difficult for you to digest, you can presoak them in filtered water with sea salt for seven hours. This process neutralizes enzyme inhibitors and makes the nuts easier to digest. After thoroughly rinsing them, you can either add them directly to your recipe or dry them in the oven at a maximum of 150 degrees or in a dehydrator for 12 to 24 hours.*

Per serving: Calories 402; Fat 28.9 g (Saturated 3 g); Cholesterol 0 mg; Sodium 523 mg; Carbohydrate 26.2 g (Fiber 5.4 g); Protein 13.1 g; Sugar 11.1 g.

Vegetables Take Sides

The sound of parents telling their children to eat their vegetables is heard in dining rooms around the world. Childhood is the best time to introduce fresh vegetables because the tastier they are when you're a kid, the likelier you are to keep coming back for more. The overcooked, tasteless vegetables you had when you were may have turned you off from veggies when you were young may have turned you off, but try the vibrant, fresh-picked produce at a local farmers' market — it may bring you around on these vitamin- and mineral-rich foods.

We know we're going out on a limb by even talking about too many vegetables in conjunction with an IBS diet. However, one of the intricacies of IBS is that it can be two opposite conditions — what's good for IBS-D may be a bomb for IBS-C. We do want people with IBS-D to eat more vegetables, but you have to take it slow. We heartily encourage those with IBS-C to increase their vegetables for the fiber and the nutrients that they may need to help treat their condition.

☞ *Green Beans Almandine*

Okay, that's just a fancy way to say "green beans with almonds." You can say it however you like, but do yourself a favor and make it — it's a fast and easy side from healing chef Colleen Robinson (www.crimsondoorhealing.com). If you can buy green beans fresh, please do; they're way more flavorful than the canned stuff. Buying fresh beans by the pound generally serves four people. If you can't get fresh, go for the Grade-A frozen ones (preferably organic) because you get the least-mushy ones that way. Speaking of mush, you can make your beans more easily digestible by chewing them to mush or overcooking them a tad so they're more broken down.

If you're avoiding slivered or sliced nuts, just toast them and grind them to a powder in your food processor and dust your beans with that. To make this simple and tasty dish even IBS-friendlier, serve it with a simple cooked rice of your choice (flip to "Reveling in Rice" earlier in this chapter for more on this lovely grain). Check out a photo of this healthy side dish in the color insert.

Preparation time: *5 minutes*

Cooking time: *10 minutes*

Yield: *4 servings*

1 pound fresh green beans, trimmed	*1 teaspoon butter*
2 to 4 tablespoons sliced or slivered almonds	*¼ teaspoon each salt and pepper, or to taste*

1 Boil a large pot of water over high heat. While you wait for it to boil, toast the almonds in a pan over medium heat for 5 to 7 minutes, stirring constantly. Remove the almonds from the heat when they're toasted and set aside.

2 Cook the green beans in the boiling water for several minutes, until they're crisp.

3 Drain the cooked beans and toss them with the almonds, butter, and a bit of salt and pepper.

Tip: Snap the pointy ends of the beans off with your fingers; if they have a stringy bit down the side, you can peel it off and get less insoluble fiber. You can cut the ends off with a knife, but you may not get the stringy bits off.

Tip: You can also toast the almonds in a toaster oven, but make sure you watch them carefully — they go from toasted to burnt very quickly.

Tip: Whether you like your almonds sliced or slivered is up to you. Sliced almonds toast more quickly, but slivered almonds are more substantial.

Per serving: Calories 73; Fat 3.2 g (Saturated 0.75 g); Cholesterol 3 mg; Sodium 159 mg; Carbohydrate 9.1 g (Fiber 4.6 g); Protein 3 g; Sugar 1.8 g.

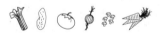

☙ *Creamed Spinach*

Thanks to our healing chef Colleen Robinson at www.crimsondoorhealing.com for showing that taking most of the dairy out of the childhood favorite creamed spinach can make it IBS- and taste bud-friendly. Spinach has more soluble fiber in its raw state, although it tends to be less digested (possibly because people don't chew their salads enough). Cooked spinach may shrivel considerably from its raw form, but it's still substantial, especially in vitamins. In the cooked state, spinach is higher in insoluble fiber and therefore more suited to IBS-C, even though it's high in iron, which can be binding. Small amounts of Parmesan are okay on the SCD, so if you're using the SCD to help control your IBS, don't worry about the cheese.

Preparation time: *10 minutes*

Cooking time: *10 minutes*

Yield: *4 servings*

1 pound fresh spinach, or two 10-ounce boxes frozen spinach, drained and chopped

2 cloves of garlic, or 1 large clove of elephant garlic

1 teaspoon olive oil

¼ cup plain soy milk

¼ teaspoon each salt and pepper, or to taste

2 teaspoons grated Parmesan cheese to garnish

1 Sauté the garlic over medium-low heat until translucent.

2 Add the spinach. For frozen spinach, mix it in with the garlic until combined. For fresh spinach, stir it into the pan with the garlic with a large spoon until it wilts to a quarter of the original size.

3 Add the soy milk and stir to warm the soy and cover the spinach. Add salt and pepper to taste, garnish with the Parmesan, and serve hot.

Vary It! *For a creamier creamed spinach, puree ¼ of the raw spinach in a blender on high speed and add it to the cooked spinach mixture when you add the soy milk. (If you're using fresh spinach, boil it for 1 minute and rinse with cold water before blending.)*

Tip: *Wash your spinach even if it comes pre-washed in a sealed bag. You want to rule out the possibility of any trace amounts of pesticides getting into your system. Fill a sink or large bowl with cool water and add 5 drops of grapefruit seed extract.*

Tip: *You can substitute 1 clove of elephant garlic for the 2 cloves of regular garlic. Elephant garlic is milder and may irritate your stomach less.*

Per serving: *Calories 49; Fat 2.1 g (Saturated 0.3 g); Cholesterol 0.8 mg; Sodium 255 mg; Carbohydrate 5.2 g (Fiber 2.6 g); Protein 4.1; Sugar 0.9g.*

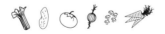

☞ Ginger Carrots

Victoria Amory (www.victoriaamory.com) brings out the flavor of carrot with ginger's earthy, fiery qualities. In IBS terms, ginger is an anti-inflammatory and anti-nausea herb, so it may be beneficial for both IBS-D and IBS-C. The vegetables are simmered for about 20 minutes, which makes them even easier to digest. Victoria suggests cutting the carrots in matchsticks or rounds for a pretty dish.

Preparation time: *15 minutes*

Cooking time: *25 minutes*

Yield: *7 servings*

4 tablespoons olive oil

One 3-inch piece of ginger, peeled and diced

1 clove of garlic, peeled and chopped

2 pounds carrots, cut into matchsticks or ¼-inch rounds

1 cup Vegetable Stock (see the recipe in Chapter 9) or low-sodium canned vegetable broth

1 tablespoon butter

½ cup parsley, chopped

1 In a large sauté pan, heat the olive oil over high heat. Add the ginger and garlic and sauté for a few seconds to release the aroma. Add the carrots and stir to coat.

2 Add the broth and bring to a boil. Reduce the heat to medium-low and cover. Simmer until the carrots are tender, about 20 minutes.

3 Remove the cover, stir in the butter and parsley, and serve hot.

Per serving: *Calories 131; Fat 9.7 g (Saturated 2.1 g); Cholesterol 4 mg; Sodium 87 mg; Carbohydrate 11.2 g (Fiber 3.2 g); Protein 1.3 g; Sugar 5.1 g.*

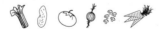

☞ Marinated Kale

Angela Elliott at www.she-zencuisine.com contributed this wonderfully healthy uncooked recipe. We know we're breaking the mold for an IBS diet by including kale that's not even cooked, so this recipe is for folks who know they can tolerate greens well or those with IBS-C who need the extra bulk and fiber. The kale here is marinated, which does break down fibers and make them more digestible. To really soften the kale up, prepare the dish the day before and let it marinate in the fridge overnight. Then you can add a side of rice, barley, or bread to make this a balanced meal especially for IBS-C.

Marinating time: *60 minutes or overnight*

Preparation time: *5 minutes*

Cooking time: *None*

Yield: *6 servings*

3 large leaves organic green leaf kale	*1½ teaspoons salt*
¼ of a sweet onion	*¼ teaspoon cayenne, or to taste*
3 tablespoons fresh tarragon	*1 teaspoon raw agave*
3 tablespoons fresh basil	*¼ teaspoon each garlic powder and chili powder, or to taste*
Juice of 1 lemon (about ¼ cup)	
3 tablespoons olive oil	

1 Gently pulse or chop the kale in a food processor and then transfer it to a bowl.

2 Add the rest of the ingredients to the kale. Toss, allow to marinate for 1 hour, and serve.

Tip: *Chopped olives make a good addition to garnish this tasty dish.*

Per serving: *Calories 84; Fat 7.1 g (Saturated 1 g); Cholesterol 0 mg; Sodium 596 mg; Carbohydrate 5.3 g (Fiber 0.9 g); Protein 1.4 g; Sugar 1 g.*

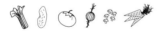

 Most people's dairy problems have to do with lactose. If you have dairy issues, avoid high-lactose cheeses, including cottage cheese, cream cheese, feta, mozzarella, ricotta, processed cheeses, and cheese spreads. Very low-lactose cheeses that you may be able to handle are cheddar, Colby, Swiss, havarti, and dry curd cottage cheese.

Bringing on the Bread

We've said it before and we'll say it again: Stay away from white bread as much as possible. It just doesn't give you the nutrients that other IBS-friendly foods do. But if you're going to eat white bread, we want you to have a good one, so in this section we give you our recipe for sourdough white bread. We recommend it because it is high in soluble fiber but doesn't contain commercial yeast, which can cause many people with yeast overgrowth to react. (See Chapter 18 for more on yeast overgrowth).

☼ Savoring Sourdough Bread

We've spoken about sourdough bread as a great soluble fiber food, so we want to make sure you have a great recipe to make your own. Sourdough bread is also called yeast-free bread, but the only reason it becomes bread at all is because of the yeast and bacteria in the air that settle on the dough! Who knew? The recipe does call for white flour, but you can make it a bit healthier by using organic white flour, which is free of any genetic modifications and chemical residues used in commercial farming or milling. Keep the extra sponge around so you don't have to make one from scratch the next time you want to bake bread.

Tools: *Bread machine (optional), wide-mouth jar with a rubber-sealed lid (such as a mason jar)*

Preparation time: *2½ hours, including rising times*

Starter time: *4 to 7 days*

Sponge time: *2 to 8 hours*

Cooking time: *45 to 50 minutes*

Yield: *1 loaf (13 servings/slices)*

4 teaspoons sugar

2 teaspoons salt

2 tablespoons olive oil, soft butter, or ghee (see the recipe in Chapter 6)

2 cups sponge (fermented starter; see the following recipes)

3 cups unbleached all-purpose flour, or more as necessary

1 Add the sugar, salt, and oil to the sponge. Mix well and (using your hands, a bread machine, or a food processor) begin to knead in the flour ½ cup at a time, using as much flour as you need to make a good, elastic bread dough.

2 Put the dough in a bowl (if it's not already in one), cover it with a towel, and set it in a warm place (70 to 80 degrees; 100 degrees is too warm). Let the dough grow to twice its original size, until poking with your finger creates a hole that doesn't spring back (this process may take 1 to 2 hours).

3 Knead the bread again and then make a loaf and place it in a 9-x-5-inch loaf pan lightly greased with olive oil or coconut oil. Cover it with a damp towel or paper towel and place it in a warm place to rise a second time for 40 minutes to an hour or until doubled in bulk.

4 Place the pan in a cold oven, set the oven temperature to 350 degrees, and bake for 45 to 50 minutes or until the crust is brown; you can turn the loaf out on a cooling rack to check the bottom for doneness, poking the bottom with a toothpick to see whether it comes out clean if desired. Cool for about 1 hour before cutting.

Per serving: Calories 254; Fat 3 g (Saturated 0.3 g); Cholesterol 0 mg; Sodium 358 mg; Carbohydrate 51.3 g (Fiber 1.5 g); Protein 7.7 g; Sugar 1.3 g.

Making the Starter

1 cup organic, unbleached all-purpose flour plus up to 3½ cups flour for feeding

1 cup water plus up to 3½ cups warm water for feeding

1 Using your blender or mixer, blend the flour and water. Pour the mixture into a wide-mouth jar and cover with a washcloth to keep out dust and bugs.

2 Keep the starter in a 70-to-80-degree environment, which allows airborne and flour-borne yeast to grow rapidly. Don't go above 100 degrees; you kill the starter.

3 Every 24 hours, pour off half the mixture and add ½ cup warm water and ½ cup flour blended together. On Day 3, start checking for lots of bubbles, the smell of beer, or a nice sour smell (these may take 7 days to develop from the time you begin the starter). When a bubbly froth develops, your starter has started and is ready for breadmaking.

4 Punch a hole in the jar lid and put the lid on the jar. Keep the starter in the fridge until you're ready to make bread. Continue to feed the starter with an extra ½ cup flour/½ cup water mixture once a week; you may have to stir the mix every day or two.

Making the Sponge

1 cup unbleached all-purpose flour

1 cup warm water

1 cup starter (see the preceding recipe)

1 Pour the starter into a mixing bowl.

2 Blend the water and the flour and add to the starter; stir well and set in a warm place for several hours to ferment until the mixture is bubbly, frothy, and sour smelling; this process may take anywhere from 2 to 8 hours or longer.

Tip: *Bread dough can rise in a temperature from 80 to 110 degrees. If you can set your stove to 95 degrees, you can use your oven and keep a uniform temperature.*

Tip: *If you're living in such sterile quarters that your starter doesn't grow within 2 hours, add ¼ packet of commercial yeast to the starter to give it a nudge.*

Tip: *Wash the empty jar and dry it. You may also want to pour boiling water over it, because you don't want other things growing in there with your pet!*

Tip: *Make your first sponge attempt in the morning to see how long it takes. If it does take 8 hours and you want to bake in the morning, set your sponge out to ferment overnight.*

Tip: *Save your leftover sponge as your starter for next time: Put it back into the jar and feed it ½ cup each of flour and warm water weekly. Keep it in the fridge as before.*

Potato Pretenders: Creating Potato-esque Side Dishes

Whether baked, mashed, or fried, potatoes in various forms are a traditional side dish that many people with IBS have on their safe lists. We offer a kid-friendly side recipe (Smashed Potatoes with Rosemary) made with real-deal potatoes in Chapter 15, but here give you some interesting takes on potato alternatives.

☞ *Fresh Fries with Raw Jicama*

These raw treats from Shannon Leone (www.rawmom.com) are shaped like French fries and have some seasoning, but they aren't fried. Jicama is a crispy, sweet, edible root that looks and feels like a turnip on the outside. It's often hidden in the vegetable section of grocery stores and passed over by most shoppers. It's high in soluble fiber, so it's considered a friendly food for IBS, especially IBS-C. Not many vegetables have more soluble fiber than insoluble fiber, but jicama is one of them, so it's a great place to start eating raw. The small amounts of chili, garlic, and onion powders are for taste and a bit of color on your fries and should not be cause for concern.

Tools: *Mandoline (optional)*

Preparation time: *5 minutes*

Cooking time: *None*

Yield: *2 servings*

1 medium jicama	1 teaspoon onion and/or garlic powder
1 tablespoon olive oil	½ teaspoon chili powder
1 teaspoon sea salt	

1 Peel the jicama and slice it into your favorite French fry shape with a mandoline or by hand with a sharp knife.

2 Mix the olive oil with the salt, onion/garlic powder, and chili powder and toss with the fries.

Vary It! *If you want your Fresh Fries coated in gravy but not coated in gluten, try them with the Rockin' Gravy recipe later in the chapter.*

Tip: *Try your fries with a squeeze of lemon or lime.*

Per serving: *Calories 191; Total fat 7.2 g (Saturated 1 g); Cholesterol 0 mg; Sodium 1182 mg; Carbohydrate 30.4 g (Fiber 16.5 g); Protein 4.1 g; Sugar 6.3 g.*

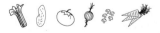

Curried Spice-Baked Sweet Potatoes

Chef Laura Pole (www.eatingforalifetime.com/) used to suffer with IBS and now applies what she learned about diet in her own recovery to her clients who have bowel inflammation. This recipe, which is featured in the color insert, is a delicious hit with lots of anti-inflammatory ingredients and ingredients that also aid digestion. It's also high in magnesium, which relaxes the smooth muscle in the colon and can help prevent or relieve symptoms of IBS-C. Laura recommends using garnet or jewel yams, which are actually sweet potatoes even though they're called yams in the grocery store; see the nearby sidebar for more on the yam–sweet potato distinction. You can use the alternate curry powder mixture shared at the end of the recipe if you want to avoid too much peppery spice.

Preparation time: *10 minutes*

Cooking time: *70 minutes*

Yield: *4 servings*

2 medium sweet potatoes, washed and pierced in the center with a fork

1 teaspoon of fresh ginger, finely grated

½ to 1 teaspoon mild curry powder

½ teaspoon turmeric

Pinch of cinnamon

⅛ teaspoon salt, or to taste

1 teaspoon coconut oil or extra virgin olive oil

1 Preheat the oven to 400 degrees. Bake the sweet potatoes in a low-sided roasting pan for 30 to 45 minutes or until soft and then remove them from the oven and allow them to cool.

2 Slice the cooled potatoes in half lengthwise and scoop out the center flesh, leaving a ¼-inch rim of sweet potato attached to the skin to help hold the skin together.

3 Mix the flesh and the remaining ingredients in a bowl until smooth and creamy. Refill the potato skins with the flesh mixture, place them on a baking sheet, and put them back in the oven until heated through and slightly golden on top — about 25 minutes. Serve hot.

Tip: *To quicken the original cooking time, cut the sweet potatoes in half lengthwise and place them face down in a roasting pan with about ½ cup water. Bake for 40 minutes.*

Tip: *Step 1 on its own produces a simple baked sweet potato great as a side dish to any meat.*

Tip: *Before putting all the curry into the bowl, check the spiciness of your curry powder. If it seems very peppery, reduce the amount to ¼ to ½ teaspoon. You can also use this alternative curry mix: ¼ teaspoon turmeric, ½ teaspoon cumin, ⅛ teaspoon each coriander and cinnamon, a pinch each of cardamom and cloves, and a pinch of cayenne (optional).*

Per serving: *Calories 69; Fat 1.2 g (Saturated 0.2 g); Cholesterol 0 mg; Sodium 109 mg; Carbohydrate 13.7 g (Fiber 2.1 g); Protein 1.1 g; Sugar 2.7 g.*

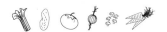

A yam by any other name still wouldn't be a sweet potato

Though many people think *yam* and *sweet potato* are basically synonyms, they're actually two different animals (well, plants):

✔ *Sweet potatoes* are yellow or orange elongated tubers with tapering ends; they're grown in the southern United States. The yellow sweet potato isn't sweet, and its cooked texture is like that of a white potato. The orange variety has vivid orange flesh and is sweet and moist when cooked.

✔ *Yams* are brown- or black-skinned tubers; they come from a tropical vine *(Dioscorea batatas)* and aren't related to the sweet potato. Yams grow in tropical climates, especially in South America, Africa, and the Caribbean, and they're usually sweeter than sweet potatoes. The flesh is off-white, purple, or red, depending on the variety.

And the Rest Is Gravy

Typical gravy is made by stirring flour into the fatty juice left over from cooking meats. But when you have IBS, you may have to set aside the gravy boat because of its floury base. This gravy recipe gives you the chance to add a little more moisture and flavor to many of the meat and vegetable recipes in this book.

☞ Rockin' Gravy

Do you want gravy with your Fresh Fries (see the recipe earlier in this chapter)? It may not be your traditional side of gravy, but this mushroom-based raw gravy from Angela Elliot's e-book *The Raw Divas Holiday Fare* (www.she-zencuisine.com) can satisfy anybody's gravy craving. Almonds have more insoluble than soluble fiber, but in nut butter form, they are easier to digest. The amount of soluble fiber in the mushrooms and flaxseed makes this a high soluble-fiber side. To keep the insoluble fiber to a minimum, strip the fibrous outer strings off the celery before chopping it very finely.

Preparation time: *15 minutes*

Cooking time: *None*

Yield: *6 servings*

¼ cup almond butter

½ cup filtered water

2 cups quartered portabella mushrooms

1 tablespoon minced onion

6 stalks celery, minced

1 teaspoon each garlic powder and onion powder

2 tablespoons Nama Shoyu

¼ teaspoon fresh black pepper, or to taste

4 tablespoons finely chopped cremini mushrooms

1 tablespoon powdered flaxseed to thicken gravy

1 Process the celery, garlic powder, onion powder, Nama Shoyu, and pepper in a blender until smooth. Transfer to a bowl.

2 Add the chopped mushrooms and powdered flaxseed until the mixture is thick and gravy-like. Warm with the warming setting of a dehydrator or in an oven on the lowest setting with the door open (if desired)

Tip: You can substitute other nut butters for the almond butter.

Per serving: *Calories 100; Fat 6.7 g (Saturated 0.7 g); Cholesterol 0 mg; Sodium 321 mg; Carbohydrate 6.6 g (Fiber 2 g); Protein 3.4 g; Sugar 2.1 g.*

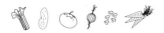

Chapter 13

Diving Into Worry-Free Desserts

In This Chapter

▶ Making IBS-friendly cake, cobbler, pie, and pudding

▶ Crowning your desserts with safe, sweet sauces

▶ Using coconut to help soothe your gut

*N*ever again will you feel like you're losing out on dessert. The tasty recipes in this chapter give you healthy desserts that are low on the white flour, fats, and sugars that may have caused you IBS grief in the past. Of course, that's if you eat them in normal servings; don't feel you have to eat them all in one sitting — go easy and share what you make. And we aren't just talking about fruit salads, either. This chapter gives you recipes for classics like chocolate cake and cherry cobbler, as well as pudding, pie, and other naughty-sounding favorites.

Satisfying your cravings with a minor indulgence is better than letting them build up into a major binge.

Like with many foods, your body's constitution plays a role in how desserts affect your stomach (read more about Ayurvedic constitutions in Chapter 2). People with Vata constitutions are able to process natural sugars like honey but should avoid white sugar because it can become a stimulant. Folks with Pitta constitutions have higher metabolisms and burn off sugar faster, so after a sugar treat, the blood sugar can soar and then plunge. Eating dessert with a main meal can help slow down the absorption of sugar and avoid the plunge. The way they handle sugar means that Pitta's have to keep their blood sugar balanced with regular meals or they can run into problems with hypoglycemia.

Filling Your Desserts with Fiber

When you're searching for ways to work soluble fiber into your desserts, look to ingredients like nuts (though you may have to blend them as in almond flour), fresh and dried fruits without the skins, non-gluten flours, and chia seeds. The fiber table in Appendix C can help you figure out which other ingredients you may want to use in your desserts; as with all eating, shoot to include soluble-fiber ingredients at least 50 percent of the time.

Having Your Cake (And Cobbler!) and Eating It Too

Most cake is made with sugar, white flour, and lots of butter or lard, ingredients that can even make sawdust tasty. But if you have IBS, the pleasures these foods elicit turn into pain when the excess fat stimulates the intestines and causes contractions, and the sugar feeds a few billion microorganisms, which leads to gas and bloating. However, you don't have to write cake off just yet; the recipes in this section show you some ingenious ways around the triggers.

As for cobbler, it's typically made with fruit and some kind of pastry or crumb topping, but we have a raw version here for those of you who are still avoiding grains. So this won't be a cakey cobbler, but it'll be delicious nonetheless.

ℭ Rich and Moist Chocolate Cake

Andrea Boje (www.myfoodmyhealth.com/OurChefs/index.php?chefid=23) is our hero for contributing this gluten- and dairy-free (but incredibly moist) chocolate cake. These factors make is safe for you if gluten and dairy are your IBS triggers. It has enough flavor and sweetness that you can enjoy it without the extra sugar in frosting. Or you can use the sugar substitute Just Like Sugar in powder form to dust the top of the cake (see the color section). Check out a photo of it in the color section.

Andrea uses Bob's Red Mill brand flours, which you can find in your local health food store. If you aren't sensitive to dairy, you can use regular milk and butter in place of the almond milk and Earth Balance margarine. (Earth Balance is a brand of margarine made from a blend of soybean, palm fruit, canola, and olive oils. It's similar to the brand Smart Balance.) For an alternate flavor, replace the coffee with an equal amount of your favorite brewed tea (such as chai or lavender). The cake will stay moist covered in the refrigerator or on the counter for a week and a half.

Tools: *Parchment paper (optional)*

Preparation time: *10 minutes*

Cooking time: *35 minutes*

Yield: *7 servings*

½ cup brown rice flour	*1 cup maple crystals*
¼ cup millet or sorghum flour	*¾ teaspoon sea salt*
¼ cup potato starch	*1 tablespoon organic vanilla*
¼ cup tapioca flour	*½ cup almond or rice milk*
½ cup plus 2 tablespoons unsweetened cocoa powder	*½ cup Earth Balance margarine, room temperature, plus more for pan greasing*
1 teaspoon xanthan gum	*1 egg, beaten*
1¼ teaspoons baking soda	*¾ cup brewed coffee, room temperature*

1 Heat oven to 350 degrees. Grease an 8-inch round cake pan with margarine or coconut oil, adding and greasing a round sheet of parchment paper if your pan tends to stick.

2 Mix the flours, potato starch, cocoa powder, xanthan gum, baking soda, maple crystals, and salt in a large bowl.

3 In another large bowl, put the vanilla, milk, margarine, and egg and mix on low speed with a hand mixer. Add the dry ingredients and continue to mix with the hand mixer. Add the coffee and blend again until mixed.

4 Pour the batter into the cake pan and smooth out the top. Bake for 30 to 35 minutes, giving the pan a half turn halfway through baking time. Remove from oven when a toothpick inserted in the center of the cake comes out clean.

5 Let the cake cool in pan for 5 minutes and then remove it and set it on a rack.

Tip: *If you can't find maple crystals, substitute an equal amount of brown sugar, organic white sugar, or turbinado sugar.*

Tip: *Store your unused portions of flour in your freezer for freshness.*

Vary It! *To make this recipe as cupcakes, follow the recipe instructions but pour the batter into a greased cupcake tin or cupcake liners. Reduce the baking time to 20 minutes. You get 12 cupcakes.*

Per serving: *Calories 205; Fat 8.6 g (Saturated 0.5 g); Cholesterol 18 mg; Sodium 290 mg; Carbohydrate 33.9 g (Fiber 2.1 g); Protein 2.4 g; Sugar 18 mg.*

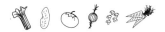

⌒ Pineapple Upside-Down Cake

Raman Prasad (www.scdrecipe.com/cookbook) contributed this American classic from his book *Recipes for the Specific Carbohydrate Diet*™ (Fair Winds Press). SCD is a diet that is safe for colitis, Crohn's disease, and IBS that avoids the carbs in grains and root vegetables that are the trigger for intestinal microorganism overgrowth. Use fresh pineapple if you possibly can; if you use canned, make sure it doesn't have any preservatives or sugars added. We prefer a fresh, ripe pineapple because the juices from the slices seep into the batter and flavor it nicely.

Preparation time: *15 minutes*

Cooking time: *30 to 40 minutes*

Yield: *15 to 20 servings*

2 cups almond flour, or more as needed for consistency

3 eggs

4 tablespoons butter, melted

½ cup honey

¾ teaspoon organic vanilla extract

¼ teaspoon cinnamon powder

½ pound fresh pineapple, thinly sliced (about 8 slices)

1 Preheat the oven to 350 degrees. Grease a 9-x-12-inch baking dish.

2 Mix the almond flour, eggs, butter, honey, vanilla, and cinnamon by hand or with a hand mixer until smooth. Add more almond flour if necessary to make sure the batter isn't too thin.

3 Layer the pineapple slices on the bottom of the baking dish. Pour in the cake batter and spread it evenly in the pan. Bake the cake for 30 to 40 minutes, or until a toothpick inserted into the center comes out clean.

Per serving: Calories 180; Fat 12.1 g (Saturated 2.8 g); Cholesterol 50 mg; Sodium 36 mg; Carbohydrate 20.9 g (Fiber 2.4 g); Protein 5.7 g; Sugar 10.9 g.

⌒ Cherry Cobbler

Cookbook author Angela Elliott (www.she-zencuisine.com) contributed this delicious raw version of the classic cobbler. It contains coconut, our favorite IBS-friendly dessert food; coconut is safe for both IBS-D and IBS-C, making this dessert safe for everybody. (Check out "Creating Coconut Cookies and Bread" later in this chapter for more treats starring coconut and info on its benefits.)

Preparation time: *15 minutes*

Cooking time: *None*

Yield: *8 servings*

1½ cups shredded coconut

1½ cups walnuts

½ teaspoon salt

⅓ cup plus ½ cup pitted dates

3 cups frozen cherries, thawed and drained

2 teaspoons lemon juice

⅛ teaspoon cinnamon

1 Combine the coconut, walnuts, and salt in a food processor. Add ⅓ cup of the pitted dates one at a time, processing to form coarse crumbs; set aside.

2 In a blender, combine 1 cup of the cherries with the rest of the dates and the lemon juice and cinnamon. Blend until it is a chunky mixture. Toss with the remaining 2 cups of cherries.

3 Put cherry mixture in a square glass baking dish. Top with crumble topping and refrigerate until ready to serve.

Tip: *You can soak the walnuts for 6 hours (see the Soaking Nuts and Seeds recipe in Chapter 8) and dehydrate them for 18 hours at 150 degrees to make them dry and crispy and easier to process.*

Tip: *For instant gratification, you can also just put the cherry mixture directly into serving dishes and top with the crumble topping.*

Per serving: *Calories 284; Fat 19 g (Saturated 5.6 g); Cholesterol 0 mg; Sodium 120 mg; Carbohydrate 44.8 g (Fiber 6.4 g); Protein 5.3 g; Sugar 35.9 g.*

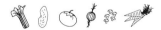

The Pies Have It! Making Pies without the Baking

When you think of pies, you probably think of lard and white flour, maybe with a bit of salt and egg (and, if your mother made six pies at a time like ours did, some white vinegar). That's not much to rave about in terms of nutritional content, except for the egg.

Folks with IBS have stomachs that just won't stand for the empty calories of white sugar, lard, and flour. They rebel. But that doesn't mean you don't still like the taste and feel of pie, so the recipes in this section show you how to have the best of both worlds. You're going to be amazed how you can satisfy your pie craving and eliminate lard, sugar, and white flour at the same time.

☞ *Vegan Lemon Meringue Pie*

Healing chef Julie Beyer provided this healthy dessert recipe. You often find coconut milk and shredded coconut listed as IBS no-no's simply because of the fat content, but that's not our experience. Those writers don't take into consideration the type of fat. Coconut *is* high in fat, but it's the easily digested kind of fat (see "Creating Coconut Cookies and Bread" later in this chapter for more on coconut). Coconut milk and shredded coconut actually make this pie friendly for IBS-D.

You may also wonder about the nuts in this recipe, but fear not: Grinding the cashews to smithereens makes them into a creamy paste. Cashew paste is thought to be soothing to the gut, not irritating. Nuts? We don't see any nuts!

Preparation time: *5 minutes*

Cooking time: *None*

Yield: *8 servings*

2 cups cashews, soaked (see the Soaking Nuts and Seeds recipe in Chapter 8)

Pinch of sea salt

4 tablespoons unsweetened coconut milk

Juice of 1 lemon (about ¼ cup)

2 to 4 tablespoons maple or agave syrup (optional)

4 to 8 tablespoons water

Lemon Meringue Pie Crust (see the following recipe)

¼ cup unsweetened shredded coconut

1 Blend the salt, coconut milk, cashews, lemon juice, syrup (if desired), and half the water in a blender until you get a thick, creamy consistency, adding the rest of the water toward the end to achieve the correct consistency without causing the filling to separate. Pour the filling on top of the crust and sprinkle with the shredded coconut. Chill the pie in the fridge for 30 minutes to allow it to firm up before cutting

Per serving: *Calories 373; Fat 28.4 g (Saturated 14.8 g); Cholesterol 0 mg; Sodium 28 mg; Carbohydrate 27.4 g (Fiber 2.4 g); Protein 11.3 g; Sugar 8.4 g.*

Lemon Meringue Pie Crust

4 tablespoons ground flaxseed

4 tablespoons brown rice protein powder

½ teaspoon stevia

1 to 2 teaspoons flaxseed oil

1 teaspoon cinnamon

1 teaspoon water

1 Mix the ground flaxseed, brown rice protein powder, stevia, flax seed oil, cinnamon, and water in a 9-inch pie plate.

2 Spread the mixture over the bottom of the pie plate.

Vary It! *For an easy, crustless upside-down alternative, spread the filling evenly in a dish and then sprinkle shredded coconut (if desired) and ground flaxseeds on top.*

Tip: *The longer you soak the nuts, the more the natural nut enzyme inhibitors break down and the creamier the texture of your filling. However, if you don't have much time, you can get a creamy, easy-to-digest paste by soaking the nuts for only 1 hour. You can soak them for less than 1 hour, but the cream has a stronger taste and is a bit less creamy.*

Tip: *To get the best results, use a good sea salt such as Himalayan Rock Salt or Harvest of France, found at your local health food store. These salts have all the minerals still in them, so they're actually good for you (unlike some others) as well as tasty. Try to get No. 3 maple syrup — it's harvested at the end of the season and is richer in minerals. But any good maple syrup works fine. We also recommend Thai Kitchen coconut milk because it's one of the few preservative-free brands.*

Per serving: *Calories 55; Fat 2.5 g (Saturated 0.3 g); Cholesterol 0 mg; Sodium 1 mg; Carbohydrate 29.9 g (Fiber 1.3 g); Protein 4.4 g; Sugar 0.1 g.*

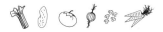

℃ Shannon's Pumpky Pie

Thanks to Shannon Leone from www.rawmom.com for this healthy, hearty confection. The sweet potatoes, blended cashews, and pine nuts are safe and soothing for IBS sufferers. This recipe may not actually include pumpkin, but the taste, especially with the pumpkin pie herbs, is very pumpky. Besides the pumpkin pie taste, allspice, cinnamon, and nutmeg are all IBS-friendly and even IBS-healing, especially cinnamon, which is a digestive aid and settles IBS cramps. This pie keeps well in the fridge for up to a week.

Preparation time: *20 minutes*

Cooking time: *None*

Yield: *8 servings*

3 uncooked sweet potatoes, washed, peeled, and chopped

1 cup raw cashews, soaked 2 hours to soften

1 cup raw pine nuts

⅓ to ½ cup raw honey

1 teaspoon organic vanilla

1 teaspoon allspice

½ teaspoon cinnamon

¼ teaspoon nutmeg

¼ teaspoon sea salt

Pumpky Pie Crust (see the following recipe)

8 to 10 whole pecans for decoration

1 Blend the sweet potatoes, cashews, pine nuts, honey, vanilla, spices, and sea salt in food processor until smooth, adding more spice or honey to taste if necessary.

2 Spoon the filling into the crust with a spatula and decorate with the pecans.

Vary It! *You can replace the honey with agave nectar if you prefer the flavor or don't have honey on your safe food list.*

Per serving: Calories 477; Fat 206.1 g (Saturated 3.5 g); Cholesterol 0 mg; Sodium 139 mg; Carbohydrate 36.9 g (Fiber 4.3 g); Protein 7.3 g; Sugar 18 g.

Pumpky Pie Crust

1 cup pecan pieces

1 cup almonds

1 cup pitted dates or raisins

1 teaspoon salt

1 Shred the sweet potatoes and then process them in a food processor until they're finely ground. Add the other ingredients and process until crumbly.

2 Flatten crust onto a 9-inch pie plate.

Vary It! *Feel free to interchange crusts in your pie making. The flax Lemon Meringue Pie Crust earlier in this chapter goes just as well with this pie.*

Per serving: Calories 249; Fat 18.7 g (Saturated 1.5 g); Cholesterol 0 mg; Sodium 291 mg; Carbohydrate 19.5 g (Fiber 4.7 g); Protein 5.5 g; Sugar 12.9 g.

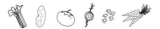

Pudding Your Best Food Forward: Enjoying Smooth Treats

Some people like crunchy desserts, and some like smooth indulgences that are less likely to stir up IBS symptoms. This section is for the smoothies in the audience — you know who you are. Just think of dipping your spoon into soft, creamy sweetness that's so good you'll want to lick the bowl.

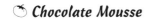

☕ *Chocolate Mousse*

We love the innovation of Raw chefs who have discovered that avocado has many more uses than guacamole! Angela Elliott (www.she-zencuisine.com) whipped up this chocolate wonder. Chocolate, the key ingredient in this recipe, is high in magnesium, which relieves cramps, and antioxidants, which neutralize toxins (see Chapter 1). Avocado is a healthy fat that most people with IBS can enjoy and it gives a rich taste to the mousse that you would only get from added fats or oils. Date syrup (see the recipe later in this chapter) is a safe sweetener, and carob powder has therapeutic uses for IBS-D (but it's also safe for IBS-C).

Preparation time: *5 minutes*

Chilling time: *30 minutes*

Yield: *4 servings*

1½ ripe avocados, peeled	*1 tablespoon organic vanilla*
¼ cup date syrup or agave	*¼ cup carob powder (optional)*
½ cup cacao powder	

1 In a food processor or blender, combine all ingredients and process or blend until smooth.

2 Chill for 30 minutes and then serve.

Tip: *Top with sliced strawberries for a contrasting color and taste.*

Per serving: Calories 196; Fat 12.5 g (Saturated 2.5 g); Cholesterol 0 mg; Sodium 7.5 mg; Carbohydrate 23.4 g (Fiber 8.6 g); Protein 3.8 g; Sugar 10.6 g.

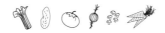

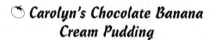

Carolyn's Chocolate Banana Cream Pudding

The name says it all! This recipe is probably already out there, but Carolyn hasn't found the original chef. It popped into her head when all she had on hand for company was frozen bananas, 100-percent raw chocolate powder (cacao), and coconut milk. And voilà: A dreamy dessert with healthy ingredients was born . . . and quickly eaten. Bananas are usually frozen ripe, so this recipe can be a treatment for IBS-D.

Preparation time: *5 minutes*

Cooking time: *None*

Yield: *2 servings*

4 small frozen bananas, cut into rounds	2 tablespoons cacao powder
4 ounces full-fat coconut milk	Strawberries or blueberries, for serving

1 Pulse the bananas, coconut milk, and cacao powder in a food processor or high-speed blender until smooth and creamy.

2 Serve with sliced strawberries and/or blueberries. Eat immediately to avoid browning.

Tip: *Cacao powder is all the rage on the Raw culinary scene, so it's getting easier to obtain at health food stores or online at stores like* www.vitacost.com.

Per serving: Calories 152; Fat 6.7 g (Saturated 5.7 g); Cholesterol 0 mg; Sodium 5 mg; Carbohydrate 25.4 g (Fiber 3.5 g); Protein 2.2 g; Sugar 12.4 g.

ᗡ *Fast, Colorful Papaya Pudding*

Thanks to Shannon Leone (www.rawmom.com) for this warp-speed offering. It's made with banana and papaya and taken from her e-book *Eating for Beauty, Health & Pleasure* (available at www.bottlinghealth.com). A ripe banana may help IBS-D, and a slightly green one is best for IBS-C. So pick a banana based on your symptoms right now. The second ingredient, papaya, is great for anyone with IBS because of its high soluble-fiber content and therapeutic amounts of digestive enzymes.

Preparation time: *8 minutes*

Cooking time: *None*

Yield: *2 servings*

½ of a large papaya, peeled and deseeded   Squeeze of lime juice

1 large banana, peeled

1 Blend the two fruits until creamy.

2 Add a squeeze of lime and serve.

Vary It! *To create a thicker pudding, add 1 tablespoon of psyllium powder to the recipe. Bonus: Psyllium powder is 75 percent soluble fiber.*

Tip: *Pair this recipe with either of the crust recipes in this chapter for a tasty pie.*

Tip: *Decorate the top of your pudding or pie with bananas, papaya, and coconut flakes.*

Per serving: *Calories 98; Fat 0.4 g (Saturated 0.1 g); Cholesterol 0 mg; Sodium 4 mg; Carbohydrate 24.8 g (Fiber 3.4 g); Protein 1.3 g; Sugar 13.9 g.*

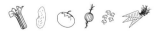

Thickening agents in the food industry are varied. *Gums* come from plant and tree *exudates* (discharges). *Algin* and *agar* come from marine plants or seaweed extracts. *Pectin* is produced from fruit and vegetable extracts. *Xanthan* gum is a fermentation product. Psyllium powder is comes from a family of plants called *Plantago*, which you probably know better as plantains.

⏱ Key Lime Mousse

This recipe, also from Shannon Leone's Raw kitchen (www.rawmom.com), is fast and so delicious that it hits the spot every time! Avocados are non-sweet fruits, a source of healing vitamin E, and a source of healthy fat that keeps joints lubricated, provides insulation around nerve sheathes, and is great for the hair and skin.

Most people with IBS can tolerate some avocado, but just be aware that eating too much of any kind of fat may trigger IBS side effects. Used in moderation, however, IBS sufferers can digest avocado; it may even have a healing effect.

Preparation time: *5 minutes*

Cooking time: *None*

Yield: *2 servings*

2 ripe avocados, pitted and peeled	*2 tablespoons raw, organic honey*
Juice of 2 limes (about ¼ cup)	*Sprig of mint for garnish*
1 teaspoon organic vanilla extract	*2 strawberries, thinly sliced, for garnish*

1 Blend the avocados, lime, vanilla, and honey in a food processor until smooth and creamy.

2 Serve in a dessert cup with a sprig of mint and very thinly sliced strawberries.

Vary It! *You can substitute 1 lemon for the 2 limes if that's all you have on hand. Add more lime or lemon juice for a stronger citrus taste. You also can use agave nectar instead of honey.*

Tip: *To save yourself time, you can purchase organic lemon juice in the health food store to keep on hand for when you don't have lemons to squeeze.*

Per serving: *Calories 407; Fat 29.3 g (Saturated 4.5 g); Cholesterol 0 mg; Sodium 18 mg; Carbohydrate 39.5 g (Fiber 23.6 g); Protein 4.3 g; Sugar 19.6 g.*

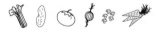

⏱ Goji Berry Tapioca

Shannon Leone's tapioca from her e-book *The Healthy Lunch Box* (available at www.rawmom.com/HealthyLunchbox) is a delight. You can find goji berries (also called wolfberries) and chia seeds in your health food store or online. Chia seeds are mild tasting and high in protein and essential fatty acids. It's also very high in soluble fiber, absorbing up to 12 times its weight in water making it an excellent way to relieve diarrhea. And if you have constipation, you can drink extra water with your dessert and turn it into the safe bulk you need.

The great thing about this recipe is that it creates some great little extras you can use for other recipes. Save the almond pulp for cookies or pie crust, and store the extra almond milk in the fridge as a tasty beverage.

Tools: *High-speed blender*

Preparation time: *15 minutes*

Cooking time: *None*

Yield: *4 servings*

½ to 1 cup goji berries	*Pinch of sea salt*
½ to 1 cup white or black chia seeds	*Drop of organic vanilla (optional)*
1 teaspoon honey, or to taste	

1 Blend the almonds and water in a high-speed blender until completely liquefied. Strain the almond milk using a fine mesh strainer, and then add the honey, salt, and vanilla (if desired).

2 Use about 1 to 2 cups per person of the almond milk for the tapioca, and store the rest in the fridge as a beverage.

3 Add the goji berries and chia seeds to the almond milk and let set for 30 minutes. Enjoy!

Vary It! *You can use agave in place of the honey.*

Per serving: *Calories 691; Fat 43.2 g (Saturated 2.8 g); Cholesterol 0 mg; Sodium 127 mg; Carbohydrate 49.2 g (Fiber 26.2 g); Protein 23.8 g; Sugar 17.1 g.*

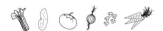

Isn't chia that seed-growing thing?

Chia (Salvia hispanica) is a member of the mint family, though you use the seeds rather than the leaves. And, yes, it's the pet that grows. Originating in Mexico, chia was part of the Aztec and Mayan diets, but the Spanish conquest hampered its cultivation. In the past few decades production has increased, especially since Ricardo Ayerza Jr. and Wayne Coates wrote *Chia: Rediscovering a Forgotten Crop of* *the Aztecs* (University of Arizona Press), the definitive book on the subject, in 2005.

Chia is 16 percent protein, 31 percent fat, and 44 percent carbohydrate (and 38 percent of that carbohydrate is fiber). It has more insoluble than soluble fiber, but its soluble fiber is denser and more absorbent than other dietary fibers, making it act more like a high soluble fiber.

☺ Vegan Khir Pudding

Healing chef Julie Beyer needed a way to use up leftover rice or noodles, so she came up with this vegan version of an Indian delight. Use non-wheat grains or noodles. Blending the cashews may make them easier to digest, making this pudding safe for both IBS-C and IBS-D.

Preparation time: *20 minutes*

Cooking time: *None*

Yield: *4 servings*

1 cup cashews, soaked in water for 4 hours and drained

1 to 1½ cups water

2 to 3 tablespoons maple syrup, or to taste

Pinch of sea salt

1 to 2 teaspoons of cardamom, or to taste

½ cup cooked brown rice or whole-grain noodles (such as rice or buckwheat noodles of your choice)

Dash of saffron (optional)

¼ cup slivered almonds (optional)

1 Blend the cashews, water, maple syrup, sea salt, and cardamom in a blender and adjust seasoning to taste.

2 Add cooked rice or noodles to cashew milk and, if desired, sprinkle with a dash of saffron and almonds as well as an extra drizzle of maple syrup.

Tip: *If you want the nutty taste of almonds but not the slivers, blend the almonds separately to a powder and then sprinkle over the finished pudding.*

Per serving: *Calories 377; Fat 25.2 g (Saturated 4.5 g); Cholesterol 0 mg; Sodium 9 mg; Carbohydrate 31.6 g (Fiber 2.5 g); Protein 11 g; Sugar 10.9 g.*

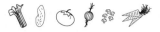

Creating Coconut Cookies and Bread

Living in Maui, Carolyn is exposed to considerable amounts of coconut. Every week at the farmer's market, she samples Lori Steer's Maui Macaroons (www.mauimacaroon.com). If she's feeling a little rumbly, just one macaroon is enough to settle her gut down. We bring that up because so much folklore surrounds the healing power of coconut macaroons for IBS-D. The meat of the coconut in the form of macaroons can relieve diarrhea.

People with IBS-C can also enjoy macaroons because they aren't binding. If you really want a coconut treatment for IBS-C, it's coconut oil. The oil in coconut helps lubricate the intestines and can relieve constipation. Even though it's a fat, it doesn't go rancid. Coconut oil is the closest to mother's milk in its medium-chain fatty acid (MCFA) content, and MCFAs are very digestible and aren't as readily stored as fat. Add a teaspoon of coconut oil once or twice a day to create a lubricating effect on the intestines. Combining coconut oil with getting enough water, exercise, fiber, magnesium, and vitamin C is very beneficial for IBS-C.

MCFAs raise metabolism, so you actually can lose weight and lower your cholesterol with coconut. MCFAs boost the immune system and fight yeast, bad bacteria and viruses. They have a huge reputation in the chronic fatigue and AIDS community.

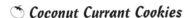

☁ *Coconut Currant Cookies*

Coconut is very healing for IBS-D and safe for IBS-C. This recipe, contributed by Jody to `www.pecanbread.com`, is SCD-safe for people with colitis and Crohn's disease, making it safe for folks with IBS as well.

Preparation time: *5 minutes*

Cooking time: *12 minutes*

Yield: *6 servings (12 cookies total)*

1 egg	*1½ cups shredded coconut*
½ cup honey	*½ cup chopped walnuts*
¼ teaspoon salt	*½ cup currants*
½ cup almond flour	

1 Preheat the oven to 350 degrees.

2 Using an electric mixer or blender, blend the egg, honey, and salt together. Add the almond flour to the mixture and mix until well blended. Add the coconut, walnuts, and currants and mix until thoroughly combined.

3 Bake for 10 to 12 minutes.

Per serving: *Calories 126; Fat 6.92 g (Saturated 1.5 g); Cholesterol 18 mg; Sodium 65 mg; Carbohydrate 15.8 g (Fiber 1 g); Protein 2.5 g; Sugar 13.5 g.*

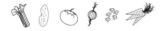

☺ *Coconut Bread*

Michelle Gay, our Australian chef at `www.eatingjourney.wordpress.com`, contributed this delicious recipe. Coconut is a very healing food for the intestines, killing intestinal infectious microorganisms; eggs are a neutral food, and the rest of the ingredients are safe and healthy. Honey does contain natural sugar, but it's a very low amount that your body can digest quickly, leaving none to feed your intestinal microorganisms. And it's also far less sugar than most dessert breads and cakes contain. If you can't find coconut flour, you can buy shredded coconut and blend it down until it's very fine. Just be sure not too blend it down too far because it turns into a paste.

Preparation time: *10 minutes*

Cooking time: *50 minutes*

Yield: *10 servings*

1⅔ cups coconut flour	½ teaspoon salt
5 eggs	1 tablespoon of gluten-free baking powder
1 teaspoon organic vanilla	¼ cup plus 1 tablespoon honey
2 teaspoons cinnamon	

1 Preheat the oven to 330 degrees.

2 Mix 1 teaspoon of the cinnamon with the salt, baking powder, and ¼ cup of the honey in a bowl.

3 Place the batter into a greased 9-x-5-inch loaf pan or an ungreased silicone bread pan.

4 Top the dough with a sprinkle of the remaining cinnamon and honey and bake for 45 to 50 minutes.

Tip: *Slice warm or cold and spread with whipped butter and honey.*

Per serving: *Calories 151; Fat 4.5 g (Saturated 2.1 g); Cholesterol 105 mg; Sodium 261 mg; Carbohydrate 36.3 g (Fiber 8.3 g); Protein 5.9 g; Sugar 8.9 g.*

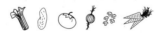

Topping Things Off: Decadent Dessert Toppers

Many people just can't eat pudding, pie, or cake without a little something to put on top. But many store-bought toppings can wreak havoc on your IBS. Beware of the whipped products that are dairy-free alternatives to whipped cream. Just because they're lactose-free doesn't mean they're IBS-friendly — in fact, they often include *casein,* a milk protein that triggers some people's IBS, and *high-fructose corn syrup,* a processed sweetener that's not a good addition to any diet. The recipes in this section give you a few options for homemade toppers that you can enjoy worry-free.

Date Syrup

If you find that you're very sensitive to sweeteners but would love to have something safe, try Angela Elliott's (www.she-zencuisine.com) Date Syrup. It's high in soluble fiber, and any insoluble fiber is blended to be more digestible, so folks with all kinds of IBS can enjoy it as they would honey: as a tea sweetener, on pancakes, or in recipes like the chocolate mousse in this chapter. You can store the date syrup in a glass jar in the refrigerator for 2 weeks, but it's better if you use it fresh.

Soaking time: *3 to 4 hours*

Preparation time: *5 minutes*

Cooking time: *None*

Yield: *Six ¼-cup servings (1½ cups total)*

20 to 25 honey or medjool dates	1 cup filtered, spring, or alkaline water

1 Pit the dates and cover them with the water in a bowl. Soak for 3 to 4 hours.

2 Blend the dates and the soaking water in a blender until smooth.

Tip: *Pour this syrup on the pancakes in Chapter 6.*

Per serving: *Calories 277; Fat 0.2 g (Saturated 0 g); Cholesterol 0 mg; Sodium 1 mg; Carbohydrate 75 g (Fiber 6.7 g); Protein 1.8 g; Sugar 66.5 g.*

☙ *Angel's Decadent Whipped Cream*

This recipe comes from Angela Elliott (www.she-zencuisine.com), author of many Raw cookbooks. The message here is that something doesn't have to be cream to be creamy! Because of the antimicrobial and lubricant effect of coconut oil and bowel stimulating effect of the oil in macadamia nuts, this recipe is very beneficial for IBS-C. Cold pressed coconut oil avoids heat processing that can destroy some of the nutrient value of this valuable nut.

Preparation time: *5 minutes*

Cooking time: *None*

Yield: *Eight ¼-cup servings (2 cups total)*

1 cup macadamia nuts, soaked in water for 4 hours and drained

½ cup water

½ cup Date Syrup (see the preceding recipe) or agave, or more to taste

1 teaspoon organic vanilla

1 tablespoon cold-pressed coconut oil

1 Blend all the ingredients in a blender until smooth and creamy in texture.

Tip: If your cream doesn't seem thick enough, blending it for a few seconds more should thicken it up.

Per serving: *Calories 206; Fat 14.4 g (Saturated 3.5 g); Cholesterol 0 mg; Sodium 1.3 mg; Carbohydrate 21.1 g (Fiber 3.1 g); Protein 1.8 g; Sugar 17.5 g.*

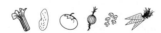

Part III
Simple Solutions for Specific Situations

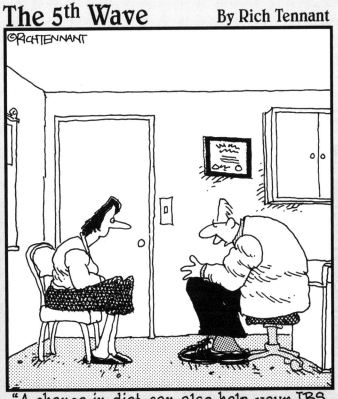

The 5th Wave   By Rich Tennant

"A change in diet can also help your IBS. The next time you're at a restaurant, go ahead and order those probiotics, and treat yourself to some digestive enzymes."

In this part . . .

*H*ere we tackle three common situations where eating for IBS can be the most challenging. Chapter 14 makes eating on the go less daunting, and Chapter 15 helps you satisfy even the pickiest IBS kid (without grossing out the rest of the family). Chapter 16 shows you how to find IBS-friendly meals when you eat out — even IBS cooks need a night off.

Chapter 14

Eating On the Go

. . . .

In This Chapter

▶ Preparing and packing meals and snacks ahead of time

▶ Controlling your IBS away from home

▶ Taking the worry out of travelling with IBS

. . . .

For many people with IBS, leaving the house can be a major challenge even on good days. We know that virtually every time you leave the house you're worried that you'll have an IBS attack. In fact, some IBS sufferers have secret maps to the bathrooms all over their cities; at least one Web site even maps clean bathrooms all over the world (that's www.sitorsquat.com if you're interested).

But the number two worry (pardon the pun) for people with IBS is what they're going to eat when they leave the house. We're not talking about what you can eat at restaurants — that's in Chapter 16. We're talking about planning your food when you're away from the house for work, school, or a visit to Grandma's. You're ready to venture out into the world after being stuck at home with your symptoms, and we want to help you plan a successful outing. In this chapter, we offer ideas and suggestions for creating a self-contained, portable survival kit you can grab whenever you head out the door. You have to take your finicky digestive system with you wherever you go, and we want to help you prepare.

Being Prepared Keeps You in Control

Yes, things were absolutely much easier when you could grab a prepared meal or snack at the coffee shop, corner store, or lunchroom. But now you have IBS — you can't just grab any old munchies if you want to stave off an attack. This section shows you how a little preparation can help you avoid getting stuck without an appropriate way to satisfy your hunger.

Eating small portions is important for controlling IBS. As you prep and pack meals ahead of time, make sure you aren't sabotaging yourself with portion size.

Preparation starts in the kitchen: Cooking meals in advance

Planning for eating on the go takes some time and dedication, but we want to help take the torture out of the chore. The plan is that in just a short couple of hours a week, you can have days of dishes ready to go. So clear the family out of the kitchen, crank up your favorite music, and get started. Just remember that you're setting this time aside to celebrate your healthy approach to food — and to living safely in the world.

Deciding what you're going to eat for the week is a great start. Create a weekly menu (see Chapter 4) and check your menu for recipes that you can make in multiples and store or freeze the extras to pack for work or school. Make sure the ingredients you need are on your shopping list. (Chapter 4 also provides tips for shopping success.)

Roast a large chicken on your cooking day and use the left over meat and vegetables to make a soup or stew that you can freeze for several meals to come.

Gather together the vegetables that you want to cut up. No matter what shape, size, or density, chopping piles of veggies all at once can be fun and therapeutic. After you've got them chopped, separate the veggies you want to blanch (to make them more digestible) and dip them in boiling water for the allotted time. You can cool and then freeze them in freezer baggies to grab when you go.

Stacking soups to save space

If you find that you're running out of space in the freezer for all your tiny tubs of soups and stews, we've got you covered. Our healing chef Colleen Robinson suggests pouring cooled soup into heavy-duty zippered plastic storage bags and stacking the bags on top of each other on a cookie sheet. Put the sheet of soups or stews in the freezer until frozen. Your final product will be flat bags of soup that you can stack in your freezer rather than a mixed bag of frozen shapes and sizes that take up much more space. If you're worried about the bags sticking together while they're freezing, put a sheet of waxed paper between the layers of soup bags. The added bonus is that when you take your soup bag to work or school, it helps keep the other food cool.

If you're chopping zucchini, you can bag some raw because it's high in soluble fiber and IBS-friendly.

A couple of dips you can make ahead are nut pâté (see the recipe in Chapter 7) and pesto (see the recipe in Chapter 11). They're not meals, but they make great pasta toppings or wrap sauces. Nut pâté doesn't freeze well, but the garlic in the recipe keeps it fresh for a week. You can freeze pesto for about 3 months.

Keeping a portable snack pack on hand

Chapter 2 helps you understand the foods that work best for you and your sensitive self. Copies of your safe food list are likely laminated and placed strategically around your home, office, and car (and if they aren't, they should be). Take a copy of your safe food list and assign numbers based on how safe those foods are for you: Put a *1* next to foods you know you can absolutely always eat safely, a *2* next to those foods that are usually very safe, and a *3* beside those foods that are safe but only under certain circumstances.

We strongly recommend that you always have a supply of at least one of your number one safe foods on your person whenever you're away from your own kitchen. For example, if applesauce is one of your top safe foods, buy small, sealed containers and keep a couple in your desk at work, a couple in your car (depending on the temperature outside), and a couple in your handbag, computer bag, or somewhere else handy. That way, when hunger hits, you have safe food to eat immediately and won't be tempted to grab a less-safe snack from the vending machine.

The following list details the foods that are easiest to pack and safest for IBS stomachs in general. You know your gut better than we do, so you can certainly add other foods you have flagged on your safe food list. If you're trying out the Specific Carbohydrate Diet (SCD, see Chapter 3), check out the extensive list of legal and illegal foods at www.pecanbread.com/c.

- ✔ **Applesauce:** You can purchase individual containers of applesauce or make your own and store it in small containers.

- ✔ **Avocados:** They come with their own container (a pretty durable shell), and you can slice them in half with a sharp knife, remove the pit, and eat them plain or with a teaspoon of lemon juice. If you're a Vata constitution (see Chapter 5), you can even sprinkle in a few drops of a mild chili sauce.

- ✔ **Bananas:** More great foods with their own baggies. As we mention in Chapter 3, unripe bananas are suitable for IBS-C and ripe ones for IBS-D.

- ✔ **Barley:** Bring some barley soup with you when you travel and cook it up when you can. Amy's brand has a tasty canned Organic Vegetable Barley Soup (www.amys.com). One can is 398 milliliters, which is about 1.5 cups of soup.

- ✔ **Beets:** Mixing cut-up cooked beets with carrots, corn, some brown rice, and a bit of lemon and olive oil can make a great snack. Add some chestnuts, and you've got a gourmet meal. All these foods are high in soluble fiber and can be packed alone or in combination.

- ✔ **Currants, figs, raisins, and prunes:** These dried fruits are great choices separately and together are a good combination for IBS-C. High in soluble fiber and stimulating to the intestines, they help to keep your bowels working when you're traveling.

- ✔ **French bread and sourdough bread:** A long stick of French bread is a great soluble-fiber food to add to any meal on the road. It can counteract insoluble fiber or fill a vacuum when you can't find anything else safe to eat. Sourdough bread isn't made from yeast, so it's a good option for folks who may be following a yeast-free diet.

- ✔ **Oatmeal:** This standby is the IBS traveler's breakfast of choice. Check out Chapter 6 for oatmeal recipes and tips on making it in your hotel room.

- ✔ **Mangos and papayas:** These fruits are high in soluble fiber, and papaya is high in enzymes, making it especially easy on the stomach. Cut them in half, scoop out the seeds and pit, and eat the goodness inside.

- ✔ **Parsnips:** If you love parsnips, mix and match them with brown rice, yams, sweet potato, carrots, beets, turnips, squash, and pumpkins.

- ✔ **Peas:** Put fresh peas in a container with some potato and yam for a great meal on the go; you can add a bit of olive oil and vinegar to help mix the flavors. All three vegetables are high in soluble fiber. If you're into cooked peas, adding butter or ghee (see the recipe in Chapter 6) gives them a rich taste.

- ✔ **Psyllium seed husks:** These bad boys may sound pretty intimidating, but they're what you find in powdered fiber supplements like Metamucil. They're a great soluble-fiber addition to your travel pack; a tablespoon or two a day when you travel helps regulate your bowels — take a tablespoon with 6 or 12 ounces of water for IBS-D and -C, respectively.

- ✔ **Quinoa:** Rice and barley aren't the only safe grains. Use cooked, cooled quinoa as a base for the safe soluble vegetables you can tolerate.

- ✔ **Rice:** It's generally safe for IBS-D and IBS-C, so you may want to have a small covered container of cooked brown rice as your personal portable soluble fiber.

Always make sure that your survival kit has a vegetable peeler. Matches (for dispelling odors caused by flaring symptoms) are another good addition.

Enjoying Common Events without Worrying About Side Effects

Most people without irritable bowels have no idea how much thought and care goes into getting out the door for those who do. As an IBS sufferer, you never know whether that pressure in your rectum is a gas or a solid, which makes planning any trip outside the house somewhat difficult. But we assure you it won't always be like that. In this section, we show you how a little forethought can help IBS sufferers function in everyday situations.

Enjoying food at the office

Even if you love your job and have a positive workplace, anywhere but home can be stressful if you have IBS. To help keep control over your situation, make sure you have lots of nourishing, nurturing foods and drinks with you when you head to work; in fact, stash a stockpile of your top safe foods at your desk so you're always prepared. We also recommend keeping a supply of soothing drinks (such as peppermint, black, and ginger tea and lemonade) as well for those times your IBS day doesn't go quite as planned.

Of course, the office-eating issue is lunch; head to "Preparation Starts in the Kitchen: Cooking Meals in Advance" earlier in this chapter for tips on cooking grab-and-go lunches in advance, and check out the recipes in Parts II and III for tons of IBS-friendly food ideas. If you miss going out to lunch with your work pals, check out Chapter 16 for some ideas on making that easier as well.

 One of Christine's favorite portable foods is cooked low-fat turkey sausages. Shop for a selection that doesn't have fillers like wheat or additives like nitrates. Cook up a bunch and let them cool and then wrap each one in tinfoil and pop them in the freezer. Christine drops one in her purse in the morning — by lunch it's a thawed and tasty protein boost.

 Feeling deprived during that 3-p.m. slump when everyone in the office is feeding dollar bills into the candy machine? Check out the dessert recipes in Chapter 13 and tuck some safe sweets in your desk at your office.

If your office is prone to pitch-ins, check out "The potluck dinner" section later in this chapter for info on navigating these parties.

Sending kids to school

Most kids just want to fit in with their friends and not stand out as different — especially at school, where standing out can be brutal. If your child has IBS, she's probably feeling the anxiety of being different on top of the anxiety caused by her condition. Try packing a discreet survival kit with things to help her feel safer at school, such as a thermos of her favorite soothing tea, soup, or stew, or some rice crackers or plain mini rice cakes. Just be sure to check the school's regulations for bringing in outside food (and you should probably forgo the matches in this case).

Preparation is the key for helping your child feel safe at school. It may take some time to settle on lunches that nourish without embarrassing. Chapter 15 shows you how to do avoidance and challenging and create a food diary with your child; after she has a better understanding of food's effect on her condition, let her help you shop for the foods she's put on her own safe list and work together to create lunches that satisfy both hunger and the need to fit in.

For kids with IBS, sitting in a classroom under scrutiny of the teacher can be upsetting. Putting her hand up to be excused to go to the bathroom can be difficult for any kid, but if your IBS kid has to raise her hand to be excused five or six times a day, that can feel like torture (and that emotional strain isn't going to help the situation any). And the bathroom isn't the only issue. Kids tend to get hungry throughout the day, and a standard tip for people with IBS is to eat smaller meals throughout the day, but your student's snack and mealtimes are limited when she's in school.

Explain your child's condition to her teacher, principal, and school nurse so that they understand what may happen in the course of the day. Her teacher may already be aware that frequent bathroom breaks have been necessary, but a sit-down meeting can drive the point home. You also want to work out a plan for necessary snacking, such as having your student keep a stash of snacks in her locker or in the nurse's office and duck out of class to keep her eating schedule on track.

Class celebrations are another challenge for kids with IBS. Having a conversation about why she can't share in the cupcakes is mandatory, and if you've already done the food diary and elimination diet with your kid, she knows that the sweet treat, no matter how delicious, can still send her to the bathroom in an unpleasant way. Teachers generally send home a note to let parents know when a cupcake or pizza day is pending. Make sure you've put a treat from Chapter 13 in your kid's lunchbag to help soften the blow.

No matter what age you are, in many ways, school and IBS do not mix well. If you are an adult with IBS going to school, you can let your instructor know that you have a condition that may require you to leave the room occasionally. Sit near the door so your comings and goings are less distracting. Your class schedule may be more flexible around your eating schedule, but you may also want to mention that you may sometimes need to bring a snack to class.

Socializing with IBS: Functioning at a function

No, we don't mean that you're going to invite your bowels to a party. Like any public event, social functions can be very stressful for people with IBS. They have to deal with tempting but potentially triggering foods, strange (and sometimes public) washrooms, and folks who may not understand their restrictions. The good news is that you can overcome these obstacles with a little preplanning.

If your event's venue is a public place, you can always call or drop by to check out the bathroom facilities to help to ease your mind. If food will be served, make sure you've eaten a safe and balanced meal beforehand. You don't want to show up hungry and be tempted to eat unidentified foods or foods you know are bad but look reaaallly good to your growling stomach. If you see foods that you know are safe for you, try them out. Otherwise, just pop a few drops of mint essential oil into a glass of mineral water and enjoy conversation rather than canapés. The following sections give you more tips for surviving more-specific kinds of shindigs.

The dreaded dinner party

We've heard so many stories about dinner party mishaps. Rule number one: If you don't know what it is, don't eat it. Period. Experts tell us that they would rather be a bit rude for turning down the creamed artichoke dip they know they can't handle than be embarrassed (and even ruder) for spending dessert in the bathroom with the fan working and matches burning.

If you've accepted an invitation to a dinner party because you're feeling like your symptoms have been behaving lately, great. However, keep in mind that they can still throw a tantrum at any moment. This setting isn't the place to test unknown foods or go back to foods that have been a problem in the past. Save testing foods for the privacy of your own home.

Many hosts ask their guests if they have any food allergies or sensitivities. Although you may be able to tell someone that you're gluten intolerant and lactose intolerant, they may not be too tolerant of you giving them your whole IBS trigger list. Instead, give them some or all of your safe food list, or rely on the following version of the safe soluble food list in Chapter 2, which we've modified here for common dinner party ingredients:

- ✔ Applesauce
- ✔ Avocados
- ✔ Bananas
- ✔ Barley
- ✔ Beets
- ✔ Brown rice
- ✔ Carrots
- ✔ Corn
- ✔ French bread

- ✔ Fresh peas
- ✔ Mangos
- ✔ Papayas
- ✔ Pasta
- ✔ Potatoes
- ✔ Rice
- ✔ Squash
- ✔ Sweet potatoes
- ✔ Yams

We haven't included any salad greens here — those have to come from your personal preferences and experiments. Fish, chicken, and lean meats are usually fine as long as they're not fried.

The potluck dinner

We love the idea of potluck dinners because you know you can find at least one food you can eat safely — the dish you bring! In addition to bringing a safe dish, have a safe snack beforehand at home and, as always, have your survival kit with you. Make sure to make plenty of your dish; you need to be able to get some even if it's the hit of the party (and if you use one of the recipes in this book, it very well may be).

If you're having a potluck lunch at work, offer to organize the menu and add a couple of safe side dishes to the sign-up sheet like steamed rice and baked yams.

At your next potluck, suggest that everyone bring copies of the written recipe for their dishes for everyone at the party. That way, you can read the ingredients and determine what's safe fare for you. It's also a great way to collect recipes. Or if this book is your book club's selection this month, meet somewhere with a big kitchen and have a cooking party where everyone gets to take home a few meals for the freezer.

Venturing Further Afield: Eating On the Road

Whether you're taking a day trip or a long holiday, you have to do your homework before you leave. The following list provides tips for keeping your tummy happy while you travel.

- ✔ **Make sure everyone's on the same page.** If they don't know already, let your travelling companions know that you have special considerations to keep in mind when travelling. If you're visiting family or friends, send them an e-mail with your safe food list and let them know that you'll be bringing some food with you and doing some of your own grocery shopping after you get there and may need to do some of your own cooking.

- ✔ **Scope out your destinations for grocery stores and health food stores that carry the foods you need.** You want to stock up on soluble-fiber staples after you reach your destination. If you're headed somewhere that may not have the ingredients you need, take them with you. For example, coconut flour may be hard to get in the middle of nowhere, so if you anticipate needing it, pack some up in a heavy-duty zipper bag that can withstand travel.

- ✔ **Prepack food in to-go portions.** You can easily find snack-sized plastic bags and containers so that you always have munchies on hand regardless of your vacation activities. (See "Keeping a portable snack pack on hand" for snack suggestions.)

  For quick, safe on-the-go meals, throw a cooked chicken leg into a baggie and head out. It comes with its own stick, and you can hold it with the baggie to keep your fingers clean. Other protein sources you can easily store in baggies are thick slices of meat (so they don't fall apart), lamb or pork chops, and even a chicken breast. Just be sure to keep them cold if you're going to be out for a while before eating them. Freezing them beforehand and popping them in your bag before you leave will keep them cool for a few hours. By the time you're ready to eat, your food will be thawed.

- ✔ **Make the best of rest stop offerings.** Nothing is worse than being on a long drive without a prepacked meal and knowing that the convenient restaurants at the travel plazas are fast-food nightmares. That's why we encourage you to take food with you when you travel. If you stop to use the restroom and want to grab a cool drink, remember that the safest thing to buy is water. And you can put a drop of peppermint essential oil in the water to soothe your travel worn intestines.

✔ **Stick to your routine as much as possible.** Try to stay on schedule with your meals and bathroom breaks. If you see a rest stop, use it. This strategy will ease your mind and stomach in the long run. If you know that your bowels typically like to empty themselves three times before you leave the house in the morning, make sure you honor this when you're on the road. You may get up earlier than your travelling companions (the same as you do at home) to relieve yourself. If you take off after only two bowel movements, you may set up a problem later. If you're traveling with IBS-C, visiting rest stops along the way gives you a chance to stretch your legs, and maybe your colon will get the message!

✔ **Take charge of your own meals.** Although it may be more work, you can be assured you have the right meals if you make them yourself. Your host may appreciate the help, and you'll know exactly what you're eating. However, keep in mind that some folks are pretty territorial about their kitchens; be sure to verify with your host in advance that it's okay for you to do your own cooking.

Chapter 15

Making Mealtime Easier for Kids with IBS

*I*n this chapter we focus on feeding safe food to tiny tummies. If your IBS kid eats less sugar, wheat, and dairy (the three big triggers), he's likely to be healthier, get fewer colds and flus, and take fewer antibiotics. And finding the right foods can play a major role in helping kids with IBS feel normal. You can even tell your kids, and it won't be a lie, that they will be healthier and miss less school if they eat an IBS diet. Wait, maybe you shouldn't say the part about school.

Figuring Out Your Kid's Trigger Foods

Your IBS-D child may already be aware that sometimes she has an urgent, painful, explosive need to go to the bathroom and may have even had an embarrassing accident or two along the way. An IBS-C child may recognize his symptoms (the pain and bloated feeling in his stomach) but not their cause. If you haven't connected your child's symptoms to the foods he or she eats, chances are the kid isn't going to make the connection either. Regardless of IBS variety, children need to understand that paying attention to food choices can lead to more comfort in their bodies and doesn't have to be a chore.

Finding fiber that satisfies your tot's tastes

We address soluble fiber in several of the chapters in Part II, but the soluble foods children favor may be different from adult choices. Applesauce, apricots, bananas, peaches, papayas, carrots, potatoes, squash, zucchini, oatmeal, rice, miracle noodles, and non-gluten pasta are some examples of safe soluble foods for kids.

Suspecting food sensitivities

In Chapter 2, we tell you about the food diary that helps adults monitor what they eat and the physical and emotional symptoms that may go along with their favorite foods. You can use the same technique to help determine which foods trigger your child's IBS symptoms. Quietly pay attention to how your child seems to feel or behave after eating a meal or a snack. The goal is to notice any patterns he has around normal mealtimes and snack times or after holidays and parties. Track your observations in a notebook. How many times a day did he visit the bathroom? Was he grouchy or complaining of pain? Was he demanding or indulging in more of a specific food (such as ice cream, cake, or bread)?

We encourage you to be subtle about recording his eating habits — no need to tell him you're watching every piece of food that he puts into his mouth!

A weekend is a great time to start your detective work because your child isn't away at school for several hours during the day and you likely have more time free to observe him.

If you prepare food for your kid, just carry on with your typical menu. Remember, you want to notice what is in his current diet that may be causing IBS symptoms (and we suspect that if your kid has an IBS reaction to certain foods, you'll start making that connection very quickly). At this stage, you're just observing and making notes.

After a few weeks of being a private detective, do a simple experiment. Pick a weekend when your child will be having all his meals at home. Plan your menu for the weekend and leave out one or two foods that your research suggests may be the IBS culprits. You may want to start with dairy and/or wheat, which are often in the top two. Instead of the typical milk-on-cereal breakfast and cheese sandwich at lunch, plan ahead for alternatives; you can check out the recipes later in this chapter or the information in Chapter 3 for ideas. Remember, you're just avoiding one or two things for a couple of days. Make notes about any changes (or lack thereof) you observe in your child's symptoms. If you see no perceivable improvements, experiment with two different foods on another weekend. But if you feel ready to introduce your kid to the avoidance and challenge experiment, read on.

Challenging foods to find the culprits

We talk about doing avoidance and challenge testing of certain foods in Chapter 2. We acknowledge that it can be a tough experiment, even for adults. After all, who wants to give up favorite foods? It can be even harder with kids because their trigger foods are often the ones they love most and will fight you tooth and nail for. When a kid craves a food, it can be like an addiction, and she won't give it up easily.

So if you want to encourage your child to do the challenge, be ready with your sales pitch. One idea is to wait until she complains about spending too much time in the bathroom or being uncomfortable from pain and bloating. If you've been monitoring her food habits and reactions (see the preceding section), present some of your detective work in a way that doesn't make her feel like you've been stalking her! Mention that you noticed her running to the bathroom after the pizza and movie night and that you've read that the ingredients in pizza can have that effect on some people. Then ask her whether she wants to do an experiment to see what foods her body does and doesn't like. Have her pick a Saturday when she can eat as much junk food as she likes and explain that you want her to avoid sugar, wheat, and dairy for six days leading up to that splurge day. During this time, you both will note how she feels emotionally and physically and keep track of her bowel movements.

We highly recommend that you do the experiment together and invite any other family members to participate. The more family members who participate in this experiment, the better. Not only does full participation make food preparation easier, but even those without IBS also feel some benefit from the exercise. In our experience, anyone who does the avoidance and challenge test comes away with a greater insight into how food affects their mind and body. The stomach ache after eating ice cream gets explained, as do the ongoing sugar cravings that can follow. It's a great opportunity to explore family health and support the kid who has IBS trouble.

Your child may be miserable for a few days while going through junk food withdrawal, but by Saturday she just may be healthier and happier than you've seen her in a long time. Make sure you check in with her during those six days to see how she's feeling and how her relationship has been with the bathroom. If you're participating yourself, you can compare notes.

When Saturday rolls around, let her eat all the pizza, soda, ice cream, sugar-coated cereal, and sweets she can stomach. The aftermath of such a day may be filled with stomachache, headache, irritability, gas, bloating, lethargy, diarrhea, or constipation. Have her write down how she feels after indulging in these foods. If it's in her own handwriting that she made seven bathroom trips after eating pizza and ice cream, she may be more likely to believe it two months down the line when she is tempted by pizza. The experiment should give you and your child some great insight into the part food plays in her health picture. In our experience, kids become very conscientious about avoiding foods that are making them feel that bad. Now, it's your job to keep the kitchen stocked with foods they can eat, and we're here to help you with that chore.

You may have to conduct the challenge adventure a few times a year to remind your child of the connection between food and her symptoms. The body remembers how to react to trigger foods, but cravings for treats have a short attention span.

Keeping a kid's food diary to connect symptoms and triggers

When your child isn't doing avoidance and challenge testing (which we discuss in the preceding section), keeping a food diary (like the adult version in Chapter 2) can help him make a connection between food and his physical and emotional symptoms. Depending on age, your child can keep a paper diary, an electronic one on his computer or cellphone, or put all the facts on a big chalkboard. Younger children can use happy faces, neutral faces, or sad faces to illustrate how they feel after eating various foods. You can even make a game out of collecting happy faces in your child's food diary; he feels like he's winning at something, and you know he really is winning because he's eating more safe food.

Keep in mind that younger kids may not be able to make the connection between food and symptoms, even with a food diary. You may have to explain that what your child eats may be what's affecting his body.

If your child is older, she's more likely to make those connections, so encourage her to do so. If she notes in her diary that she was terrified her guts would explode at the birthday party, help her to reason that this reaction happened after eating the birthday cake.

Helping Your Kid (And the Family) Cope Emotionally with IBS

Being diagnosed with something like IBS is stressful for your child and for the family. Kids especially take their cues from you on how upset they should be about this condition. The more you highlight your child's IBS, the more he feels like it makes him stick out. The more worried you are, the more likely he is to think he has a serious illness.

Your job as a parent is to keep life as normal as possible. Downplay the fact that your child is different or sick as much as possible. You have to acknowledge the fact that he has symptoms and do whatever you can to help give him relief, but that doesn't mean it needs to be a production. Be conscious of labeling him as sensitive, different, and so on, because those labels can hurt (and stick). And make sure you respect your child's privacy; for example, don't talk about his bowel movement in front of his friends or siblings.

That said, don't pay so little attention to your child's IBS that he feels alone. Try to keep chatting with your IBS child. If he doesn't feel like you understand, he may close up and avoid talking about his bathroom experiences and symptoms, feeling like he has to deal with them on his own.

Remember that one child's IBS affects other kids in the family as well. Suddenly, brother is getting more attention and special food treatment, which if left unchecked may lead to resentment (especially if the non-IBSers feel like they're having to throw out their cheese puffs to accommodate the IBS kid's new restrictions). Make sure everyone is getting attention, information about the new changes, and healthy snacks, and check out the following section for more on keeping everybody feeling well fed.

Creating As Little Headache As Possible in the Kitchen

One of the most important steps to take when you have an IBS sufferer in the house is to make sure that your kitchen is stocked with IBS-friendly food. Everyone has seen (or been) the kid who stands in front of the full fridge — door wide open — and proclaims that there is nothing to eat. Multiply that with the feelings of deprivation that come when a kid's favorite foods are deemed unsafe, and you can understand why loading your kitchen with fabulous IBS-safe foods and keeping the unsafe foods out of sight is crucial for making your child's IBS journey a little easier. We show you how to create an IBS-friendly kitchen in Chapter 4.

Have several types of IBS-safe snacks available to encourage your kid to eat different things each day. Munching on the same thing day after day can lead to food sensitivities, and providing lots of options helps your IBS child feel less restricted — like she's making a choice rather than not having any choices.

We already hear you say that making special food for your kid with IBS seems like a lot of extra work, but we encourage you to have a look at the recipes and tips in this book and consider introducing some new IBS-friendly dishes in the whole family's diet.

While the family is transitioning into this new way with food, have everyone write their names on the packages of one or two of their favorite snacks or foods. This way, everyone (parents, siblings, and your child with IBS) has foods that nobody else will touch. And because kids can be territorial, bogarting their own snacks may actually take their minds off the fact that those snacks are different.

What about siblings who don't have IBS challenges? They're going to insist on eating their favorite foods no matter what. We suggest some creative healthy snack swapping (such as fruit leather for a chocolate bar; Carolyn's Chocolate Banana Cream Pudding (see Chapter 13) instead of chocolate ice cream, and apple chips for potato chips). Chapter 7 is full of snacks that the whole family can enjoy and Chapter 13 has safe desserts to snack on. Great snacks show siblings that the fact that one person has IBS isn't going to force them to gag down inedible food!

Involving Kids in Shopping

Letting your little IBS sufferer help you shop for his foods is a great way to help him feel like he has choices in spite of his restrictions. Work together to come up with safe snack and meal favorites.

Before heading to the market, make sure your child has had a satisfying snack or meal to diminish his cravings for unfriendly foods. All shoppers know that shopping hungry tends to make people want to grab everything in sight. We suggest putting aside time to make the first shopping excursion a fun and thorough one. Leave the rest of the family at home for this one so you can both focus your attention on finding foods that fit.

At the store, give your kid as much control as possible when choosing IBS-friendly foods. Teach him how to read nutrition labels; a great rule of thumb is that if you can't pronounce the ingredient, you should keep it off the IBS-friendly list. See how quickly he can identify the sugar, wheat, and dairy on the labels, because he's most likely avoiding these ingredients. You may want to do some detective work beforehand and have a list of IBS-friendly products to direct him towards.

Making IBS-Friendly Foods for Your Kids

If your kid is like most kids, her favorite foods are probably French fries, hot dogs, milk, PB&J, and sugar-coated cereals. We've tried to include recipes in this section that are safe substitutes (though not necessarily exact replacements) for these standbys, and you can also adapt any of the recipes in this book for your child.

Breakfasting for kids

What do kids usually eat for breakfast before they go off to a stressful or exciting day at school? You may already be curbing the morning ritual of acidic orange juice and milk-drenched, sugar-coated wheat cereal, but a lot of the available alternatives aren't much friendlier. This section gives you recipes to replace your kid's trigger-loaded breakfast with friendlier fare. Check out Chapter 6 for more breakfast recipes.

Beef in a Pillow

We were inspired to create Beef in a Pillow using two kid-friendly and IBS-friendly foods: eggs and beef. Neither ingredient has the insoluble fiber that can irritate your gut, but both do have some fat. Be sure to drain the cooked beef well as the recipe calls for to help keep some of that fat out of your system. The egg fat comes in the yolk; if you're concerned about the fat irritating the intestines, you can substitute two egg whites for one egg, although the yolk is the most nutritious part of the egg.

Preparation time: 5 minutes

Cooking time: 10 minutes

Yield: 4 servings

2 tablespoons coconut oil	4 eggs
¼ pound free-range lean ground beef	½ teaspoon salt

1 Heat a medium skillet over medium heat and add 1 tablespoon of the coconut oil. Add the ground beef, cooking thoroughly while breaking it up into small chunks. Remove from the skillet and sit on paper towels to drain off the beef fat.

2 Beat the eggs and salt in a bowl.

3 In a clean, hot pan, heat the rest of the coconut oil and add the eggs. As the eggs begin to set (about 3 minutes), sprinkle the cooked beef into the center of the omelet. Flip the omelet in half, slide it halfway down the pan, and flip it over for another minute of cooking.

4 Remove the pan from the heat and cover for a few minutes so the center of the omelet finishes cooking. Cut into four servings and serve.

Per serving: Calories 174; Fat 14.1 g (Saturated 8.3 g); Cholesterol 229 mg; Sodium 377 mg; Carbohydrate 0.4 g (Fiber 0 g); Protein 11.8 g; Sugar 0.4 g.

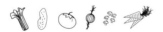

☺ Eggs in a Basket

This recipe is basically poached eggs on bread, but Eggs in a Basket makes it sound a little more fun. Eggs are a safe food for IBS; add them to an IBS-safe bread (such as the homemade sourdough in Chapter 12), and you have a winning combination. You can toast or not toast the bread depending on your child's preference.

Preparation time: 5 minutes

Cooking time: 5 minutes

Yield: 2 servings

2 eggs

2 slices of sourdough bread (store-bought, or see the recipe in Chapter 12)

2 teaspoons butter or ghee (see the recipe in Chapter 6)

Dash of paprika (optional)

1 Put 3 to 4 inches of water in a deep skillet (with a lid) and place on high heat. Crack each egg into a separate small cup; when the water in the skillet boils, gently slip the egg into the water and cover immediately.

2 Turn off the heat and cook until the eggs are just slightly runny, about 3 minutes. While the eggs are cooking, toast the bread (if desired), spread butter or ghee on each piece, and then cut a hole in the center of each piece. After the eggs are done, use a slotted spoon to put each egg in the hole of one piece of bread. Garnish with a dash of paprika (if desired).

Per serving: Calories 172; Fat 9.7 g (Saturated 4 g); Cholesterol 222 mg; Sodium 227 mg; Carbohydrate 12.3 g (Fiber 0.9 g); Protein 5.9 g; Sugar 1.8 g.

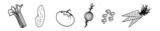

☺ Sheila's Tea Biscuits

This recipe contributed by Sheila to www.pecanbread.com for tea biscuits gives kids a safe biscuit option that also includes that childhood standby, peanut butter. These biscuits are safe for colitis and Crohn's disease, so they're safe for kids with IBS. We recommend Organic Maranatha Peanut Butter because the nuts are grown in a dry climate and not exposed to the dampness that can cause mold to grow on peanut crops in wet climates.

Preparation time: 5 minutes

Cooking time: 15 minutes

Yield: 7 servings (14 biscuits total)

2⅓ cups almond flour

½ cup creamy peanut butter

3 eggs

¼ cup plain yogurt (or water)

½ teaspoon salt

1 teaspoon honey (optional)

½ teaspoon baking soda

1 Preheat the oven to 325 degrees. Mix the almond flour and peanut butter well and set aside.

2 Beat the eggs and then mix in the yogurt or water, salt, honey (if desired) and baking soda. Add the egg mixture to the flour mixture and beat until it firms up.

3 Roll heaping tablespoons between barely wet hands, keeping a bowl of water nearby to rewet your hands as necessary. Place biscuits on a buttered baking sheet and flatten to about ¾ inch in height. Bake for approximately 15 minutes or until lightly browned. Cool and enjoy.

Vary It! *Add about ½ cup of raisins after all other ingredients are mixed well.*

Tip: *Enjoy with butter and homemade strawberry jam.*

Per serving: *Calories 250; Fat 21.2 g (Saturated 3 g); Cholesterol 64 mg; Sodium 262 mg; Carbohydrate 8.6 g (Fiber 1.8 g); Protein 11 g; Sugar 1.6 g.*

Munching lunches for little munchkins

Brown-bagging kids' lunches can be a challenge regardless of age because of their food restrictions and the added limitations of getting foods to school or day care. In this section, we give you some lunch alternatives that won't tempt your kids to go for the mystery meat.

Nuts are being regulated out of school lunches, so peanut butter sandwiches and snacks will soon be a thing of the past. What's left for snacks, you ask? Shannon Leone, author of *The Healthy Lunch Box* (available at www.rawmom. com/HealthyLunchbox), offers these suggestions from an article she wrote for www.naturallysavy.com:

- ✔ Loads of fresh fruits and berries
- ✔ Freshly ground sesame seeds mixed with a bit of honey
- ✔ Manna bread (sprouted grain breads)
- ✔ Rice and sushi loaded with veggie strips
- ✔ Vegetable crudités
- ✔ A cool pack with a smoothie
- ✔ Bean salads (made with chick peas, sprouted lentils, and so on)

- ✔ Rice cakes
- ✔ Veggie pâté

Black 'n' White Chicken Nuggets

This great kids' recipe, which is featured in the color section, comes from Colleen Robinson at www.crimsondoorhealing.com. It gives them the chicken nuggets they love minus the wheat batter, additives, and deep frying that can upset their tummies. They can even help make it! The sesame seeds do have some insoluble fiber, but you can grind them down in a food processor to make them more IBS-friendly.

Tools: *Parchment paper (optional)*

Preparation time: *10 minutes*

Cooking time: *20 to 25 minutes*

Yield: *4 servings*

½ cup black sesame seeds

½ cup white sesame seeds

¼ cup honey

2 egg whites, beaten

1 tablespoon tamari or low-sodium soy sauce

1 teaspoon water

¼ teaspoon each salt and pepper

4 boneless, skinless 6-ounce chicken breasts, cut into nugget-sized chunks

2 teaspoons olive oil

1 Preheat the oven to 400 degrees. Put half of the black sesame seeds in a large plastic zipper bag and repeat with a separate bag for the white sesame seeds.

2 In a medium bowl, whisk or fork-beat the honey, egg whites, tamari or soy sauce, water, salt, and pepper. Add the chicken and stir with a slotted spoon until all the chicken pieces are evenly coated. Remove the chicken with the slotted spoon, allowing the extra liquid to drip off the chicken.

3 Put half the chicken in the black sesame seed bag and the other half in the white sesame seed bag. Seal the bags and shake, shake, shake until the chicken is all coated in seeds, adding more seeds if you need to.

4 Cover two cookie sheets with a very thin coating of olive oil or parchment paper. Using a clean slotted spoon, take the chicken chunks out of the bags and put them on the cookie sheets, making sure the chunks don't touch each other to ensure faster cooking. Bake for 20 to 25 minutes or until a chunk cut open has no pink in the center.

Tip: *Honey makes a tasty dipping sauce if it's on your safe list.*

Per serving: *Calories 749; Fat 46.9 g (Saturated 8.3 g); Cholesterol 70 mg; Sodium 1196 g; Carbohydrate 51.9 g (Fiber 6.2 g); Protein 33.5 g; Sugar 18.3 g.*

Pita Pizza

Kids long for pizza, a classic treat, reward, and party food. Here's a recipe from Colleen Robinson (www.crimsondoorhealing.com) that puts pizza control in the hands of your children. These basic instructions are for 1 serving, but you can easily multiply by adding an extra pita per person.

This dish, which is featured in the color section, is as IBS-friendly as you make it because pretty much all of the ingredients are optional; leave off any trigger ingredients to avoid reactions. You can use either the tomato sauce or soy cream cheese (or both, if that's what floats your boat) as your topping base, and add the toppings here or anything else you have in your fridge. (Try chopped broccoli.) If you can handle cheese, choose an SCD variety such as brick cheese, white cheddar, or Colby.

Preparation time: *10 minutes*

Cooking time: *15 minutes*

Yield: *1 serving*

1 piece of non-wheat pita bread

1 tablespoon tomato sauce

4 medium mushrooms, sliced

¼ cup SCD-safe medium cheddar cheese

⅛ teaspoon each dried basil and dried oregano

1 Preheat the oven to 350 degrees (for a softer crust) or turn on the broiler (for a crispier crust).

2 Spread the pita with a small amount of tomato sauce. Sprinkle on the mushrooms, a bit of cheese as a highlight rather than a blanket, and the dried basil and oregano. Put the pizza on a cookie sheet and bake or broil until the mushrooms are a little wilted and any cheese is melted/browned to your liking.

Vary It! *You can use soy cream cheese in place of the tomato paste, and feel free to add whatever cheese and toppings you prefer from your safe foods list.*

Tip: *Kids enjoy cleaning spinach and other leafy greens when they get to put the greens in a towel and whirl it around their heads to dry them.*

Per serving: *Calories 269; Fat 10.7 g (Saturated 6 g); Cholesterol 30 mg; Sodium 256 mg; Carbohydrate 31.7 g (Fiber 1.1 g) Protein 12.7 g; Sugar 3.8 g.*

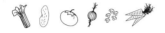

Colorful Kids Pasta Salad

You cook the pasta — the kiddies put the salad together. Everybody wins. This family-friendly favorite comes from Colleen Robinson (www.crimsondoorhealing.com) and lets everybody get involved with their dinner. Use gluten-free, Orgran Rice & Corn Vegetable Pasta, which comes in multicolored animal shapes. You can also use gluten-free Tinkyada Organic Brown Rice Pasta, but then you have to change the name to Kids Pasta Salad — just as tasty, but less fun. Peas are high in soluble fiber and make this dish very IBS-friendly.

Preparation time: *5 minutes*

Cooking time: *10 minutes*

Yield: *4 servings*

One 8.8-ounce package dried pasta, cooked and drained

1 cup frozen peas, thawed under running water

One 12-ounce can of tuna packed in water, drained

1 tablespoon lemon juice

½ tablespoon olive oil

¼ teaspoon each salt and pepper, or to taste

1 Place the cooked pasta in a big bowl; have the kid(s) add in the peas and tuna and stir.

2 Put the lemon juice and olive oil in a small jar and let the kid(s) shake it and pour it over the pasta mixture. Add salt and pepper to taste.

Per serving: *Calories 443; Fat 9.8 g (Saturated 1.8 g); Cholesterol 15 mg; Sodium 228 mg; Carbohydrate 51.8 g (Fiber 3.8 g); Protein 34.7 g; Sugar 3.4 g.*

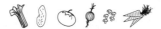

Dining in

Certain dishes are just plain kid-friendly. Fish sticks and macaroni and cheese are a couple of kid cravings you may have to watch out for with IBS tots. So our healing chef Colleen Robinson has adapted these faves to enhance their friendliness. After your IBS kid knows that he can still eat "normally," the impact of IBS on his diet may lessen a little.

Fried-Free Fish for Four

Colleen Robinson (www.crimsondoorhealing.com) presents this simple-to-make, kid-friendly recipe. To increase its IBS-friendliness, use breadcrumbs from homemade sourdough bread (see Chapter 12 for the recipe).

For those of you who are scared of baking fish, tilapia is your friend. It's a firm, user-friendly fish that holds its moisture well and doesn't easily fall apart, dry out, or get mushy or mealy. You can also use whatever fish looks good at the store — salmon, tuna, and cod are other good options.

Tools: *Parchment paper*

Preparation time: *15 minutes*

Cooking time: *20 minutes*

Yield: *4 servings*

Four 8-ounce tilapia fillets	*1 teaspoon dried parsley*
1 egg white, beaten	*½ teaspoon dried sage or basil*
½ to 1 cup dry breadcrumbs or panko breadcrumbs (see Chapter 11 for the recipe)	

1 Rinse the fish under cold running water and pat dry with a paper towel. Preheat the oven to 350 degrees.

2 In a bowl big enough to fit the fish pieces in, combine the breadcrumbs or panko and the herbs. Dip the fish into the egg white and then into bread crumbs, turning to coat. Place the coated fish on a cookie sheet covered with parchment paper and sprayed with a cooking spray.

3 Bake for 20 to 25 minutes or until the outside is a dark golden brown and the inside flakes when you stick a fork into it, turning after about 10 minutes so both sides get crispy.

Vary It! *For even more kid points, cut the fish into 4-inch fish sticks before coating in the egg and breadcrumbs. Bake for 15 minutes because the smaller portions cook faster — and get to the table faster.*

Tip: *Serve with Oven Baked Yam (or Potato) UnFries (see the recipe in Chapter 7).*

Per serving: *Calories 604; Fat 10 g (Saturated 4 g); Cholesterol 236 mg; Sodium 562 mg; Carbohydrate 29.6 g (Fiber 2 g); Protein 98.4 g; Sugar 2.6 g.*

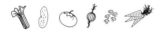

☉ Happy Mac 'n' Cheese

Colleen Robinson (www.crimsondoorhealing.com) knows kids (and, heck, adults) love macaroni and cheese, so she gave us this IBS-friendly version of the classic comfort food. This dish is far less likely to trigger your tyke's IBS than the boxed stuff or the lactose-heavy, fat-laden traditional version.

If all cheese is a trigger for you, skip this recipe, but otherwise the cheese options here are generally well-tolerated, naturally low in lactose, and approved for the SCD. SCD-legal cheeses include cheddar, Colby, Swiss, Havarti, and an occasional bit of Asiago; Colleen likes a combo of 4 ounces of cheddar, 3 ounces of brick cheese or Colby, and 1 ounce of Asiago, but you can mix it up depending on your child's preferences and trigger foods. If your kid has wheat problems, you can leave off the breadcrumbs or try spelt or rye breadcrumbs.

Preparation time: *10 minutes*

Cooking time: *30 minutes*

Yield: *4 servings*

8 ounces dry short rice or wheat pasta (such as elbow macaroni, penne, shells, or fusilli)

½ tablespoon butter

1½ tablespoons flour

1 teaspoon powdered mustard

2½ cups plain soymilk

1 teaspoon paprika

8 ounces grated cheddar cheese

1 teaspoon dry parsley, or 1 tablespoon fresh

½ cup breadcrumbs or panko crumbs (see the recipe in Chapter 11) (optional)

½ teaspoon salt

1 Bring a large pot of water to a boil. Cook the pasta according to package directions, subtracting 1 minute from the cooking time to allow for oven time later. Drain and rinse with cold water to stop the pasta from cooking.

2 Turn the broiler on and place the oven rack about ⅓ of the way from the top.

3 In a large pot, melt ½ tablespoon of butter over medium heat. Sprinkle in the flour and powdered mustard and whisk or fork-mix for about a minute to cook the flour so it doesn't taste pasty in the sauce. Stir in the soymilk slowly in a gentle pour, whisking like mad so the flour mixture distributes evenly and doesn't get lumpy. Add ½ teaspoon of the paprika.

4 Crank the heat up to high to bring the sauce mixture to a boil and then lower the heat to low until the sauce is barely bubbling. Simmer to thicken (3 to 5 minutes), stirring a lot.

5 Sprinkle in the cheese by handfuls, stirring as you add each handful, until it melts and the sauce is smooth and gooey. Add the cooked pasta and turn the heat to medium-low, stirring for a couple of minutes to heat the pasta and make sure it's well coated.

6 Pour the cheesy pasta into an 8- or 9-inch baking dish sprayed with cooking spray. Sprinkle the breadcrumbs over the top (if desired) and then the remaining paprika and the parsley.

7 Place the pan under the hot broiler and broil until the crumbs are golden brown or the pasta is toasty-brown, keeping the oven door cracked so the dish doesn't overheat. Remove it from the oven and let it sit for about 5 minutes to allow everything to set nicely.

Tip: *Rice pasta is a great option here. Christine recommends Tinkyada Organic Brown Rice Pasta, which comes in many shapes and sizes.*

Tip: *Try miracle noodles if your child doesn't seem to be able to digest grains. Miracle noodles are a soluble fiber product.*

Per serving: *Calories 578; Fat 24.1 g (Saturated 13.3 g); Cholesterol 63 mg; Sodium 827 mg; Carbohydrate 63.6 g (Fiber 3.72 g); Protein 24.4g; Sugar 6.5 g.*

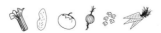

⟲ Smashed Potatoes with Rosemary

Chef Victoria Amory (www.victoriaamory.com) contributed this recipe that's a bit like making mud pies (or at least, you can tell the kids it is), and they're like potato pancakes when they're done! Little ones love to do the smashing part of the job, which is essential for exposing as much potato as possible to the high heat, resulting in a super crisp shell encasing creamy potatoes. When the potatoes are soft, use a meat mallet, the back of a spoon, or even your fist to smash or press the potatoes into patties (just watch the heat if you're going the hand route — the taters did just come off the stove). A drizzle of olive oil, a sprinkle of sea salt, and a pinch of rosemary is all it takes to elevate them to dinner party status.

Tools: *Parchment paper*

Preparation time: *15 minutes*

Cooking time: *35 minutes*

Yield: *6 servings*

2 pounds white, red, or purple baby potatoes

2 sprigs fresh rosemary, needles stripped and chopped

2 cloves garlic, peeled and chopped

6 tablespoons olive oil

⅛ teaspoon each salt and pepper

1 Heat the oven to 350 degrees. In a stock pot filled with salted water, boil the potatoes for about 15 minutes until a fork can be inserted into one with slight resistance.

2 In a bowl, combine the rosemary, garlic, olive oil, salt, and pepper. Using a slotted spoon, transfer the potatoes to a cutting board and invite kids to smash them with the back of a large spoon to form a disk. An inch in thickness is good to shoot for, but your kids may not be into symmetry.

3 Place the disks on a rimmed cookie sheet lined with parchment paper and brush the flavored olive oil on top. Roast in the oven until golden and crispy, about 15 to 20 minutes

Per serving: *Calories 258; Fat 13.7 g (Saturated 1.8 g); Cholesterol 0 mg; Sodium 200 mg; Carbohydrate 30.9 g (Fiber 2.8 g); Protein 2.9 g; Sugar 1.3 g.*

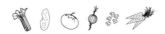

Don't desert dessert

It's a treat to know that your kids can eat and enjoy some safe sweets that don't involve 10 to 27 teaspoons of sugar like some sodas and milkshakes do. We include a special kid-friendly dessert here, but they'll be just as pleased to eat any of the desserts from Chapter 13.

⏱ Frozen Fruit Pops

This great treat from Colleen Robinson (www.crimsondoorhealing.com) is for kids who may be missing the high-sugar frozen treats their friends seem to enjoy. If fresh fruit is a trigger food for your child, the skins are likely the problem, and this recipe eliminates the skins *and* the worry. Use whatever fruit you have on hand; mango is a favorite of Carolyn's from her perch in paradise in Maui.

Tools: *Popsicle sticks*

Preparation time: *5 minutes*

Freezing time: *30 minutes to 2 hours*

Yield: *Five 3-ounce pops*

2 cups fresh mango	1 teaspoon brown sugar or agave (optional)
1 teaspoon lemon juice	½ cup water

1 Puree the fruit and lemon juice in a food processor until it's super-smooth; taste and sweeten with the brown sugar or agave if necessary. Pour into small cups or large ice cube trays and place them in the freezer until they get slushy (15 to 45 minutes, depending on cup size and the temperature of your freezer).

2 When slushy, insert the popsicle sticks and let them finish freezing, up to 2 hours.

Tip: *You can buy plastic frozen popsicle molds with the sticks included and you won't have to wait to put in the sticks.*

Vary It! *You can use other fresh fruits in place of the mango such as peaches, nectarines, apricots, and pears, peeled and cored or pitted.*

Per serving: *Calories 47; Fat 0.2 g (Saturated 0 g); Cholesterol 0 mg; Sodium 2 mg; Carbohydrate 12.4 g (Fiber 1 g); Protein 0.4 g; Sugar 10.7 g.*

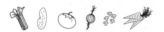

Chapter 16

Finding Safe Dishes When You're Dining Out

In This Chapter

▶ Working to ensure a successful restaurant outing

▶ Scrutinizing fast food

▶ Knowing what to order at different kinds of restaurants

*B*eing cooped up at home and eating the contents of your kitchen may be safe for you and your bowels, but continually missing out on Friday-night dinner with friends can be gut-wrenching. We're pretty confident that if you follow the eating guidelines we give you in this book, you're going to feel more at peace with your gastrointestinal tract (GIT). And when you've got a handle on what foods feel friendly, you may just find that some of your favorite restaurants are safer than you thought.

A big part of eating out is splurging on your favorite treat, but ordering that breaded mozzarella stick appetizer and eating it guiltily can send your IBS into a frenzy before you can say "Check, please!" So we suggest that you allow the experience of eating out to be the treat and save the splurges for a time when you know that your body is immune to reaction, or that reaction isn't going to compromise your plans for the rest of the night.

In this chapter, we give you plenty of tips to ensure your restaurant experience is a positive one that doesn't leave you spending dessert in the restroom.

Planning Ahead for an Enjoyable Experience

When you're feeling up to a meal on the town, a bit of planning can make for a great time. As you're healing and dealing with your IBS, we want you to enjoy yourself, so the planning tips in this section show you that you have more control in your life and dining experiences than you thought you had. You may need some practice to get up the nerve to ask for what you want and how you want it in a restaurant, but having the guts to order your sauces on the side will have your gut thanking you.

Check out the washroom facility beforehand so you encounter no surprises if you have an emergency while you're there. Is it a one-seater that you may have to wait for if it's occupied? Does it look like the kind of place you want to spend a significant amount of time in if necessary? Is it equipped with a ventilation fan and plenty of toilet paper? Is it situated far enough away from a common area so that you won't be worried about smells and sounds leaking out? Knowing your bathroom options ahead of time can help you determine how adventurous you're willing to be.

Eating out when you have IBS-D

You may recognize this common scene: You're enjoying a birthday party with friends at a local restaurant. After a dinner of cheeseburgers and fries, the waiter shows up with some sort of chocolate ice cream explosion smothered in whipped cream and nuts. You can't say no to the birthday boy's ice-cream toast, so you take a spoonful — and then another, and then about 17 more. You enjoy the festivities for a while until you start to feel the familiar rumblings; despite your best attempts to reason with your intestines, you're forced to flee to the restroom while the rest of the party finishes the sundae.

Although simply avoiding the temptation of cheeseburgers and ice cream seems like a no-brainer, this story is a classic tale for people with IBS. You get lulled into the magic of the party and feel like the stomach gods simply won't let you have an attack. But the stress and excitement of a party can also put your body on high alert, actually making you more susceptible to an attack. Here are some steps you can take at restaurant shindigs to avoid goading your guts into turning on you:

- ✔ **Consult your safe food list as a reminder of the reality of your current safe food choices.** If you haven't compiled a safe food list yet, we encourage you to head to Chapter 2 now to do so. A food list is a great way to remind yourself of which foods work for you and which ones you've already challenged and dismissed from your diet. Because IBS triggers vary so widely from person to person, we can't give you a one-size-fits-all crib sheet of foods to avoid, but making your own is entirely worthwhile and in fact could be a huge key to staying in the attack-free zone.

- ✔ **Pick a restaurant that has a lot of variety on the menu.** The more variety a menu offers, the more likely you are to find something that works for you. Plus, many restaurants these days are more conscious of the healthy choices their customers are making and have adjusted their menus to reflect that. But before you rush off to a drive-through, please read "Avoiding Fast Food" later in the chapter for a caveat about the so-called healthy options some fast food places offer.

✔ **Review restaurant menus online.** This way, you can have some idea ahead of time of what food choices seem safer than others. When searching for a new restaurant, always be conscious of words like *creamy, crispy* (may mean fried), and *rich* in the menu descriptions; these terms mean to lure in folks craving a decadent treat, but they may serve as a trigger warning to you.

✔ **Call the restaurant ahead of time and ask whether the chef can prepare specific ingredients in a safer way for you.** For example, many restaurants have items like chicken strips that they may be able to grill for you instead of breading and frying. Get the chef's name and her permission to tell the waiter that she's confirmed the kitchen can prepare your dish according to your request. Although chain restaurants often have staff trained to deal with special requests, we find that smaller family-owned restaurants are also often happy to oblige when you make specific requests.

✔ **Write down what you plan to order and stick to that decision.** Don't be tempted by those visions of chicken fries dancing in your head when you see what all your friends are ordering. If you have to, close your eyes when the waiter wheels the dessert tray to your table. And don't sample from your friends' plates. Just because you didn't order it doesn't make it safe!

✔ **Order takeout to take a practice run with the food.** Of course, the conditions and environment are different from a dinner out with friends, but at least you can test the food in the safety of your own dining room.

✔ **Let your companions know what's up ahead of time.** Sure, admitting to friends that you have IBS is embarrassing (although IBS affects about 20 percent of the population, so you may find that someone else in the group suffers too). But telling friends upfront that you have some stomach sensitivities and may be making special requests of the kitchen is less embarrassing than telling them through the wall of the washroom stall in the restaurant.

✔ **Don't eat and drive!** We're largely kidding here, but if being the group's driver adds extra stress to your evening, meet your friends at the restaurant. That way, if a bathroom emergency comes up, you can make your apologies and leave rather than strand everybody else at the table while you take care of business.

✔ **Instead of BYOB, try BYOR (bring your own rice).** Having a soluble-fiber side on hand can help you diffuse a less-than-ideal restaurant meal. If rice isn't on the menu of the restaurant you're visiting, call ahead and ask if you can BYOR because you have food sensitivities. Some kitchens will even heat it up for you.

✔ **Learn the art of substituting.** As you get into a natural rhythm of eating for IBS and get used to your safe food list, you'll discover uses for food that you didn't think about before. Think about the job you need a food to do in your meal. For example, a bun typically holds a hamburger and fixings, but if you're avoiding bread, then you need a substitute. So if you're craving a burger, ask the restaurant to wrap it in romaine lettuce (if that's on your safe food list) rather than a wheat bun. If lettuce isn't on your list, ask for a burger without the bun and transfer it to a thin rice cake at your table. If that isn't appealing, just eat your burger with a knife and fork.

Eating out when you have IBS-C

People who have IBS-C aren't blindsided by the sudden bathroom rush that can hit IBS-D sufferers in the middle of the meal. We know eating out with IBS-C presents its own challenges because it seems like you simply can't do enough to prepare, so we hope the following tips help you hit the town:

✔ **Don't overdo it if you're having a bout of constipation.** We're not suggesting that you don't eat at all, but do realize that whatever you eat goes into your already-plugged gastrointestinal tract (GIT), so getting carried away isn't going to help your evening.

✔ **To prepare for an event, be extra vigilant about drinking extra water, up your fiber intake, and get lots of exercise.** This is the normal advice we give for IBS-C, and it may just work well enough for you to enjoy your evening.

✔ **Wear clothing that is loose and comfortable, especially around your waist.** If you have IBS-C, you likely have a closet full of stretchy pants that don't restrict your stomach. But make sure you have a couple of comfortable and flattering outfits that you can wear when socializing. The "I have nothing to wear syndrome" feels even worse when your tight pants are a painful reminder of your days without relief.

✔ **Keep soothing tea with you.** If you feel discomfort during your meal and you've found the tea that soothes your stomach, always keep several bags on hand. Ask your server for a pot of hot water, and they usually oblige. Just pop your teabag into the pot and sip through the discomfort.

✔ **Avoid your trigger foods even if you're feeling good.** As tempting as that questionable dish may look, you don't want to risk setting off your IBS on your night out.

Avoiding Fast Food

The point of fast food restaurants is to feed you quick, tasty food. Although fast food places may be modifying their menus to attract people looking for healthier meals, they're doing so within their prefabricated, prepared, and quickly cooked format. Any investment they may be making to provide healthier options is likely more of a marketing ploy than a health plan.

As an IBS sufferer, you have to see through the hype and consider what constitutes a safe meal for you. As painful a step as it may be, we suggest you steer clear of anything with a fast food feel, drive-through access, or mascots. If your family insists on a trip to a burger-iffic chain, do your homework first. Compare your food list to the lists of ingredients on the Web sites of the restaurants in question. Most restaurant chain Web sites have a tab or link labeled something like "Nutrition" for this information.

You can quickly search a particular Web page for specific words without having to slog through everything. In your browser toolbar, just click Edit and then choose the Find on this Page option to search that page for ingredients that bug you.

At first glance, you can easily find the basic ingredients: a burger patty, a bun, and a couple of condiments. But dig a little deeper. What's in the burger? What's in the bun? How many ingredients are in the condiments, sauces, and side dishes?

A basic burger at Joint A says it's 100 percent beef with salt and pepper seasoning. But not all burgers — even different offerings from the same restaurant — are created equal. A different burger at the same restaurant has a list of 25 ingredients including milk, wheat, soy, MSG (under one of its many pseudonyms), and several types of sugar. Certain sauces that go on some burgers have about 30 different ingredients, including wheat, different forms of sugar, high fructose corn syrup, and a few unpronounceable items that sound more like chemicals than food (probably because they are).

This advice comes straight from a fast food worker: If you want to be sure the restaurant makes your burger plain, tell them you have an allergy. Many burgers are already prepared, packaged, and ready to drop in your drive through bag; a plain order often means workers just scrape the toppings off one of these premade patties.

What about the healthier options like grilled chicken breasts? We were shocked to find that a grilled chicken breast at one fast food restaurant involved nearly 50 ingredients. And that didn't include the bun! Many preservatives, sugars, yeasts, and flavorings all go into that grilled chicken breast (which may actually be made from chicken rib meat).

Getting a glimpse into the kitchen

We've done a bunch of the detective work for you about what may be going on in the kitchen of your favorite eateries, and you may be surprised (as we were) to find that lots of restaurants take shortcuts that can spell trouble for your intestines. Here are some restaurant habits to be aware of when dining out:

✔ **Making items from mixes:** Many restaurants don't make everything fresh on site. Shocking! Instead, they use mixes for sauces, gravies, scrambled eggs, desserts, and toppings that can be full of preservatives and other nasties your stomach can't tolerate. Ask your server to ask the chef for clarification on what's in the sauces before you order them.

✔ **Warming frozen food:** Christine was pretty surprised to get a peek into a kitchen at a local diner to find the cook pulling a giant bag of breaded chicken strips out of the freezer and dumping them in the deep fryer. Ask your waiter to find out whether the chef makes his own dishes (especially appetizers). If you see food on a menu that you've also seen in the freezer at a big-box store, the chances are it's not handmade and may be full of additives and ingredients that you can't tolerate.

✔ **Adding unexpected extras:** Christine is often surprised by what the chef puts on the plate as a sauce or garnish despite it not being in the menu. Her rule of thumb is to ask for any sauces or toppings on the side. Asking for the condiments on the side gives you control of what goes into your mouth! Sometimes her dinner companions cringe when she asks, but they've learned that it's a better alternative to her sending back the whole plate when it's smothered in a béarnaise sauce that wasn't mentioned on the menu.

 Read what's in the parentheses and brackets beside certain ingredients on the ingredient list. These are the sub-ingredients (and sometimes sub-sub-ingredients) of the main ingredients. Don't assume you know what seasoning is — next to one seasoning, we found 19 different ingredients.

Finding IBS-Friendlier Food in Your Favorite Restaurant

Going out to eat doesn't have to be a source of torture, although we know it can be. People with IBS have to have creative solutions to their dining dilemmas, so here we share some tried and true tricks of the trade. You may be surprised to find you have more options than you thought for dining out with IBS. Just remember that in general your basic foods to avoid are those that include dairy, wheat, and sugar, and check out the tips for dining out in general in the section "Planning Ahead for an Enjoyable Experience" earlier in this chapter.

We give you tips for enjoying lots of ethnic cuisines in this section, but French cooking is really one to stay away from. It has so many pâtés, cheeses, breads, and creamy sauces that we don't know how to make it safe.

If you think your waiter isn't listening, say you have a serious food allergy so the cooks legitimately leave the problem ingredients out instead of just scraping, say, the mayo off your dish. Or if you've arranged to have your chicken cooked without being breaded first, feel free to spell it out to your waiter that no breadcrumb should come in contact with your chicken. Carolyn has been known to mention that a certain food will surely kill her if she eats it. Gets their attention every time!

Mastering the meat-and-potatoes breakfast

If you find yourself eating the most important meal of the day in a restaurant, you may have to dig a little as you search the menu for a safe breakfast. The offerings are usually, bacon, fried eggs, cereal, coffee, donuts, and bagels — nothing there to get your day off to a good start when you have IBS. But if you look a little further on the menu you can order oatmeal without the brown sugar, poached or soft boiled eggs without the bacon, and even a small steak (grilled, not fried) without the fried hash browns.

Making Mexican work for you

Most Mexican restaurants start you out with chips and salsa; the chips are usually corn, which is likely safe, and you may be able to handle mild salsa, but pass on the hot salsa and people who challenge you to a chili pepper eating contest!

Many dishes come with or actually incorporate tortillas, which are generally corn or flour (which means wheat) — make sure you get the corn variety if you have wheat sensitivities.

Cheese can be shaky, but ask what type of cheese they use; if it's on your safe food list, it may work for you. Lean portions of chicken, beef, and pork are also safe.

Many Mexican menus have complex dishes that have meat, beans, cheese in a wrap covered in sauce and more melted cheese. Such an adventure may not work for you, but fajitas are a great alternative. They often consist of simply grilled meat and vegetables with tortillas and condiments on the side so you can build your own dish. If you don't want to be tempted by sour cream, ask for a safer alternative, such as more guacamole or mild salsa. If the flour tortilla doesn't work for you, ask for romaine or iceberg lettuce leaves to stuff with your fajita mixture, or just use a knife and fork instead.

Inviting Italian back to the table

Although you may consider lasagna, garlic bread, and wine comfort food, your bowels may not agree. Bread, wheat pasta, and sauces made with creams can pose a real hazard to your IBS; you especially want to stay away from the stuffed pastas that can be too creamy, cheesy, and dense for your sensitive system. Pizza probably isn't the best choice for you either, although you may be able to remove the meat and vegetables and enjoy the crust (if you're not wheat sensitive), sauce, and a safe cheese.

But never fear — you may still be able to find some great, friendly options at the local Italian eatery. Veal, chicken, and fish are common in Italian cuisine, and many restaurants that are conscious of their customers' dietary needs will happily grill the meat instead of cooking it in a sauce. Most Italian restaurants serve *risotto,* which is a rice dish, so they likely have rice on hand; try ordering plain rice with a basic tomato sauce. Or if tomato isn't on your safe list, make it risotto in clear broth.

Also ask about the soup of the day — it's often made with simple ingredients. Salads and side dishes of cooked vegetables like potatoes and broccoli may be available plain — always ask for sauces on the side so you can control the amounts.

Staying safe with Chinese

A meal of Chinese is exciting because you have lots of choices, but one big drawback is that the biggest flavor enhancer in Chinese food is MSG, which is often built into the sauces that you order.

Pay close attention to what your server says. If you've asked him for your food to have no MSG, he may repeat back "No added MSG," which likely means you're still getting some MSG in your sauces, soups, and prepared items like egg rolls.

Favorites like egg rolls, spring rolls, and wontons are usually meat and/or vegetables wrapped in a flour pastry and deep fried. They're tasty (that's why they're favorites), but they may not be the best choice for your IBS. Sweet-and-sour pork is breaded, deep fried, and smothered in a sugary sauce, which can present all sorts of triggers. And don't forget that Chinese staple soy sauce — it contains wheat and sugar that may set off your symptoms.

Your best dish may be a simple bowl of steamed rice with stir-fried meat, chicken, or fish and vegetables. Some Chinese soups can be quite simple; for example, egg drop soup is a broth with threads of egg and peas (just make sure it doesn't also include MSG). You may also be able to get some plain rice noodles on the side or that you can dip into your soup. Moo shu meals can be another good choice because they come with lettuce leaves that you can fill with the marinated meat and vegetable mixture.

Treating yourself to Thai

Thai food is one of our very favorites because it's got lots of mild flavor and is generally light, but watch out for some pitfalls. Many appetizers include fried items, and they're big on coconut, peanut sauce, and cooking oils, which are in almost all their entrées and may be potentially problematic ingredients. Pad Thai, for example, has peanuts plus sesame and canola oils.

Luckily, you can get some much better options. Grilled marinated squid and prawns have less fat than fried appetizers. Satay, substituting the peanut sauce with fresh lime, is another great choice. Most Thai noodles served are made from rice and boiled or steamed, so they should be safe as well. Steamed rice is preferable to Thai Fried Rice, which is sautéed in oil.

Tom Yum Gai, is a very light flavorful broth featuring Asian mushrooms and lemongrass. Finally, we suggest you take the fresh tropical fruit over the deep-fried bananas for dessert — many Thai restaurants offer an exotic selection including mango, papaya, and pineapple.

Enjoying Japanese food

Yes, we know we told you to avoid sushi because of the safety of raw fish, and we stick to that. You can, however, have vegetable sushi, or even sushi with cooked fish. The avocado roll and California roll are good choices, but avoid the tempura roll or fried salmon skin roll. Most menus list all the ingredients of each roll so you can scan the list for your safe ingredients. Keep a safe distance from the wasabi green hot sauce — it may light a fire in your intestines. For a safe sushi dip, look for wheat-free soy sauce in the larger restaurants.

Japanese cuisine isn't all about sushi, though. Rice is a staple of Japanese fare, so you can simply order teriyaki beef or chicken with a side of rice. Japanese soups can be a very safe IBS choice. Soba (buckwheat) noodle soup, egg drop soup, or miso soup are three common offerings that you may want to try. Just be sure to ask about MSG if the restaurant uses prepackaged soups instead of preparing them fresh.

Surviving steak- and chophouses

You don't have to give up the steakhouse! They may be more expensive, but you can have a well-prepared yet simple grilled steak, fish, or chicken and side order of cooked vegetables and call it a great night.

The first items that appear to the table are ice water and the bread basket, but if you stay away from both, you should be fine. For most people, ice water chills the stomach and may cause cramping. French bread is an acceptable soluble side, so if you need one and it's great French bread, go ahead.

Don't be afraid of doggie bags so you can eat lightly and take the rest home and enjoy it later. We recommend freezing your leftovers right away and eating them a few days later so that you aren't overloading on certain foods.

Be aware of salad bar offerings. Many people have reported IBS reactions after having been to a salad bar. Turns out many restaurants with large buffets and salad bars use a preservative spray on the vegetables to keep them looking fresh and crisp, which is likely what's causing the problems. Just check with the restaurant staff to see whether a particular place uses the spray.

Part IV
The Part of Tens

The 5th Wave

By Rich Tennant

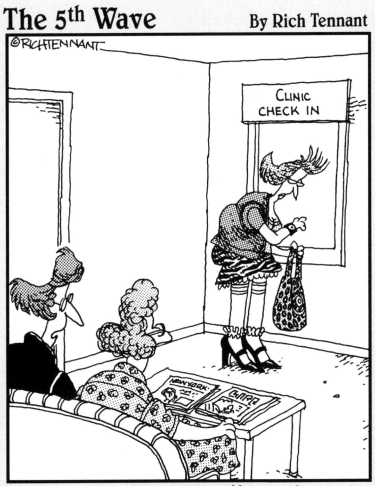

"I can't believe her IBS is affecting her body any worse than her sense of style is."

In this part . . .

*W*e do our best in this part to provide you with some simple solutions to increase your success with your individualized IBS diet.

Chapter 17 helps you make foods friendlier for your IBS gut. Chapter 18 focuses on yeast, one important and often underacknowledged factor in IBS. Chapter 19 gives you solid reasons to avoid ten particular foods, and in Chapter 20 we help you eat your way out of some common eating traps that you may find yourself in.

Chapter 17

Ten Tips for Making Foods Friendlier to Your Tummy

In This Chapter

▶ Preparing and eating your food in ways that minimize symptoms

▶ Having the right eating attitude

*Y*ou simply have to eat to survive, even when the only available food may result in a trip to the bathroom or a bout of cramps and gas. This chapter gives you some tips to increase the odds of you eating a decent meal even under less-than-ideal circumstances.

Cook Your Fruits and Vegetables

In the raw state, fruits and veggies are packed with insoluble fiber, which can be agitating if you tend towards IBS-D (but you may need it if you have IBS-C). If raw fruits and vegetables give you problems, you can cook them to make them behave better in your gut.

Cooking breaks down the cell walls of plants, making them less rigid and less irritating to your sensitive gut. Some well-tolerated cooked vegetables for IBS-D are zucchini, potatoes, and yams. Fruits are a little more forgiving than vegetables; raw pineapple, kiwi, papaya, and figs have plant enzymes that help your digestion when you eat small amounts. Friendly cooked fruits include apples, pears, pumpkin, and plums with the skin removed for IBS-D and the skin intact for the extra fiber for IBS-C.

But you don't have to take our word for it . . .

We're not the only people who believe cooked food is easier on the stomach. Chinese medicine teaches that raw vegetables take longer to digest than cooked ones because the stomach has to warm the food before it can break it down. Cold food has to get up to your body temperature (98.6 degrees for the average person) to begin digestion, so cooking vegetables can be like predigestion, doing some of the work that your body may not have the energy to do.

Quickly boiling or steaming vegetables can start the process for you.

Additionally, during the macrobiotic diet boom many years ago some people said the brown rice, vegetable, and seaweed diet was healing for people with cancer because the fact that all the food was cooked put less strain on the digestion. For more on the macrobiotic lifestyle, check out Verne Varona's *Macrobiotics For Dummies* (Wiley).

Puree Your Foods

If you favor the flavor of a Raw food diet but can't handle its digestion, you can puree your foods in a high-speed blender. This process breaks down cell walls and reduces the load of insoluble fiber, making foods more digestible. Many people report that eating puréed food does help them get some nutrition while going through a bad patch of IBS.

Pureeing is different from juicing because it keeps some of the fiber from the vegetables, whereas juicing removes all the fiber from the vegetable. Head to the following section for more on juicing.

Pureeing cooked food may not seem as appetizing because a steak is no longer a steak if you don't have to cut it with a knife, but whizzing it in a food processor for a few seconds to break down the meat fibers may help you digest it better. Cooked and pureed yams, cauliflower, and carrots are tasty, even though they may remind you of baby food.

If you do puree your food, make sure that you just eat a teaspoon or so at a time and hold the food in your mouth for a few seconds to let your saliva start the digestion process.

Juice Your Fruits and Vegetables

If you want to take insoluble fiber completely out of the fruit and veggie equation, try juicing, which leaves the nourishment but gets rid of all the fiber and especially the insoluble fiber that may set off your intestines. You can turn your juice into a healing drink by adding peppermint leaves, ginger, or fennel to help support your gastrointestinal system. For some tasty juice options, try the recipes in Chapter 8.

Have a Side of Soluble Fiber

Whether you're eating out or eating in, you can make a questionable main dish more IBS-friendly if you have a side of soluble fiber handy. Rice is one of your best soluble side choices, especially in a restaurant, and cooked or steamed rice is great to keep in your fridge all the time. Applesauce and bananas are other good sources of soluble fiber.

Keep bananas around in different stages of ripeness. You can treat IBS-D with a green banana and IBS-C with a ripe one.

The latest soluble safety net to hit the shelves is chia seeds. Chia absorbs twelve times its weight in water and turns into a soluble jelly that can help bind up your IBS-D or break through your IBS-C. A teaspoon in your smoothie or stirred in water can be a useful remedy before, during, or after your meal. Remember to take it with a large glass of water if you have IBS-C and only a few ounces of water for IBS-D.

Consider the Fit for Life Strategy

In 1985, Harvey and Marilyn Diamond wrote *Fit for Life* (Warner Books, Inc.), which was based on the premise that you shouldn't mix certain food groups. It suggested that combining foods like protein with foods like fruit causes incomplete digestion of both because protein requires more acidic gastric juices than fruit does. By paying attention to what foods you eat together, you may take some of the pressure off your digestive juices.

Although this program may not be the right way to eat for everyone, we've seen people have success with it. If nothing else, it may be a way to give your digestive system a break from its usual way of dealing with food. Here are some of the main *Fit for Life* rules with some commentary from us:

> ✔ **Eat fruits by themselves.** Fruit passes through your digestive system very quickly and should be allowed to do so without interruption from other foods needing more acidic digestive juices. If you eat fruit with protein, the meat can hog all the digestive powers you have, leaving the fruit to ferment in your belly. Fermenting fruit can open the door to

yeast (see Chapter 18) and cause gas and bloating in your gastrointestinal tract (GIT).

You may have trouble digesting fruit because of the fructose whether or not you eat it by itself.

- ✔ **Eat carbs and proteins separately.** Much like fruit, these items can ferment in your stomach because you don't have enough digestive juices to go around.

- ✔ **Never drink water with meals.** Drinking water with your meals dilutes the enzymes and acids that help you to digest your food completely and properly. This rule doesn't apply to drinking liquid soups, or to drinking a teaspoon or two of apple cider vinegar with 4 ounces of water at a meal to enhance digestion.

- ✔ **Avoid dairy products.** The Diamonds believed that we did not digest dairy products in general and made them out of bounds. We do agree that you should avoid dairy products, with the possible exception of some safe cheeses and yogurts that we talk about in Chapters 3 and 6.

Change Up Your Drink Routine

The best way to make your drinks IBS-friendly is to make sure they don't contain alcohol, caffeine, or carbonation. Caffeine can annoy your colon if you have IBS-D; carbonation is gas, and you don't want more gas in an already gassy stomach. Alcohol is a laxative and feeds intestinal organisms; check out Chapter 19 for more on why you should avoid these substances.

So what do you drink instead? You can make safe and soothing teas from chamomile, peppermint, ginger, and fennel. Brew the tea and leave it to cool before keeping it covered in the fridge for a delicious summer treat. Sweeten it with stevia, and you have a sweet, friendly, and soothing beverage. We suggest taking a bottle of cooled tea with you rather than bottled water if you're going to dinner — a few sips of peppermint tea can soothe your stomach while you're waiting for the food to be served. You can also put one drop of essential oil of peppermint in a bottle or jug of water and have a delicious drink in seconds.

Watch Fatty Meats (And Grill, Don't Fry)

Greasy burgers and fried chicken slow down your digestive system for hours and cause IBS cramping and abdominal pain. If you eat animal protein, go lean.

If you can, talk to your neighborhood butcher about the cuts of meat that are leanest; you can typically get extra-lean ground beef. If chicken is your thing, try grilled chicken breast rather than fried chicken wings. (And of course, you should be getting free-range, hormone-free meat to avoid the chemicals.)

When grilling, keep the fire to a minimum; burned meat may be kind of tasty, but the charcoal is hard to digest. We like the indoor countertop grills that drain the fat from your food while you're cooking. You can grill vegetables and meat at the same time and have a full tasty meal while using just one appliance. Just don't be tempted to slather oil on your grill — you don't need to when a quick spritz will do.

Defuse Dairy

If you have difficulty digesting lactose, you can try lactose-free dairy products or lactase enzyme pills that aid in dairy digestion. Check out Chapters 3 and 6 for both cheese suggestions and yogurt recipes that may be easier on your gut. You can also try warming your milk, which makes it more digestible than cold milk and less likely to cause constipation, or go for organic milk and non-homogenized milk, which are also easier to digest. You may also find limiting your dairy portion size helpful; head to the following section for more on portion control.

Minimize Serving Size

You may remember a time when you had an enormous Thanksgiving dinner and your stomach and intestines felt like a cyclone had hit them. Many people who don't have and have never heard of IBS have had those symptoms just because they ate a meal the size of a small car. IBS-friendly foods come in small portions; you may even get away with something that you don't think is good for your IBS if you only eat a little bit. A good guideline is that your meat serving should be about the size of a deck of cards (and not one of those giant novelty decks, either); many single servings by today's standards can easily feed three people.

Think Food Friendly

Monitoring your thoughts is a powerful exercise for people who have IBS. You may have a column in your food diary to keep track of what you're thinking when you're eating so you can easily see the correlation between your thoughts and your IBS symptoms.

We've said it before, but we'll repeat it: When you're thinking negative thoughts as you eat something, you're associating that thought with the food. So when you reach for a food that you're concerned may be a trigger for your IBS, stop for a moment and consider how often thoughts like the following take you in a negative direction:

- ✔ I know if I eat this item I'll pay for it later.
- ✔ I don't care whether I get a bad reaction from eating this food.
- ✔ I shouldn't eat this dish.

As you think these thoughts, even without having food around you, can you feel how uncomfortable it feels? You may even feel a gripping sensation in your stomach or feel it tightening as if you're holding your breath. But now practice thinking positive thoughts about food:

- ✔ This treat is so delicious.
- ✔ This dish is really one of my favorite things to eat.
- ✔ I'm so happy to be eating this snack.

We don't expect you to believe these new thoughts right away, but we do ask you to practice thinking positive or even neutral thoughts while you eat. The more you tell your body that what you're eating is good, the more your body believes you. Of course, this exercise doesn't apply to eating a pint of rocky road ice cream after a plate of ribs washed down by a quart of beer. It's part of the comprehensive IBS healing program that you are developing.

Chapter 18

Ten Ways to Keep Yeast in Check

In This Chapter

▶ Understanding yeast overgrowth's symptoms and effects

▶ Getting rid of yeast

▶ Treating other conditions without contributing to a yeast problem

*Y*east has been around forever; it's not some mystery bug just now discovered. The real mystery is why it's not recognized as a trigger for IBS. It lives happily and harmlessly in your gut as tiny little yeast buds playing tag with good bacteria and even the occasional parasite. But yeast turns into a rampaging monster when the conditions in your gut are right. Trouble can start when you take antibiotics that kill all the good bacteria in your gut that serve as a barrier to keep yeast in check. If you feed yeast with lots of sugar and carbs and nothing to check its growth, it turns into an invading army of threads.

How can a thread be dangerous? The problem isn't *a* thread — it's a billion threads that together can irritate and even penetrate the gut lining. This penetration causes a recognized medical condition called *leaky gut* that allows the absorption of yeast toxins into the blood stream. You can read more about yeast in Chapter 1, but here we give you ten ways to keep yeast under wraps so you don't have to deal with these conditions. They're not all cooking or eating tips, but together they can help you manage your yeast situation and therefore your IBS.

Quickly Identifying a Yeast-Related Flare-Up

Answering the following seven fungal questions can give you a heads up on what's causing those gut symptoms that you think are untreatable IBS. If you answer yes to two or more bullets, it's likely yeast, which means it's treatable and you're ahead of the game. Several sections later in this chapter help get you on the antifungal path.

- ✔ **Have you recently taken antibiotics?** Whether it's one dose or dozens of doses, the effect of antibiotics is that they kill off intestinal bacteria and leave lots of room for yeast to grow. Most people with yeast overgrowth recall that their symptoms started after a long course of these killing drugs.

- ✔ **Do you crave sugar?** Yeast is like the Borg in *Star Trek:* a mass mind that has taken over your body. Whatever it wants, it gets, and what it wants is sugar and carbs (foods that may trigger your IBS on their own). The number of microorganisms in your intestines is ten times your body cell count, so if you have yeast overgrowth, you may be outnumbered and outvoted when it comes to ordering that pizza and milkshake. After you starve and kill your abnormal yeast population, outside of having hypoglycemia or diabetes, you may find you don't crave sugar anymore.

- ✔ **Do you feel worse on wet, damp days or in moldy places?** Addams family aside, most people prefer sunny, warm, dry environments, so we're not talking about feeling great when you're vacationing in Arizona. If you find yourself sneezing up a storm on rainy days or in your damp basement, one reason may be that mold spores are irritating your nasal passages because your nose is already being poked with marauding yeast just like your gut. These micropunctures in your nasal passages allow molecules of chemicals and allergens to be absorbed, causing you to react to mold, dust, pollens, and animal dander, as well as to perfumes and cleaning products. Carolyn has had depressed patients and clients who've seen their depression worsen on damp days. Treating their yeast and eliminating mold in their environment turned their depression around and took away their rainy-day melancholy.

- ✔ **Do you feel you have extremely low energy?** When you have yeast overgrowth, your energy is low because of all the time your immune system has to spend defending against 178 different yeast toxins. Now that's an energy drain! One really potent yeast toxin is *acetaldehyde,* which can damage all the tissues in the body, including the brain. Another factor: When yeast is having a party in your gut, it produces alcohol in your body. For some folks, it's enough to make them feel drunk and even show up on a breathalyzer test or a blood alcohol reading. It sounds bizarre, but it's a documented condition called Drunken Syndrome in Japan. Maybe that's why people with yeast problems tell us they feel like they have a perpetual hangover. Of course, your energy drain may also be affected by the exhaustion that goes along with trying to figure out what's wrong with you and find a doctor who actually listens to all your symptoms instead of just diagnosing you with depression and handing over a prescription for an antidepressant. How depressing is that?

✔ **Are you bothered by vaginal burning, itching, or discharge?** Not quite a game-show question, or even cookbook conversation. Nevertheless, yeast ends up in these orifices, too. Most doctors think that yeast is only a pesky inflammation, but we know different. It can also be an intestinal overgrowth that comes from the intestine and crawls down your rectum and anus into the vagina. Yuck! That's why you can also have rectal itch along with vaginal itch.

✔ **Do you have frequent sinus infections?** The Mayo Clinic reported in one study several years ago that 97 percent of chronic sinus infections were fungal-related. What do doctors use to treat sinus infections? Antibiotics! And what causes fungal overgrowth? Antibiotics! It's a vicious cycle that you can break only by understanding the origins of yeast overgrowth and treating yeast as an underlying cause.

Any mucus membrane in your body can have yeast overgrowth. Stick out your tongue. If it's coated with white, that can be a dead giveaway that you have yeast overgrowth. A yeast infection in your esophagus can contribute to heartburn and gas, which sometimes can make such a stretching pain around your diaphragm or upper stomach that you think you're having a heart attack.

✔ **Do you suffer from burning, itching, or tearing of the eyes and ears?** Carolyn tells her clients that when you have an itchy, tearing eye discharge, you probably have yeast up to your eyeballs and it's high time you did something about it!

Yeast can grow from your sinuses through the Eustachian tube that runs from your nose to your ear, causing itchy ears. One of the first cases of yeast infection that Carolyn saw in her practice was a 10-month-old boy who had been on eight courses of antibiotics for ear discharge found at birth. His mother was a nurse, and even though she said the discharge smelled yeasty, nobody listened. Finally, she had a swab taken of the discharge; sure enough, it was yeast, and the antibiotics were only making the problem worse.

Making Sure Your Doctor Considers All Courses of Action

Doctors simply don't learn about yeast overgrowth in medical school. Most either think of yeast problems as either *vaginitis* (vaginal inflammation) or the worst case scenario that it's infecting your blood and is life threatening and only happens in the hospital from IV antibiotics, cancer chemotherapy, or AIDS. You may have to suggest the third option: that what you have is an overgrowth of yeast in your intestines.

Even if your doctor does understand the intestinal option, he may think the treatment is simply a matter of giving you an antifungal drug like Nystatin or Diflucan for a week or two. You can use an antifungal, but the best results come from a long-term diet, *probiotics* (supplements that replace good bacteria), and natural antifungals.

Starving Yeast

Like annoying party guests, if you feed yeast, it will come, and if you don't feed it, it will go. Simple. Okay, not exactly simple, but doable. All you have to do is begin a very strict anti-yeast diet. For the first few weeks, avoid sugar, dairy, gluten grains (rye, wheat, and barley), most fruit, and fermented foods. (You may notice that this plan looks an awful lot like the elimination diet for determining IBS triggers in Chapter 2.) What's left? Plenty: dozens of vegetables, some fruit, gluten-free grains (millet, rice, amaranth, kamut, quinoa, and oats), fish, and antibiotic- and hormone-free chicken, turkey, lamb, and beef.

After the second or third week of a yeast-free diet, you should begin to feel much better. And we promise that you will feel better enough to make up for having endured this diet! But in the meantime, don't be discouraged if you feel worse before you feel better. During the first week, you may feel some aggravation of symptoms as the dying yeast floods the system with its toxic byproducts. The most common of these *die-off* symptoms are rashes, headache, shifting bowel movement, and aches and pains.

After several weeks on a strict diet, reintroduce foods, one by one, to get an indication of whether you have any reaction to that food. You can also take bentonite clay, which we talk about later in this chapter and in Chapter 1, to absorb toxins and lessen the die-off that you may otherwise experience.

If you reintroduce a food that your body doesn't like (and we're not talking taste buds here), you may find that it's a food allergy or an IBS trigger. Or you may just start feeling awful simply because you've eaten a sugar or carb food that grows yeast in your newly cleaned gut. If your yeast has irritated the lining of your gastrointestinal tract, you may also have a leaky gut, which means that undigested foods can leak through the injured intestinal wall into the blood stream and set up a reaction with the immune system.

Replacing Yeast

Add *lactobacillus acidophilus* bacteria to your diet in the form of organic yogurt without added sugar. Lactobacillus acidophilus is a good bacteria, called a probiotic, that helps build up the normal bacteria in the bowel as the yeast are killed off and leave vacancies in the intestines and vagina. This bacteria is a friendly one that produces lactic acid that poisons yeast and keeps it in check.

You can also take lactobacillus acidophilus capsules. The criteria for choosing a good lactobacillus acidophilus is one that has 2 to 10 billion live organisms in each capsule; make sure that amount is guaranteed through the expiration date. You usually take the capsules on an empty stomach at least one hour before or two hours after food. Most people take them before bed and allow the lactobacillus acidophilus to populate their bowel overnight.

Though we're happy that the yogurt companies have jumped on the probiotic bandwagon, please be aware of the other ingredients in probiotic yogurts, specifically sugar. If you're on mission to purge yeast from your system, eating any kind sugary yogurt, probiotic or not, isn't going to help matters at all — it just feeds the yeast.

Killing Yeast in the Gut

You can begin getting yeast under control by eating antifungal foods that are natural yeast killers; garlic, onions, coconut milk, and coconut oil are a few of the most common ones. You can also add antifungal herbs such as hops and Pau d'Arco (also called Lapacho or Taheebo) taken in the form of herbal tea.

A comprehensive treatment for killing yeast and eliminating yeast toxins includes psyllium powder, bentonite clay liquid, and liquid caprylic acid (caproyl). Put one teaspoon to one tablespoon of each in 2 ounces of water in a bottle with a lid. Shake and drink quickly so the psyllium doesn't turn immediately into a gel. Then drink another 8 to 10 ounces of water. Drinking extra water is very important; otherwise, psyllium can cause constipation by absorbing water from your gut.

Start with one detox shake a day and then, under a naturopath's supervision, increase to two daily. Your doctor will help you decide if you should continue the treatment for two or three weeks and how often you repeat it. If you use this treatment, make sure to take it one hour before or at least two hours after eating or taking supplements. Otherwise, the shake pulls the goodness out of your meal or supplement.

Treating Yeast Where It Lies

Yeast problems may start in the intestines, but they can cause aggravation in various parts of the body if the yeast spreads. The following list gives you some tips for dealing with these secondary yeast sources:

✔ **Vagina/penis:** Vaginal yeast can be treated locally with douches or suppositories. You can buy all sorts of drugstore antifungal vaginal creams and suppositories over the counter, but they may not work unless you also do the yeast-free diet and probiotics.

You can use boric acid (found in your local drugstore) in a vaginal douche. It comes in powdered form and is also used as an eyewash, so it's considered safe for vaginal use. Add one teaspoon per pint of warm water. Boric acid is also conveniently made into suppositories (such as Yeast Arrest). Another type of douche can be made with diluted sugar-free yogurt or by inserting a small tampon soaked in yogurt.

Yeast can form a redness and irritation around the head of the penis. You can treat it with vaginal antifungal cream or rinse it with a boric acid wash or diluted yogurt. But diet and probiotics are also a must.

✔ **Sinuses:** You can treat yeast in the sinuses with a neti pot. Health food or yoga supply stores carry *neti pots,* items specifically designed with a spout that fits into one nostril and allows saline water to flow through the sinuses and out the other nostril. Add one drop of tea tree oil for an antifungal effect. It will take some practice to master the use of the neti pot, but the results are great. If you don't have access to a health food store, you can also have your pharmacist order NeilMed Sinus Rinse and use it in the same way as a neti pot.

The recipe for rinsing the sinuses is ¼ teaspoon of noniodized sea salt in 1 cup of boiled water — cool and use in a neti pot or in a NeilMed syringe.

✔ **Nails:** Fungal nails are difficult to treat, especially if you don't treat the whole body. Some of the drugs used to treat fungal nails are very harsh; some natural treatments include rubbing tea tree oil or oregano oil into the nails once or twice per day.

Avoiding Overuse of Antibiotics

As a society, Americans use way too many antibiotics. Bacteria are becoming resistant to most current antibiotics, which leads researchers to create stronger drugs, which kill even more of the good bacteria in your body and give yeast a chance to take hold.

The best way to keep yeast in check is to stop using antibiotics unless absolutely necessary. So think twice before your doctor gives you an antibiotic for your cold or flu. Most colds and flus are viral, and antibiotics don't kill viruses anyway! The antibiotic won't be helping your symptoms, and it may very well be contributing to a yeast problem. Save the antibiotics for when you really need them; in the next three sections, we give you a host of natural remedies for colds and flus. Carolyn is an expert in natural cures and staying healthy; her health program, Future Health Now! and remedies from her e-book *Future Health Now! Encyclopedia* (available online at www.drcarolyndean.com) can help you stay on top of life.

Treating Infections with Supplements

The best way to avoid taking medications and ending up in the hospital is to stay healthy. Sounds silly, right? But with the right tools such as supplements, you can avoid unnecessary medications that can lead to side effects and more meds for the side effects. Consider taking some of the following supplements to help you stay healthy.

- ✔ **Vitamin D:** Taking 2,000 international units (IU) daily is a proven cold and flu prevention.

- ✔ **Vitamin C:** Take a daily dose of 500 milligrams; increase the amount to 1,000 milligrams every 1 to 2 hours during infection.

- ✔ **Vitamin A:** A daily dose of 20,000 IU strengthens mucus membranes against infection.

- ✔ **Zinc:** Chew zinc lozenges, 10 milligrams several times a day, to kill throat infection.

- ✔ **Ionic silver:** Silver liquid in nanogram size is a natural antibiotic, and research shows it can kill just about anything. Follow the dosing instructions on the label. Like with many products, quality fluctuates from brand to brand; we trust Natural Immunogenics, Sovereign Silver.

Helping with Herbs

Herbal helpers have been around for centuries, and here are some of our favorites for treating colds and flus. Remember to stop yourself before you put sugar in your herbal tea; you may not be using antibiotics, but you still don't want to feed yeast. Keep it natural!

- ✔ **Garlic:** Place a small clove or half a clove of garlic in your mouth and let it sit without chewing. Swallow it with water when it starts breaking down in your mouth. A great side benefit is that vampires will keep their distance (but so will human folk)! You can also use it as a natural antibiotic, antiviral, and antifungal.

- ✔ **Sage:** Steep sage for 20 minutes to make a tea that treats cough.

- ✔ **Fenugreek:** Steeping fenugreek for 5 minutes brews a tea that helps reduce mucus.

- ✔ **Ginger:** To treat a sore throat and swollen neck glands, grate two tablespoons of ginger and boil it in 3 cups of water to make a gargle. You can also use it as a poultice by saturating a hand towel and wrapping it around your throat.

✔ **Herbal antibiotics:** Use wild oregano oil, garlic, or echinacea herbal antibiotics as drops, tablets, or tea at least three times a day for colds or flus.

✔ **Mullein and lobelia:** These little-known herbs are great for chest congestion — just take ½ teaspoon of each in hot water three times a day. They can also be used as a chest poultice for pleurisy, bronchitis, or pneumonia.

Healing with Homeopathy

Homeopathy is a form of medicine that uses mostly plants and mineral extracts that are diluted in alcohol or water to infinitesimal amounts. When used correctly, it has no side effects, does not interact with medications, and can be used safely by pregnant women and infants. Here are a few options:

✔ **Oscillococcinum** is probably the most ridiculous name for a flu remedy that you'll ever hear (so we call it Oscillo instead). It works for many people when used at the first signs of a cold or flu — it has proven about 70 percent effective in clinical trials to boost the immune system against viruses. Take one vial of pellets three times a day at the onset of symptoms. Some people use it as a preventative when they travel or are in crowds, or throughout the flu season on a weekly basis. Considering that flu vaccines are only about 8 percent effective and may have side effects, this remedy is an important addition to your medicine cabinet.

✔ **Gelsemium** treats colds and flus caused by overwork and exhaustion.

✔ **Dulcamara** helps knock out colds and flus that develop at the end of summer and into fall.

✔ **Aconite** can be used to nip cold and flu symptoms in the bud at their first signs.

✔ **Ferrum phos** also takes care of symptoms at the beginning of a cold.

✔ **Kali bich** treats colds and sinusitis with tough, stringy mucus.

Chapter 19

Ten Tempting Trigger Foods You May Want to Avoid

In This Chapter

▶ Recognizing that certain foods can be IBS nightmares

▶ Watching out for hidden sources of triggers

*W*hen you have IBS, sometimes you flare and sometimes you're flying. Whatever end of the spectrum you're on, the last thing you want to do is make your IBS worse. The following sections list the top foods you may have heard that people with IBS steer clear of if they want the closest thing to a happy-stomach guarantee. But, we're here to tell you that you may not be that IBS person. So tread carefully through these foods knowing that everyone is different, and you may not be the one these foods are going to attack.

Steering Clear of Artificial Sweeteners

Whether or not you have IBS, you may have replaced some sugary items in your diet with an artificial sweetener in an effort to avoid sugar (perhaps as a calorie-counting measure). However, these artificial sweeteners can have as much of an effect on your IBS as sugar does. Although studies may show these substances to be scientifically safe, many people still report reactions.

Artificial sweeteners come in several varieties:

✔ **Aspartame:** Sold under the brand names Equal and NutraSweet, *aspartame* is a chemical that breaks down into methanol and formaldehyde when you drink it. Reports have been made to the U.S. Food and Drug Administration (FDA) that related aspartame to two dozen illnesses and conditions like headaches, nausea, and stomach disorders. When you drink a can of aspartame-sweetened cola, the dual effects of carbonation and the chemical can cause gas and bloating in your stomach, so we recommend you avoid it.

- ✔ **Sucralose:** Sucralose, which you may know by the brand name Splenda, can affect thyroid function and your ability to absorb minerals like magnesium which are crucial to your intestinal health. Reports of stomach pain, diarrhea, and anxiety are also linked to the use of sucralose.

- ✔ **Saccharin:** You may be familiar with saccharin as Sweet'N Low. Use of saccharin is linked to diarrhea, headaches, and breathing problems. We remember our parents dropping pellets of saccharin in their tea many times a day for many years even after health warnings showed up on the packages.

- ✔ **Sorbitol:** Sorbitol is a sugar alcohol found in many products made for diabetics. This sugar alcohol passes into the intestines where it ferments, and you know what happens with fermentation; bubbles form and fill the container with gas. When that container is your intestines, you're dealing with discomfort and diarrhea. We strongly suggest staying away from any sorbitol products as we know that even small amounts can cause discomfort in your system.

You are more likely to find sorbitol in chewing gum and candies which are small items because in larger amounts (10 grams), sorbitol is also a laxative. In fact, sorbitol is also sold by pharmaceutical companies as a laxative.

Guarding your health

Don't be caught off guard because you're feeling good! Even if you've gone weeks or months since your last flare-up, you have to stay vigilant about your food intake. We don't mean to sound negative — we really want you to enjoy your healthy feeling colon! — but just be alert, because if you're feeling pretty good you may decide to eat something on your not-so-safe list.

Don't assume that a risky food is now suddenly safe just because you eat it one or two days with no effects. That's an easy trap to fall into — that first day, you feel fine after snacking on a favorite food that's been on your forbidden list

for ages, so the next day, you reason that you don't need to deprive yourself and you delve in again with no ill effects.

Day three is about the time you need to worry about getting smug. By day three, continued eating of the previously forbidden food may start to overload your system and set off the alarm in your bowels. To avoid this situation, just remember that how much you eat is also an important component of IBS. You may be able to eat small amounts of certain trigger foods and not pay the price, but too much of that good thing may send your bowels into a tizzy. We aren't recommending deprivation, just caution.

Distancing Yourself from Dairy

Dairy is the first food group to avoid when you have a symptom flare-up. Dairy-digesting enzymes are most active and plentiful in infancy and decline after weaning, so many adults don't have enough of those lactase enzymes to digest dairy products. Even when you're flying along without problems, we recommend that you only eat dairy once every three days, but introduce it in reasonable ways — don't pound back a cheesecake to celebrate the liberation of your colon.

Waving Good-bye to Wheat

You may have eaten wheat three times a day for decades and not even given it a second thought, but your bowels have calculated every wheat particle and are coming up with an overload. Some theorists believe that if you don't chew your food well, undigested wheat can be absorbed through the gut wall (although this situation tends to happen more to folks with leaky gut, a condition we describe in Chapter 18). The undigested wheat molecules can set up antigen/antibody reactions in your blood stream and cause widespread symptoms.

One way to weaken wheat's hold on you is to stop eating it altogether for two weeks. Then you may be able to eat it once every three days, but let your bowels be the judge of that. Any kind of rumbling in any part of your gastrointestinal tract (GIT) may be a sign to back off the wheat. We often hear of people who report a feeling of heartburn but ignore it because it doesn't involve a terror trip to the toilet. Then a morning wheat muffin sends rumblings farther into the GIT; the ensuing panic alone can be enough to set off an attack.

Saying "Sayonara, Sushi"

When you have a sensitive stomach, the last thing you need is to expose yourself to the parasites that are fairly common in raw fish. If they're microscopic, and some of them are, nobody's going to notice them decorating your raw tuna or salmon. And don't count on the heat from the wasabi to kill any lurking bacteria — that's a myth.

Eating cooked or vegetable sushi may not keep you out of the woods either. Even if the sushi chef keeps a spotless work area, raw fish bits can creep over into cooked fish.

Soy sauce is another sushi caution — most soy sauces are wheat based (see the preceding section) and can launch an IBS missile.

Pushing Away Popcorn

You may be tempted to grab a $12 tub of popcorn at the movie theater, but even if fat isn't an issue for you, this stuff has the fat power to launch its own IBS attack. In fact, a large tub of buttered movie popcorn can have as much as 125 grams of fat. That's more than double the recommended daily amount for an adult with a high-functioning GIT.

"But what about that light-butter microwave popcorn, or my air popper?" you ask. Those options may be better on the fat front, but fat isn't the only issue with popcorn: It's simply impossible to chew down the insoluble fiber particles of popcorn that can irritate a sensitive gut. Have you ever found popcorn casings lodged between your teeth days after having eaten popcorn? Imagine those bits lurking in your colon. If something has survived in your mouth for three days without ever showing signs of being digested, you simply don't want to go near the stuff if you have IBS.

Trashing Trail Mix and Ditching Dried Fruit

Christine doesn't remember tasting a trail mix that didn't have a moldy taste (and to her, Brazil nuts always taste moldy anyway). Trail mixes are great lab experiments for growing bacteria and fungus because nuts, especially peanuts grow mold and fruit provides a sugary meal for bacteria. This fact is especially true of the big bags that the whole family puts their unsterilized hands into. And the bulk bins at the store are worse; who knows who's been ignoring the signs and dipping in for a snack?

The germ factor aside, the foods that make up trail mix can cause problems on their own. Nuts can produce gut-irritating shards if you don't chew them completely and thoroughly. The sugar in dried fruit draws fluids into the intestine and can cause a flushing of diarrhea because your body doesn't distinguish fruit sugar from plain old sugar. Plus, some dried fruit still includes fruit skins, which are high in insoluble fiber and irritating to an IBS gut.

Marooning MSG and Other Unpronounceable Ingredients

Granted, the acronym *MSG* is pretty pronounceable, but try saying its full name (monosodium glutamate) five times fast. Labeling often doesn't help because MSG is hidden in various foods like seasonings, flavorings, hydrolyzed foods, bouillon cubes, cans of broth, and barley malt. Now that you're familiar with its aliases, keep away from it! MSG reactions may include stomach upset, nausea and vomiting, and diarrhea, among other non-intestinal symptoms.

When it comes to monitoring IBS-safe ingredients, if you can't say it, you can't eat it! Okay, that's a bit extreme, but honestly, the harder an ingredient is to pronounce, the more likely it is to be so chemically souped up that your intestines won't be able to handle it.

Canning Caffeine and Alcohol

Caffeine is a stimulant, as coffee drinkers the world over can attest; unfortunately for folks with IBS, their bowels are what get stimulated. Caffeine irritates the intestines, acting as a laxative for some people who just don't need that interference. Watch out for hidden sources of caffeine; you know coffee and soda, but don't forget about energy drinks. One patient we know dramatically improved his morning IBS-D symptoms just by cutting out his day-starting energy drink.

No science currently indicates that alcohol triggers IBS, but there's common sense. Drinking too much alcohol can have a direct impact on your GIT, causing nausea, vomiting, and diarrhea. So we're still pretty clear about telling people with IBS to avoid it.

Forgetting Fast Food Sauces, Condiments, and Gravies

You can be sure that most fast food sauces and gravies are land mines for IBS — they have ingredients that aren't even labeled, including MSG (see

"Marooning MSG and Other Unpronounceable Ingredients" earlier in this chapter), aspartame, colorings, dyes, emulsifiers, and all kinds of other awful stuff. Actually, we're pretty sure they come in huge vats with skulls and crossbones on the sides (or at least they should).

This holds true for not-so-fast food restaurants as well. Many popular chain and privately owned restaurants use mixes for their gravies and sauces to save time in the kitchen. And check to see if your local diner actually mashes real cooked potatoes or adds milk to a powdered mixture.

Flipping the Switch on Fatty Foods

Fat in food naturally stimulates intestinal contractions to help move your meal along from one end to another. It also stimulates the release of bile from the gall bladder to digest the fat in the small intestine. Both actions are necessary for food digestion and absorption, but in a sensitive gut that can trigger diarrhea and/or cramps. We recommend lean beef, which most people can tolerate, but you want to avoid fatty meats and anything deep-fried. The skin of poultry can be a problem, but you can remove it and enjoy fat-free chicken or turkey. Also be aware of the fat in many dairy products (although a reaction to them may be more related to lactose and added sugars).

Chapter 20

Ten Strategies for Avoiding Common Eating Traps

*T*he traps we present in this chapter may seem obvious to you, but the nature of traps is that you can't really see them all the time, and everybody has at least one blind spot. We're stripping away the camouflage and putting up police tape around these common pitfalls so you can identify them from a mile away.

We can help keep you from accidentally falling into these traps, but after you know about them, you have to make the choice to avoid them. One proven way to help you make more positive choices and avoid traps is to use *Emotional Freedom Techniques* (EFT), a self-help tool sometimes referred to as *emotional acupressure*. EFT can provide you with a sense of calm and relaxation so that decision-making feels easier when you face challenges and choices that feel difficult to make. Christine is an expert EFT Practitioner and provides information about EFT for IBS on her Web site (www.christinewheeler.com).

Find Safe Ways to Socialize with Friends

IBS is a lonely condition that many people never tell their friends they have. We're not suggesting that you post it in your online dating or social networking profile, but coming clean may help your friends understand why you always have to wash your hair or rearrange your sock drawer on Friday nights instead of coming out for pizza and beer.

Being social is more about the people you're with and less about the food you're eating. Consider telling your friends that you want to hang out with them but suspect you have some food sensitivities and are staying away from beer and pizza (or whatever the food of choice may be). Then suggest another place whose menu you feel safe with. If they insist on the pizza parlor, you can try having a snack before you go (so your starving stomach isn't tempted by the pepperoni special) and ordering a safe salad and mineral water when you're there.

Another option: Invite everyone over to your place and prepare the snacks yourself. You get the best of both worlds: quality time with your buddies and food you don't have to worry about. You may even start a new tradition.

Use the Sniff Test to Avoid Taking that One Little Bite

Any number of people (including you) may be trying to twist your arm to eat one little bite of wheat, dairy, sugar — you name it. Of course, for many people that one little bite quickly turns into eating the whole thing. Even if you can stop yourself after one bite, that amount can still be enough to set off a serious reaction depending on your level of sensitivity and the trigger in question; people who have celiac disease can be sidelined by a crumb of gluten. But resistance can still be tough when your favorite coworker shows up with a pan of her homemade brownies and you have to decide between hurting her feelings and risking an IBS episode.

One seemingly silly but surprisingly satisfying solution is to do the sniff test. The sense of smell is so powerful that one good whiff of the desired delicacy may be all you need to satisfy your craving.

Don't Assume One Small Indulgence Is a Huge Problem

If you do succumb to taking just one teensy bite of something you know you shouldn't have (see the preceding section), don't throw in the towel just yet. You may be tempted to reason, "Well, I've already blown it, so why not finish the whole cake if I'm already going to have an attack?", but that makes about as much sense as saying, "I already got my feet wet in the rain, so why not just jump in the shower fully clothed?" With IBS, the amount you eat can play a pivotal role. If you eat a small portion of a food you know your bowels shouldn't have, you haven't sealed your (or your colon's) fate.

We think that the big problem is that most people eat that first small portion with a large helping of guilt. If you savor the small portion — make it last and enjoy the heck out of it — you may not even want any more because you're so perfectly satisfied. And, with all those positive neurotransmitters that you stimulate by thinking happy thoughts about your food, your body may just digest that small portion without it bothering you.

Remind Yourself that IBS Doesn't Recognize Special Occasions

Thanksgiving, New Year's, Halloween, their sister's birthday — for many people, these special days are just another chance to prove to themselves that they can't eat cheese dip or chocolate cake. Your bowels don't distinguish special occasions, except for the fact that they may be even more tense with the stress of the holiday, so you have to train yourself not to either, at least when you're talking about diving into a buffet of triggers. Unless spending a family function in the bathroom is preferable to spending it with your family. . . .

Start Taking Care of Your IBS Today

Refusing to eat for your IBS doesn't mean you don't have IBS, so don't put off determining and implementing a diet that supports your health. We understand that part of what you're putting off is the feeling of deprivation and loss of freedom to eat what you want, but you're also putting off feeling better. So today, go shopping to fill your cupboards, fridge, and freezer with food you've tested to be tasty and safe; check out Chapter 4 for our kitchen-stocking suggestions You may even want to do some baking from the desserts in Chapter 13 so you have something ready when that decadent urge hits! If you haven't done elimination testing to determine what foods do and don't work for you, head to Chapter 2 to get started.

Create a Healthy Environment for Yourself

An unhealthy environment for IBS can come in many forms — maybe you're surrounded by more unhealthy foods than healthy ones, or your friends and family treat your IBS like it's a figment of your imagination. Unfortunately, the stress of these situations can make your condition worse, so you really want to work to build a positive atmosphere.

We hear from so many people with IBS who are struggling to maintain a healthy diet for themselves while still preparing all the meals for family members who don't have IBS. In Chapter 4, we tell you how to stock your kitchen to maximize your success, and Chapter 15 gives you tips on getting the entire family on board with one member's IBS diet.

A harder trap to avoid is feeling like those around you don't respect your IBS symptoms. Many folks feel so weak and guilty because others treat their IBS like some sort of silly, inconvenient made-up problem that they feel forced to eat unfriendly foods and suffer the effects later just so they don't draw attention to their illness. Chapter 4 also shows you how to minimize your IBS guilt and anxiety, and in *IBS For Dummies* (Wiley), we discuss having the IBS Talk with friends and family to explain the reality of your condition and let them know what you need from them.

Don't Keep Triggers in the House

It's as simple as that. If you crave something that worsens your symptoms, you have a much better chance of avoiding that stuff if you don't have it around. Otherwise, you know it's there, every cell in your brain knows it's there, and no part of you gets any peace until you get a piece of it. Then you have a war in your gut.

But banning tasty triggers is a bit harder when you share a kitchen with non-IBS family members, roommates, or houseguests, so you have to have some strong strategies in place to decrease your risk of temptation. In Chapter 4, we give you some tips on separating your foods from those of your IBS-free family. Putting your name on your special food packages, putting those packages on separate shelves, and keeping tempting but unfriendly foods on higher shelves out of reach are great ideas. Neither of us is very tall, but both of us have tall husbands who enjoy hiding things out of our physical reaches and lines of vision. We have to admit, it works!

Resist the Temptation to Skip Meals

Who knew that not eating at all is one of the biggest eating traps for IBS? When you allow yourself to get too hungry, you don't have the calories present to keep your body at its healing peak or to perform at your mental and emotional best. For example, as Christine worked on this chapter late one afternoon, she noticed that she was starting to get irritable and having trouble coming up with bright ideas and witty comments. She realized she'd been so immersed in her work that she'd forgotten to eat.

Folks can get so caught up in work, the Internet, and TV that they live in a virtual world without thinking of the very real needs of their physical bodies. To get you back into the habit, set a timer to tell you to eat every 3 to 4 hours and follow regular meal times.

If you're deliberately skipping meals because you really don't know what you can safely eat, stop. Having your gut rumble every time you start thinking of food is scary, but you need to eat. In Chapter 5, we list our top soothing recipes; these foods can be helpful even when your symptoms are flaring, so reassure yourself that not all food is going to set you off and work your way back into eating with one of these options.

 If you're at the stage of skipping meals because you're worried about the effects of food, start with the smoothie recipes in Chapter 8. You need to have some nourishment, and smoothies are a quick, safe, and delicious way to get it.

Don't Succumb to Emotional Eating

Emotional eating is a catchy term used to describe eating when you're emotionally upset but not physically hungry. If you regularly turn to food to feed your feelings, emotional eating is a food trap that may be feeding your IBS symptoms. When you feed your feelings, you aren't eating consciously and conscientiously; maybe you zone out and simply eat without caring or even being aware of what you're putting in your mouth. You aren't feeding your body, but your body still has to process the food.

When you find yourself heading for the kitchen ask yourself, "Am I physically hungry or just bored, tired, sad, needy, or irritable and looking for something to fill the gap?" Keep your food diary on the counter at the entrance to your kitchen and start writing about the snack or meal that you want and what you are feeling. If it's physical hunger, by all means, eat. If it's not, write down what emotion is driving the bus.

Pay Attention to How You Feel As You Eat

A common thread that runs through many eating traps is the feelings eating can generate. Why is resisting taking a bite of your brother's homemade triple-chocolate ganache so difficult? Because you have the added stress of worrying about hurting his feelings. When you do take a bite out of guilt, the panic at undoing your eating rules can be enough to set off an attack that the food itself may not have triggered. We don't tell you this to make you feel even guiltier but rather to give you an awareness of how your thoughts affect your whole body when you're eating.

As soon as you take a bite of some forbidden food and have a negative thought, you need to spit that morsel out immediately! You have our permission to do this unsightly act because after you do it once or twice, you start to recognize the importance of how you feel and what you're thinking when you eat. If you check in with your body and find your tummy is tight and you can't take a deep breath, that's not the time to be eating much of anything. If you find yourself in that tense, tight state too much, think about the magnesium solutions in Chapter 1 for calming your body and turning off the tension.

Part V
Appendixes

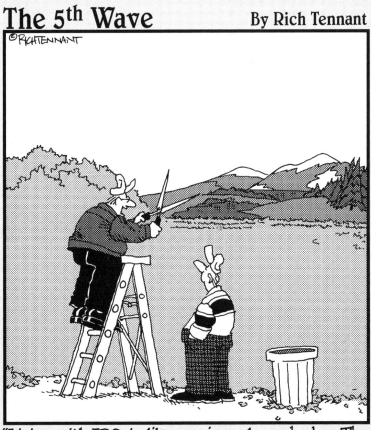

In this part . . .

This part is where we give you all the supplemental information we couldn't fit in the rest of the book. Appendix A provides metric unit conversions for those of you who operate on the metric system. In Appendix B, we help you substitute safer foods for common triggers. Because soluble and insoluble fiber are such important parts of eating for IBS, we chart the fiber contents of lots of foods in Appendix C to help you make more-informed decisions. Finally, Appendix D shows you how to identify potential trigger foods masquerading as other ingredients or in unexpected places.

Appendix A

Metric Conversion Guide

*N**ote:* The recipes in this cookbook were not developed or tested using metric measures. You may experience some variation in quality when converting to metric units.

Table A-1	Common Abbreviations
Abbreviation	*What It Stands For*
C, c	cup
g	gram
kg	kilogram
L, l	liter
lb	pound
mL, ml	milliliter
oz	ounce
pt	pint
t, tsp	teaspoon
T, TB, Tbl, Tbsp	tablespoon

Table A-2	Volume	
U.S Units	*Canadian Metric*	*Australian Metric*
¼ teaspoon	1 milliliter	1 milliliter
½ teaspoon	2 milliliters	2 milliliters
1 teaspoon	5 milliliters	5 milliliters
1 tablespoon	15 milliliters	20 milliliters
¼ cup	50 milliliters	60 milliliters
⅓ cup	75 milliliters	80 milliliters
½ cup	125 milliliters	125 milliliters
⅔ cup	150 milliliters	170 milliliters
¾ cup	175 milliliters	190 milliliters
1 cup	250 milliliters	250 milliliters
1 quart	1 liter	1 liter
1½ quarts	1.5 liters	1.5 liters
2 quarts	2 liters	2 liters
2½ quarts	2.5 liters	2.5 liters
3 quarts	3 liters	3 liters
4 quarts	4 liters	4 liters

Table A-3	Weight	
U.S. Units	*Canadian Metric*	*Australian Metric*
1 ounce	30 grams	30 grams
2 ounces	55 grams	60 grams
3 ounces	85 grams	90 grams
4 ounces (¼ pound)	115 grams	125 grams
8 ounces (½ pound)	225 grams	225 grams
16 ounces (1 pound)	455 grams	500 grams
1 pound	455 grams	½ kilogram

Table A-4	Measurements
Inches	*Centimeters*
½	1.5
1	2.5
2	5.0
3	7.5
4	10.0
5	12.5
6	15.0
7	17.5
8	20.5
9	23.0
10	25.5
11	28.0
12	30.5
13	33.0

Table A-5	Temperature (Degrees)
Fahrenheit	*Celsius*
32	0
212	100
250	120
275	140
300	150
325	160
350	180
375	190
400	200
425	220
450	230
475	240
500	260

For any temperature conversions you need that don't appear in Table A-5, use the following handy formulas:

- ✔ **Celsius to Fahrenheit:** (Degrees Celsius × ⅘) + 32 = degrees Fahrenheit
- ✔ **Fahrenheit to Celsius:** (Degrees Fahrenheit – 32) × ⅝ = degrees Celsius

Appendix B

Sensible Trigger Food Substitutes

When you've figured out which foods trigger your IBS symptoms, your first question is probably, "Well, what can I have instead?" (If you haven't determined your trigger foods yet, Chapter 2 helps you do so.) To answer your question, this appendix provides some common IBS trigger foods and possible replacement ingredients. Experiment with putting some of these ingredients into your favorite recipes. Thank you to Lori Alden and her Web site www.foodsubs.com for some great substitution suggestions; for even more, check out the site.

IBS is an individual condition; the ingredients we suggest here are generally safer than the original, but you have to do your own testing to figure out what you can tolerate.

Substituting Milk

In North America, milk is a staple on cereal, in baking, and as a drink on its own. For some people with IBS, though, milk is a troublesome substance because they're sensitive to lactose or the milk protein *casein.* The following alternatives may help you milk the most out of your recipes; you can easily substitute them one to one.

- **Lactose-free milk:** If your problem with milk is lactose intolerance, most dairies offer lactose-free versions of their milks.

- **Goat's milk:** For some people, goat's milk is easier to digest than cow's milk. But be forewarned that it has a distinct flavor.

- **Oat milk:** Oat milk has a slightly sweet taste and may be a good replacement for low-fat milk unless you're gluten sensitive.

- **Soy milk:** Some people find soy hard to digest, but this option may be worth trying. It has a nutty taste and is better for baking than for cooking.

- **Rice milk:** This low-protein sweet milk works well in desserts.

✔ **Almond milk:** A high-protein sweet milk, almond milk is best used in desserts and is also tasty in coffee and on cereal. Check out the Essential Nut Milk recipe in Chapter 8 to try it out for yourself.

✔ **Water:** You may not believe it, but water can whip up into something miraculous. It makes your scrambled eggs creamier and gives bread a thicker texture and a lighter crust.

Changing Up Cheese

Because cheese is from the dairy family, certain types of cheese may trigger your IBS. We're not promising that all these cheese substitutions taste, melt, or bake like your typical cheddar or mozzarella, but they may well be better than no cheese at all.

Depending on your level of cheese tolerance, you may be able to use some of the "real" cheeses approved for the Specific Carbohydrate Diet (SCD). Check out the list in Chapter 3. Also, be sure to read labels because some cheese substitutes may contain casein or caseinates, which are derived from milk and may upset your system if you're lactose intolerant.

✔ **Goat or sheep cheese:** Try cheeses made from the milk of animals other than cows. Some people find that they can digest goat cheese more easily than cheese made from cow's milk. Goat and sheep cheese are easy to find in your local supermarket.

✔ **Vegetarian cheese substitutes:** Vegetarian cheese can be made from soybeans, rice, almonds, or hemp seeds. These faux cheeses are formulated to taste and act like the real deal, including melting. But experiment to find what works for you because some can be bland and rubbery.

Trading Eggs

Most people can digest egg whites, but the fat in the egg yolk is troublesome for some. (As a guideline, a typical egg contains 2 tablespoons of white and 1 tablespoon of yolk.) Here are some ways you may be able to get around your egg dilemma (and we don't mean the old "Which came first?" question).

✔ **Egg whites only:** In most recipes calling for one egg, you can substitute two egg whites instead.

✔ **Flax meal:** Grind flaxseed to the consistency of cornmeal and mix about 2 tablespoons of it with ⅛ teaspoon of baking powder and 3 tablespoons of water to replace one egg in a recipe.

✓ **Tofu (not genetically modified):** For a yummy breakfast scramble, crumble the firm kind and sauté with herbs, onions, mushrooms, vegetarian cheese, or a cheese approved for the SCD.

✓ **Silken tofu (Non-GMO):** Substitute ¼ cup of silken tofu for each egg.

✓ **Egg substitutes:** These products are mostly egg whites but may contain fillers and flavorings that don't pass muster on your safe food list. Use ¼ cup of substitute per egg; for baking, try 3 tablespoons of substitute and 1 tablespoon of oil.

✓ **Gelatin:** To replace one egg in a recipe, dissolve 1 tablespoon of unflavored gelatin in 1 tablespoon of cold water and then add 2 tablespoons of boiling water and beat vigorously until frothy.

✓ **Banana:** Substitute ½ of a mashed ripe banana plus ¼ teaspoon of baking powder for each egg.

Swapping Out Sugar

The list of problems stemming from the overuse of refined sugars is long, but the main IBS issue is that it encourages the overgrowth of yeast and abnormal bacteria. In Appendix D, we give you 93 names for sugar; we can't promise nearly as many substitutes for sugar here, but we do have a few up our sleeves.

✓ **Date sugar:** Substitute 1 cup of date sugar for each cup of granulated sugar.

✓ **Powdered milk:** Replace up to ¼ of the granulated sugar in a recipe with the same amount of powdered milk.

✓ **Maple syrup:** You may be able to substitute ¾ cup of maple syrup and ¼ teaspoon of baking soda for each cup of granulated sugar in a recipe, but reduce another liquid in the recipe by 3 tablespoons.

✓ **Rice syrup:** Try substituting 1¾ cups of rice syrup for each cup of granulated sugar called for in a recipe, but reduce another liquid in the recipe by ¼ cup.

✓ **Molasses:** Molasses gives your final product a strong molasses flavor. Replace each cup of granulated sugar with 1⅓ cup of molasses and 1 teaspoon of baking soda, but reduce another liquid in the recipe by ⅓ cup and lower the oven temperature by 25 degrees.

✓ **Stevia:** Stevia is the most natural sweetener we know of. Made from stevia leaves, it may actually be good for your health. It's many times stronger than sugar, so tread carefully. The strengths of various brands differs wildly, so we can't give a specific exchange.

✓ **Just Like Sugar**: This sugar substitute has the consistency of sugar but is made from chicory and has zero calories. Replace sugar with an equal amount of Just Like Sugar.

✓ **Agave:** Agave is another natural sweetener; swap 1¾ cups of agave for each cup of granulated sugar in a recipe. Be sure to reduce another liquid in the recipe by ¼ cup.

Replacing White Flour

White flour is wheat flour with the bran removed. The insoluble fiber in bran can be a problem for a sensitive gut, but both flours have gluten that may be an underlying cause for your IBS symptoms.

Each bullet includes the conversion for replacing one cup of all-purpose white flour with the alternative flour in your recipes.

With flours, you can buy a few cups in bulk to try them out before committing to a whole container.

✓ **Brown or white rice flour:** One loosely packed cup

✓ **Chickpea flour:** ¾ cup

✓ **Corn flour:** 1 cup

✓ **Kamut flour:** 1 cup

✓ **Millet flour:** 1 cup

✓ **Potato flour:** ½ cup

✓ **Quinoa flour:** 1 cup

Appendix C

Soluble and Insoluble Fiber Charts

*W*e talk about fiber and its solubility throughout this book, and you may have some idea how much soluble or insoluble fiber is ideal for your individual IBS. Because most food labels don't break the fiber count into soluble or insoluble, we've found a chart released by the U.S. Department of Agriculture (USDA) that gives an estimate of the soluble and insoluble fiber in 70 different, common foods.

We suggest using these charts as a guideline rather than the gospel because all of the sources we researched had different fiber numbers for similar foods. These numbers can give you an idea of whether the foods you're choosing are more soluble than insoluble, and that can help you make decisions about your diet.

There's more to your IBS diet than just fiber. In Chapter 2, we talk about insoluble fiber as a trigger for IBS but confess that, much like a wild horse, fiber is a very difficult trigger to tie down, with contradictory values in different charts. Our advice is to not rely on fiber as the main driving force of your IBS diet. Instead, use these fiber charts to guide your fiber intake, but be sure to also find out about your body type and food preferences so you're sure to know your individual preferences based on who you are, not on some general guidelines.

Tables C-1 through C-6 provide the soluble and insoluble fiber estimates of 70 common foods. We say estimates because we want you to use these as guidelines in making food choices. Many foods have similar amounts of soluble and insoluble fiber, which still makes them IBS-friendly. Also note that a lot of the insoluble fiber in many fruits is concentrated largely in the skin.

Table C-1	Baked Goods	
Food	**Soluble Fiber Content in Grams**	**Insoluble Fiber Content in Grams**
Bagel, plain, frozen	1.29	2.46
Bread, rye, with caraway seeds	1.98	3.07
Bread, rye, seedless	2.84	4.46
Bread, wheat, firm	4.63	6.19
Bread, wheat, soft	2.13	3.38
Bread, white, firm	1.36	2.66
Bread, white, soft	0.53	1.54
Bread, white, reduced-calorie, firm	8.64	9.67
Bread, white, reduced-calorie, soft	8.46	9.47
Bread, whole-wheat, firm	5.21	6.71
Bread, whole-wheat, soft	4.76	6.01
Buns, hamburger/hotdog	1.44	1.99
Tortilla, corn	4.39	5.50
Tortilla, flour (wheat)	0.85	2.37

Table C-2	Cereal Grains and Pastas	
Food	**Soluble Fiber Content in Grams**	**Insoluble Fiber Content in Grams**
Brown rice, long-grain, cooked	2.89	3.33
Cornmeal, yellow	3.32	3.94
Cornstarch, wholesale	0.08	1.08
Flour, all-purpose, bleached	1.50	3.04
Grits, instant, cooked	1.48	1.55
Grits, quick, cooked	1.14	1.26
Oatmeal, instant, cooked	1.14	2.58
Oatmeal, regular, cooked	1.23	1.65
Spaghetti, cooked	1.33	2.06
White rice, long-grain, cooked	0.34	0.34

Table C-3	Fruits	
Food	*Soluble Fiber Content in Grams*	*Insoluble Fiber Content in Grams*
Apple (Red Delicious), raw, ripe, with skin	1.54	2.21
Avocado (California, Haas), raw, ripe	3.51	5.53
Avocado (Florida, Fuerte), raw, ripe	5.48	6.72
Banana, raw, ripe	1.21	1.79
Grapefruit, white, raw, ripe	0.32	0.89
Grapes (Thompson seedless), raw, ripe	0.36	0.60
Guava, raw, ripe	11.81	12.72
Mango, raw, ripe	1.08	1.76
Nectarine, raw, ripe, with skin	1.06	2.04
Orange (Navel), raw, ripe	0.99	2.35
Orange juice, retail, from concentrate	0.03	0.31
Peach, raw, ripe, with skin	1.54	2.85
Peach, raw, ripe, w/o skin	1.16	2.00
Pear, raw, ripe, with skin	2.25	3.16
Pineapple (smooth Cayenne), raw, ripe	1.42	1.46
Plum, raw, ripe, with skin	1.76	2.87
Prune, pitted	3.63	8.13
Raisins, seedless	2.17	3.07
Watermelon, raw, ripe	0.27	0.40

Table C-4	Legumes	
Food	*Soluble Fiber Content in Grams*	*Insoluble Fiber Content in Grams*
Beans, canned, with pork and tomato sauce	4.02	5.40
Chickpeas, canned, drained	5.79	6.19
Cowpeas, canned, drained	4.11	4.53
Lentils, dry then cooked and drained	5.42	5.86
Pinto beans, canned, drained	5.66	6.65
Red kidney beans, canned, drained	5.77	7.13
Split peas, dry then cooked and drained	10.56	10.65

Table C-5	Cooked Vegetables	
Food	*Soluble Fiber Content in Grams*	*Insoluble Fiber Content in Grams*
Broccoli, fresh, microwaved	2.81	4.66
Carrots, fresh, microwaved	2.29	3.87
Corn, yellow, from cob, farm market	2.63	2.87
Corn, yellow, from cob, grocery store	4.12	4.25
Green beans, fresh, microwaved	2.93	4.31
Lima beans, immature, frozen, microwaved	4.21	5.23
Peas, green, frozen, microwaved	2.61	3.54
Potato, French Fries, fast food	3.44	4.11
Potato, white, baked, with skin	1.70	2.31
Potato, white, boiled, without skin	1.06	2.05

Table C-6	Raw Vegetables	
Food	*Soluble Fiber Content in Grams*	*Insoluble Fiber Content in Grams*
Broccoli	3.06	3.50
Cabbage, green	1.79	2.24
Carrot	2.39	2.88
Cauliflower	2.15	2.62
Cucumber, with peel	0.94	1.14
Green pepper, sweet	0.99	1.52
Lettuce, iceberg	0.88	0.98
Onion, mature	1.22	1.93
Spinach	2.43	3.20
Tomato, red, ripe	1.19	1.34

Appendix D

Surprising Sources of Major Triggers

. . . .

*F*ood sensitivities and IBS triggers are hard to avoid when problem ingredients hide out in places you never expect to find them. How can you eliminate something from your diet when you don't even know that it's in your food? Yelling "Come out, come out, wherever you are!" doesn't work on food, so we offer this appendix to help you uncover some of the secret hideaways of sugar, gluten, lactose, and casein.

Sussing Out Sugar

If eliminating sugar from your diet is important for your individualized IBS treatment, you need to know where all the sugar is lurking. Manufacturers of packaged food have been known to use different types of sugar in their sweet concoctions to spread the sugary ingredients throughout the ingredient list.

The first ingredient on the label list is the most prominent single ingredient in the product. But if manufacturers include sugar through many different ingredients, they may be able to load the product with sugar without tipping off casual label readers who assume that if sugar was the main ingredient, it would be first on the list.

To hunt down all the sugar in your pantry, check your labels carefully for these other words:

- Amasake
- Apple sugar
- Barbados sugar
- Bark sugar
- Barley malt or barley malt syrup
- Beet sugar
- Brown rice syrup
- Brown sugar
- Cane juice or sugar
- Carbitol
- Caramelized foods
- Carmel coloring
- Carmel sugars
- Concentrated fruit juice
- Corn sweetener or syrup
- Date sugar
- Dextrin
- Dextrose
- Diglycerides
- Disaccharides
- D-tagalose
- Evaporated cane juice
- Florida crystals
- Fructooligosaccharides (FOS)
- Fructose
- Fruit juice concentrate
- Galactose
- Glucitol
- Glucoamine
- Gluconolactone
- Glucose, glucose polymers, or glucose syrup
- Glycerides
- Glycerine
- Glycerol
- Glycol
- Hexitol
- High-fructose corn syrup
- Honey
- Inversol
- Invert sugar
- Isomalt
- Lactose
- Levulose
- Light or lite sugar
- Malitol
- Malt dextrin
- Malted barley
- Maltodextrins
- Maltodextrose
- Maltose
- Malts
- Mannitol
- Mannose
- Maple syrup

- Microcrystalline cellulose
- Molasses
- Monoglycerides
- Monosaccarides
- Nectars
- Pentose
- Polydextrose
- Polyglycerides
- Powdered sugar
- Raisin juice
- Raisin syrup
- Raw sugar
- Ribose rice syrup
- Rice malt

- Rice sugar or sweeteners
- Rice syrup solids
- Saccharides
- Sorbitol
- Sorghum
- Sucanat or sucanet
- Sucrose
- Sugar cane
- Trisaccharides
- Turbinado sugar
- Unrefined sugar
- White sugar
- Xylitol
- Zylose

Getting to the Gluten

Avoiding gluten is a must for people with celiac disease, but it's also a great guideline to follow if you have IBS symptoms that you've associated with anything on the following list.

Never fear if you discover your favorite product on this list. You can find gluten-free versions of many products at gluten-free stores and online.

- Beer
- Bread and breadcrumbs
- Biscuits
- Cereal
- Communion wafers
- Cookies, cakes, cupcakes, donuts, muffins, pastries, pie crusts, brownies, and baked goods
- Cornbread
- Crackers

- ✔ Croutons
- ✔ Gravies, sauces, and roux
- ✔ Imitation seafood (for example, crab)
- ✔ Licorice
- ✔ Marinades (especially teriyaki)
- ✔ Pasta
- ✔ Pizza crust
- ✔ Pretzels
- ✔ Soy sauce
- ✔ Stuffing

Digging for Lactose

You may have an IBS reaction to lactose and dairy products regardless of whether you're officially lactose intolerant. Double check your food labels for signs of lactose, including milk, whey, cream, and milk solids, and watch out for the following foods:

- ✔ Biscuits
- ✔ Boiled sweets
- ✔ Cake (especially cake containing cream filling)
- ✔ Cheese
- ✔ Chocolate
- ✔ Cream
- ✔ Ice Cream
- ✔ Instant mashed potatoes
- ✔ Mayonnaise
- ✔ Milk
- ✔ Peanut butter
- ✔ Some pharmaceutical pills
- ✔ Salad dressing
- ✔ Yogurt

Catching Up to Casein

Casein is a protein found in all types of milk and used as a binder in many foods. It is also used in the production of plastics, nail polish, paint, glue and cosmetics. Some casein aliases you may find on your food labels include *milk solids, sodium caseinate, caseinogen,* and *caseinate.* In addition, you typically find casein in the following foods:

- Bakery glazes
- Breath mints
- Chicken sausages
- Coffee whiteners/creamers
- Fortified cereals
- Frankfurters
- High-protein beverage powders
- Ice cream
- Infant formulas
- Luncheon meats
- Nutrition bars
- Pâtés
- Processed meats
- Salad dressings
- Soy products
- Vienna sausages
- Whipped toppings

Index

• *C* •

• *E* •

Notes

Business/Accounting & Bookkeeping

Bookkeeping For Dummies
978-0-7645-9848-7

eBay Business
All-in-One For Dummies,
2nd Edition
978-0-470-38536-4

Job Interviews
For Dummies,
3rd Edition
978-0-470-17748-8

Resumes For Dummies,
5th Edition
978-0-470-08037-5

Stock Investing
For Dummies,
3rd Edition
978-0-470-40114-9

Successful Time
Management
For Dummies
978-0-470-29034-7

Computer Hardware

BlackBerry For Dummies,
3rd Edition
978-0-470-45762-7

Computers For Seniors
For Dummies
978-0-470-24055-7

iPhone For Dummies,
2nd Edition
978-0-470-42342-4

Laptops For Dummies,
3rd Edition
978-0-470-27759-1

Macs For Dummies,
10th Edition
978-0-470-27817-8

Cooking & Entertaining

Cooking Basics
For Dummies,
3rd Edition
978-0-7645-7206-7

Wine For Dummies,
4th Edition
978-0-470-04579-4

Diet & Nutrition

Dieting For Dummies,
2nd Edition
978-0-7645-4149-0

Nutrition For Dummies,
4th Edition
978-0-471-79868-2

Weight Training
For Dummies,
3rd Edition
978-0-471-76845-6

Digital Photography

Digital Photography
For Dummies,
6th Edition
978-0-470-25074-7

Photoshop Elements 7
For Dummies
978-0-470-39700-8

Gardening

Gardening Basics
For Dummies
978-0-470-03749-2

Organic Gardening
For Dummies,
2nd Edition
978-0-470-43067-5

Green/Sustainable

Green Building
& Remodeling
For Dummies
978-0-470-17559-0

Green Cleaning
For Dummies
978-0-470-39106-8

Green IT For Dummies
978-0-470-38688-0

Health

Diabetes For Dummies,
3rd Edition
978-0-470-27086-8

Food Allergies
For Dummies
978-0-470-09584-3

Living Gluten-Free
For Dummies
978-0-471-77383-2

Hobbies/General

Chess For Dummies,
2nd Edition
978-0-7645-8404-6

Drawing For Dummies
978-0-7645-5476-6

Knitting For Dummies,
2nd Edition
978-0-470-28747-7

Organizing For Dummies
978-0-7645-5300-4

SuDoku For Dummies
978-0-470-01892-7

Home Improvement

Energy Efficient Homes
For Dummies
978-0-470-37602-7

Home Theater
For Dummies,
3rd Edition
978-0-470-41189-6

Living the Country Lifestyle
All-in-One For Dummies
978-0-470-43061-3

Solar Power Your Home
For Dummies
978-0-470-17569-9

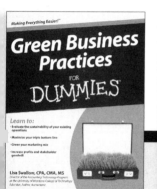

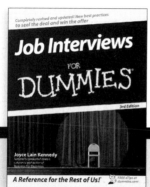

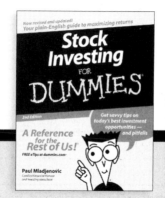

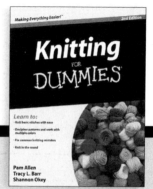

Internet

Blogging For Dummies,
2nd Edition
978-0-470-23017-6

eBay For Dummies,
6th Edition
978-0-470-49741-8

Facebook For Dummies
978-0-470-26273-3

Google Blogger
For Dummies
978-0-470-40742-4

Web Marketing
For Dummies,
2nd Edition
978-0-470-37181-7

WordPress For Dummies,
2nd Edition
978-0-470-40296-2

Language & Foreign Language

French For Dummies
978-0-7645-5193-2

Italian Phrases
For Dummies
978-0-7645-7203-6

Spanish For Dummies
978-0-7645-5194-9

Spanish For Dummies,
Audio Set
978-0-470-09585-0

Macintosh

Mac OS X Snow Leopard
For Dummies
978-0-470-43543-4

Math & Science

Algebra I For Dummies
978-0-7645-5325-7

Biology For Dummies
978-0-7645-5326-4

Calculus For Dummies
978-0-7645-2498-1

Chemistry For Dummies
978-0-7645-5430-8

Microsoft Office

Excel 2007 For Dummies
978-0-470-03737-9

Office 2007 All-in-One
Desk Reference
For Dummies
978-0-471-78279-7

Music

Guitar For Dummies,
2nd Edition
978-0-7645-9904-0

iPod & iTunes
For Dummies,
6th Edition
978-0-470-39062-7

Piano Exercises
For Dummies
978-0-470-38765-8

Parenting & Education

Parenting For Dummies,
2nd Edition
978-0-7645-5418-6

Type 1 Diabetes
For Dummies
978-0-470-17811-9

Pets

Cats For Dummies,
2nd Edition
978-0-7645-5275-5

Dog Training For Dummies,
2nd Edition
978-0-7645-8418-3

Puppies For Dummies,
2nd Edition
978-0-470-03717-1

Religion & Inspiration

The Bible For Dummies
978-0-7645-5296-0

Catholicism For Dummies
978-0-7645-5391-2

Women in the Bible
For Dummies
978-0-7645-8475-6

Self-Help & Relationship

Anger Management
For Dummies
978-0-470-03715-7

Overcoming Anxiety
For Dummies
978-0-7645-5447-6

Sports

Baseball For Dummies,
3rd Edition
978-0-7645-7537-2

Basketball For Dummies,
2nd Edition
978-0-7645-5248-9

Golf For Dummies,
3rd Edition
978-0-471-76871-5

Web Development

Web Design All-in-One
For Dummies
978-0-470-41796-6

Windows Vista

Windows Vista
For Dummies
978-0-471-75421-3

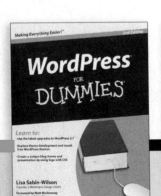
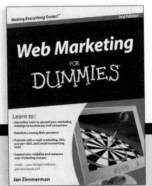
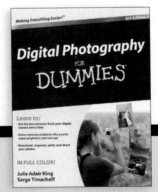
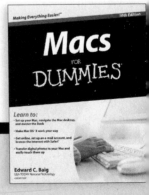